Stomatognathic Diseases: State of the Art and Future Perspectives

Stomatognathic Diseases: State of the Art and Future Perspectives

Editor

Agostino Guida

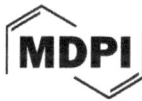

Basel • Beijing • Wuhan • Barcelona • Belgrade • Novi Sad • Cluj • Manchester

Editor
Agostino Guida
"AORN A. Cardarelli"
Hospital
Naples
Italy

Editorial Office
MDPI AG
Grosspeteranlage 5
4052 Basel, Switzerland

This is a reprint of articles from the Special Issue published online in the open access journal *Journal of Clinical Medicine* (ISSN 2077-0383) (available at: https://www.mdpi.com/journal/jcm/special_issues/C1483T40T0).

For citation purposes, cite each article independently as indicated on the article page online and as indicated below:

Lastname, A.A.; Lastname, B.B. Article Title. *Journal Name* **Year**, *Volume Number*, Page Range.

ISBN 978-3-7258-1727-6 (Hbk)
ISBN 978-3-7258-1728-3 (PDF)
doi.org/10.3390/books978-3-7258-1728-3

© 2024 by the authors. Articles in this book are Open Access and distributed under the Creative Commons Attribution (CC BY) license. The book as a whole is distributed by MDPI under the terms and conditions of the Creative Commons Attribution-NonCommercial-NoDerivs (CC BY-NC-ND) license.

Contents

About the Editor vii

Agostino Guida and Saman Warnakulasuriya
Stomatognathic Diseases: State of the Art and Future Perspectives
Reprinted from: *J. Clin. Med.* **2022**, *11*, 6525, doi:10.3390/jcm11216525 1

K. Lakshmi Priya, Jaideep Mahendra, Little Mahendra, Anilkumar Kanakamedala, Khalaf F. Alsharif, Maryam H. Mugri, et al.
Salivary Biomarkers in Periodontitis Post Scaling and Root Planing
Reprinted from: *J. Clin. Med.* **2022**, *11*, 7142, doi:10.3390/jcm11237142 5

Yeqing Yang, Junkai Zeng, Chong Jiang, Jiawen Chen, Ci Song, Ming Chen and Buling Wu
METTL3-Mediated lncSNHG7 m^{6}A Modification in the Osteogenic/Odontogenic Differentiation of Human Dental Stem Cells
Reprinted from: *J. Clin. Med.* **2023**, *12*, 113, doi:10.3390/jcm12010113 17

Xin Yi Leong, Divya Gopinath, Sakil M. Syeed, Sajesh K. Veettil, Naresh Yedthare Shetty and Rohit Kunnath Menon
Comparative Efficacy and Safety of Interventions for the Treatment of Oral Lichen Planus: A Systematic Review and Network Meta-Analysis
Reprinted from: *J. Clin. Med.* **2023**, *12*, 2763, doi:10.3390/jcm12082763 34

Angela Militi, Mirjam Bonanno and Rocco Salvatore Calabrò
It Is Time for a Multidisciplinary Rehabilitation Approach: A Scoping Review on Stomatognathic Diseases in Neurological Disorders
Reprinted from: *J. Clin. Med.* **2023**, *12*, 3528, doi:10.3390/jcm12103528 55

Małgorzata Mazurek-Mochol, Karol Serwin, Tobias Bonsmann, Małgorzata Kozak, Katarzyna Piotrowska, Michał Czerewaty, et al.
Expression of Interleukin 17A and 17B in Gingival Tissue in Patients with Periodontitis
Reprinted from: *J. Clin. Med.* **2023**, *12*, 4614, doi:10.3390/jcm12144614 73

Gaetano Scotto, Vincenzina Fazio, Salvatore Massa, Lorenzo Lo Muzio and Francesca Spirito
COVID-19 and Oral Lichen Planus: Between an "Intriguing Plot" and the "Fata Morgana Effect"
Reprinted from: *J. Clin. Med.* **2023**, *12*, 4829, doi:10.3390/jcm12144829 82

Dorin Nicolae Gheorghe, Francesco Bennardo, Margarita Silaghi, Dora-Maria Popescu, George-Alexandru Maftei, Marilena Bătăiosu and Petra Surlin
Subgingival Use of Air-Polishing Powders: Status of Knowledge: A Systematic Review
Reprinted from: *J. Clin. Med.* **2023**, *12*, 6936, doi:10.3390/jcm12216936 89

Patrick Hoss, Ole Meyer, Uta Christine Wölfle, Annika Wülk, Theresa Meusburger, Leon Meier, et al.
Detection of Periodontal Bone Loss on Periapical Radiographs—A Diagnostic Study Using Different Convolutional Neural Networks
Reprinted from: *J. Clin. Med.* **2023**, *12*, 7189, doi:10.3390/jcm12227189 112

Armina Rushiti, Chiara Castellani, Alessia Cerrato, Marny Fedrigo, Luca Sbricoli, Eriberto Bressan, et al.
The Follow-Up Necessity in Human Papilloma Virus-Positive vs. Human Papilloma Virus-Negative Oral Mucosal Lesions: A Retrospective Study
Reprinted from: *J. Clin. Med.* **2024**, *13*, 58, doi:10.3390/jcm13010058 123

Alexandra Gaál Kovalčíková, Bohuslav Novák, Oksana Roshko, Eva Kovaľová, Michal Pastorek, Barbora Vlková and Peter Celec
Extracellular DNA and Markers of Neutrophil Extracellular Traps in Saliva from Patients with Periodontitis—A Case–Control Study
Reprinted from: *J. Clin. Med.* **2024**, *13*, 468, doi:10.3390/jcm13020468 . . . . **135**

Dario Di Stasio, Agostino Guida, Antonio Romano, Massimo Petruzzi, Aldo Marrone, Fausto Fiori and Alberta Lucchese
Hepatitis C Virus (HCV) Infection: Pathogenesis, Oral Manifestations, and the Role of Direct-Acting Antiviral Therapy: A Narrative Review
Reprinted from: *J. Clin. Med.* **2024**, *13*, 4012, doi:10.3390/jcm13144012 . . . . **147**

About the Editor

Agostino Guida

Agostino Guida, DMD, PhD, MSc in Oral Medicine and Oncology, Specialist in Oral Surgery. He is a Consultant for the A.O.R.N. "A. Cardarelli" Hospital, Naples, Italy. His clinical and research activity embraces oral surgery, oral oncology, oral medicine, periodontology, and dental implants.

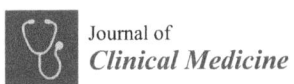

Editorial

Stomatognathic Diseases: State of the Art and Future Perspectives

Agostino Guida [1,*] and Saman Warnakulasuriya [2]

[1] U.O.C. Odontostomatologia, A.O.R.N. "A. Cardarelli", 80131 Naples, Italy
[2] Faculty of Dentistry, Oral & Craniofacial Sciences, King's College London, London SE1 9RT, UK
* Correspondence: agostino.guida@aocardarelli.it

Citation: Guida, A.; Warnakulasuriya, S. Stomatognathic Diseases: State of the Art and Future Perspectives. *J. Clin. Med.* **2022**, *11*, 6525. https://doi.org/10.3390/jcm11216525

Received: 31 October 2022
Accepted: 2 November 2022
Published: 3 November 2022

Publisher's Note: MDPI stays neutral with regard to jurisdictional claims in published maps and institutional affiliations.

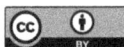

Copyright: © 2022 by the authors. Licensee MDPI, Basel, Switzerland. This article is an open access article distributed under the terms and conditions of the Creative Commons Attribution (CC BY) license (https://creativecommons.org/licenses/by/4.0/).

The World Health Organization (WHO) considers oral heath to be a key indicator of overall health, as it is linked to physical well-being and quality of life [1]. As the stomatognathic system consists of teeth, jaw bones, tongue, oral mucosa lining the mouth (including gingival tissues and lips), muscles involved in chewing and swallowing, salivary glands, and temporomandibular joints, there is a wide range of conditions that may undermine oral health: dental caries and periodontal (gum) disease leading to tooth loss, a wide range of oral mucosal diseases and oral cancer, xerostomia due to hypofunction of salivary glands, oro-facial pain, noma (necrotizing ulcerative stomatitis), and birth defects (such as cleft lip and palate).

The most common malignant condition that affects the oral cavity is oral squamous cell carcinoma (OSCC) [2], which arises from the mucosal lining of the oral cavity. On a global scale, more than 350,000 new incident cases of OSCC have been estimated, resulting in over 150,000 deaths in 2020 [3]. Despite clinical and therapeutic advances, the 5-year overall survival rate of oral cancer remains at 60%; the survival of patients with initial stages of OSCC stands at 80–90%, while it drops to under 50% for advanced-stage patients. It is apparent that the overall survival is low since most cases are diagnosed at advanced stages. Periodic surveillance and early detection by oral visual examination make up the foundation for effectively downsizing disease burden and possibly reducing the incidence of invasive cancer and related mortality [4]. In recent years, scientific literature also indicates how low-cost imaging techniques may represent a key strategy for non-invasive screening or the early detection of oral cancer [5–11].

Innovative therapeutic pathways which have proved themselves for cancers in other anatomical sites show limited results for OSCC. The lack of effectiveness of novel therapeutic approaches is partly due to the fact that the molecular biology of OSCC is not fully understood [12,13]. There are gaps in our knowledge of the natural history of OSCC, and not all oral potentially malignant disorders (OPMDs) undergo malignant transformation [14]; some remain stable, and some affected sites can revert back to health [15]. Moreover, OSCC can apparently develop from normal mucosa which may contain significant molecular aberrations that increase the likelihood of cancer [16–18]. Despite there being no consequentiality between OPMDs and OSCC, as well as between different grades of oral epithelial dysplasia, it has been reported that the risk of progression to oral cancer may increase in proportion to the severity of the dysplasia grade [19,20].

Some of the chronic oral inflammatory conditions are potentially malignant disorders too. Based on follow-up studies, there is now evidence of a low (1–2%) but significant risk of oral lichen planus (OLP) turning malignant with time [21–23], while the risk of the malignant transformation of chronic hyperplastic candidosis is still largely being debated [14]. Recent literature highlights potentially ground-breaking novelties for the diagnosis and follow-up of these chronic mucosal conditions, in terms of imaging and computer-assisted algorithm analyses [10,24].

The impact of tooth loss on global health is heavily linked to the resulting poor quality of life. The main cause of tooth loss in adults is periodontal disease. Periodontal disease is estimated to affect around one billion people worldwide (14% of the global adult population) [1]. Periodontitis is an inflammatory disease induced by an imbalance among bacterial virulence, microbiota dysbiosis, and a host defenses/inflammation [25]. Recently, scientific literature highlights the contribution of chronic inflammation to noncommunicable diseases, such as diabetes and obesity, as well as cardiovascular and neurological diseases. The link between these diseases seems to be low-grade inflammation (LGI) induced by pathogenic oral microbiota [26]; LGI causes a low-grade chronic systemic production of cytokines. LGI is a recognized risk factor for cardiovascular, cerebrovascular, and neurodegenerative diseases and cancer. Limited evidence also suggests that LGI increases the risk of insulin resistance and thus type 2 diabetes. LGI may be assessed through an evaluation of hematological (e.g., CRP, ESR, fibrinogen) or cell biomarkers (e.g., WBC and platelet counts), but this condition cannot be consistently defined or measured yet. Regarding the link between periodontitis and LGI, the most accredited hypothesis is that periodontitis may play a role in inducing/maintaining systemic LGI, and likewise LGI could promote periodontitis as an independent risk factor. Furthermore, the concept of LGI could explain the proved correlation among periodontitis and cardiovascular conditions or even degenerative neurologic conditions (e.g., Parkinson's disease and Alzheimer's disease).

As we briefly explored, despite their different origins, the pathologies of different organs comprising the stomatognathic system share common characteristics, the most important of which is that they may be heavily linked to common risk factors and general health conditions [1].

The Global Burden of Disease Study 2019 showed that oral diseases cause distress to around 3.5 billion people in total. Among these, the International Agency for Research on Cancer (IARC) evaluates that OSCC causes over 150,000 deaths each year. Furthermore, most oral conditions share risk factors with the main noncommunicable diseases (cardiovascular diseases, cancer, chronic respiratory diseases, and diabetes) and the scientific literature highlights the double link between periodontitis and conception/fertility [27]. The relationship between oral and general health is corroborated through shared risk factors such as tobacco use, alcohol consumption, and unhealthy diets unbalanced in carbohydrates. In addition to the aforementioned link between periodontitis and diabetes, the high consumption of sugars is seen as a common risk factor for diabetes, obesity, and dental caries. The WHO underlines how unhealthy lifestyles are alarmingly increasing at the global level. Furthermore, burning mouth syndrome (BMS) may be a probable link between mental health and oral health, and this peculiar oral condition is as a result of psychiatric distress in some cases. The aetiopathogenesis of this disease is complex and may be multifactorial, as local, systemic, and psychological factors are considered to be involved in generating symptoms. A recent publication points to the idea that enhanced pain perception in BMS could be linked to a higher frequency of white matter hyperintensities (WMHs) in the brain [28]. The literature indicates that psychotherapy and behavioral feedback may help to eliminate BMS symptoms [29].

With particular regard to frail older patients, the WHO recently included them in a resolution for global oral health [1], underlining how there is a strong link between oral diseases (OSCC, periodontal disease, and tooth decay) and conditions of social, cultural, and sanitary vulnerability, within the framework of an aging global population. Furthermore, conditions such as noma shall not be forgotten, as it mainly affects developing countries, especially children with poor health/quality of life or malnutrition.

Oral conditions are largely preventable and show dramatically better prognosis when treated at early stages. OSCC survival rates drop from 90–80% at stages I and II to around/less than 60–50% when treated at stages III-IV [9]. Primary (education on healthy lifestyle) and secondary (early diagnosis) prevention strategies are key factors for reaching success in reducing the burden of oral diseases which, according to the WHO, have to be integrated with primary health care. Furthermore, there is a necessity to gather data in order to determine oral health indicators and "best buys" and to implement cost-effective interventions for the population.

Researchers investigating oral health and disease from all round the globe must prosecute their part. *The Journal of Clinical Medicine*'s Special Issue, titled "Stomatognathic Diseases: State of the Art and Future Perspectives", aims to contribute to this purpose, providing a platform for research papers on oral health with particular reference to its connection with systemic conditions.

Author Contributions: Conceptualization, A.G. and S.W.; writing—original draft preparation, A.G.; writing—review and editing, S.W. All authors have read and agreed to the published version of the manuscript.

Funding: This research received no external funding.

Informed Consent Statement: Not applicable.

Conflicts of Interest: The authors declare no conflict of interest.

References

1. World Health Organization. Oral Health. Available online: https://www.who.int/health-topics/oral-health (accessed on 28 August 2020).
2. Scully, C.; Bagan, J. Oral squamous cell carcinoma overview. *Oral Oncol.* **2009**, *45*, 301–308. [CrossRef] [PubMed]
3. Sung, H.; Ferlay, J.; Siegel, R.L.; Laversanne, M.; Soerjomataram, I.; Jemal, A.; Bray, F. Global Cancer Statistics 2020: Glo-bocan Estimates of Incidence and Mortality Worldwide for 36 Cancers in 185 Countries. *CA Cancer J. Clin.* **2021**, *71*, 209–249. [CrossRef] [PubMed]
4. Bouvard, V.; Nethan, S.T.; Singh, D.; Warnakulasuriya, S.; Mehrotra, R.; Chaturvedi, A.K.; Chen, T.H.-H.; Ayo-Yusuf, O.A.; Gupta, P.C.; Kerr, A.R.; et al. IARC Perspective on Oral Cancer Prevention. *N. Engl. J. Med.* **2022**. [CrossRef]
5. Liu, J.L.; Walsh, T.; Kerr, A.R.; Lingen, M.; Brocklehurst, P.; Ogden, G.; Warnakulasuriya, S.; Scully, C. Diagnostic tests for oral cancer and potentially malignant disorders in patients presenting with clinically evident lesions. *Cochrane Database Syst. Rev.* **2012**. [CrossRef]
6. Walsh, T.; Liu, J.L.; Brocklehurst, P.; Glenny, A.-M.; Lingen, M.; Kerr, A.R.; Ogden, G.; Warnakulasuriya, S.; Scully, C. Clinical assessment to screen for the detection of oral cavity cancer and potentially malignant disorders in apparently healthy adults. *Cochrane Database Syst. Rev.* **2013**. [CrossRef]
7. De Wit, J.G.; van Schaik, J.E.; Voskuil, F.J.; Vonk, J.; De Visscher, S.; Schepman, K.P.; Van der Laan, B.; Doff, J.J.; Van der Vegt, B.; Plaat, B.; et al. Comparison of narrow band and fluorescence molecular imaging to improve intraoperative tumour margin assessment in oral cancer surgery. *Oral Oncol.* **2022**, *134*, 106099. [CrossRef]
8. Ota, A.; Miyamoto, I.; Ohashi, Y.; Chiba, T.; Takeda, Y.; Yamada, H. Diagnostic Accuracy of High-Grade Intraepithelial Papillary Capillary Loops by Narrow Band Imaging for Early Detection of Oral Malignancy: A Cross-Sectional Clinicopathological Imaging Study. *Cancers* **2022**, *14*, 2415. [CrossRef] [PubMed]
9. Guida, A.; Maglione, M.; Crispo, A.; Perri, F.; Villano, S.; Pavone, E.; Aversa, C.; Longo, F.; Feroce, F.; Botti, G.; et al. Oral lichen planus and other confounding factors in narrow band imaging (NBI) during routine inspection of oral cavity for early detection of oral squamous cell carcinoma: A retrospective pilot study. *BMC Oral Health* **2019**, *19*, 70. [CrossRef]
10. Guida, A.; Ionna, F.; Farah, C.S. Narrow-band imaging features of oral lichenoid conditions: A multicentre retrospective study. *Oral Dis.* **2021**. [CrossRef]
11. Di Stasio, D.; Lauritano, D.; Loffredo, F.; Gentile, E.; Della Vella, F.; Petruzzi, M.; Lucchese, A. Optical coherence tomography imaging of oral mucosa bullous diseases: A preliminary study. *Dentomaxillofacial Radiol.* **2020**, *49*, 20190071. [CrossRef]
12. Johnson, N.W. Cancer Biology and Carcinogenesis: Fundamental Biological Processes and How They Are Deranged in Oral Cancer. In *Textbook of Oral Cancer: Prevention, Diagnosis and Management*; Warnakulasuriya, S., Greenspan, J.S., Eds.; Springer: Basel, Switzerland, 2020; pp. 399–425.
13. González-Moles, M.; Warnakulasuriya, S.; López-Ansio, M.; Ramos-García, P. Hallmarks of Cancer Applied to Oral and Oropharyngeal Carcinogenesis: A Scoping Review of the Evidence Gaps Found in Published Systematic Reviews. *Cancers* **2022**, *14*, 3834. [CrossRef] [PubMed]
14. Warnakulasuriya, S.; Kujan, O.; Aguirre-Urizar, J.M.; Bagan, J.V.; González-Moles, M.; Kerr, A.R.; Lodi, G.; Mello, F.W.; Monteiro, L.; Ogden, G.R.; et al. Oral potentially malignant disorders: A consensus report from an international seminar on nomenclature and classification, convened by the WHO Collaborating Centre for Oral Cancer. *Oral Dis.* **2020**, *27*, 1862–1880. [CrossRef] [PubMed]
15. Speight, P.M.; Epstein, J.; Kujan, O.; Lingen, M.W.; Nagao, T.; Ranganathan, K.; Vargas, P. Screening for oral cancer-a perspecive from the Global Oral Cancer Forum. *Oral Surg. Oral Med. Oral Pathol. Oral Radiol.* **2017**, *123*, 680–687. [CrossRef] [PubMed]
16. Farah, C.S.; Shearston, K.; Nguyen, A.P.; Kujan, O. Oral Carcinogenesis and Malignant Transformation. In *Premalignant Conditions of the Oral Cavity*; Springer: Singapore, 2019; pp. 27–66. [CrossRef]
17. Monteiro, L.; Mello, F.W.; Warnakulasuriya, S. Tissue biomarkers for predicting the risk of oral cancer in patients diagnosed with oral leukoplakia: A systematic review. *Oral Dis.* **2021**, *27*, 1977–1992. [CrossRef] [PubMed]

18. Thomson, P.J.; Goodson, M.L.; Smith, D.R. Profiling cancer risk in oral potentially malignant disorders-A patient cohort study. *J. Oral Pathol. Med.* **2017**. [CrossRef]
19. Chaturvedi, A.K.; Udaltsova, N.; A Engels, E.; A Katzel, J.; Yanik, E.L.; A Katki, H.; Lingen, M.W.; Silverberg, M.J. Oral Leukoplakia and Risk of Progression to Oral Cancer: A Population-Based Cohort Study. *JNCI J. Natl. Cancer Inst.* **2019**, *112*, 1047–1054. [CrossRef]
20. Odell, E.; Kujan, O.; Warnakulasuriya, S.; Sloan, P. Oral epithelial dysplasia: Recognition, grading and clinical significance. *Oral Dis.* **2021**, *27*, 1947–1976. [CrossRef]
21. González-Moles, M.; Ramos-García, P.; Warnakulasuriya, S. An appraisal of highest quality studies reporting malignant transformation of oral lichen planus based on a systematic review. *Oral Dis.* **2020**, *27*, 1908–1918. [CrossRef]
22. Ramos-García, P.; González-Moles, M.Á.; Warnakulasuriya, S. Oral cancer development in lichen planus and related conditions-3.0 evidence level: A systematic review of systematic reviews. *Oral Dis.* **2021**, *27*, 1919–1935. [CrossRef]
23. Idrees, M.; Kujan, O.; Shearston, K.; Farah, C.S. Oral lichen planus has a very low malignant transformation rate: A systematic review and meta-analysis using strict diagnostic and inclusion criteria. *J. Oral Pathol. Med. Off. Pub. Int. Assoc. Oral Pathol. Am. Acad. Oral Pathol.* **2021**, *50*, 287–298. [CrossRef]
24. Lucchese, A.; Mittelman, A.; Lin, M.-S.; Kanduc, D.; Sinha, A. Epitope definition by proteomic similarity analysis: Identification of the linear determinant of the anti-Dsg3 MAb 5H10. *J. Transl. Med.* **2004**, *2*, 43. [CrossRef] [PubMed]
25. Rizzo, A.; Bevilacqua, N.; Guida, L.; Annunziata, M.; Carratelli, C.R.; Paolillo, R. Effect of resveratrol and modulation of cytokine production on human periodontal ligament cells. *Cytokine* **2012**, *60*, 197–204. [CrossRef] [PubMed]
26. Cecoro, G.; Annunziata, M.; Iuorio, M.T.; Nastri, L.; Guida, L. Periodontitis, Low-Grade Inflammation and Systemic Health: A Scoping Review. *Medicina* **2020**, *56*, 272. [CrossRef] [PubMed]
27. Nwhator, S.; Opeodu, O.; Ayanbadejo, P.; Umeizudike, K.; Olamijulo, J.; Alade, G.; Agbelusi, G.; Arowojolu, M.; Sorsa, T. Could periodontitis affect time to conception? *Ann. Med. Health Sci. Res.* **2014**, *4*, 817–822. [CrossRef] [PubMed]
28. Adamo, D.; Canfora, F.; Calabria, E.; Coppola, N.; Leuci, S.; Pecoraro, G.; Cuocolo, R.; Ugga, L.; D'Aniello, L.; Aria, M.; et al. White matter hyperintensities in Burning Mouth Syndrome assessed according to the Age-Related White Matter Changes scale. *Front. Aging Neurosci.* **2022**, *14*. [CrossRef]
29. Salerno, C.; Di Stasio, D.; Petruzzi, M.; Lauritano, D.; Gentile, E.; Guida, A.; Maio, C.; Tammaro, M.; Serpico, R.; Lucchese, A. An overview of burning mouth syndrome. *Front. Biosci.* **2016**, *8*, 213–218.

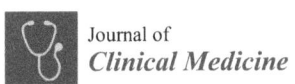

Article

Salivary Biomarkers in Periodontitis Post Scaling and Root Planing

K. Lakshmi Priya [1], Jaideep Mahendra [1,*], Little Mahendra [2], Anilkumar Kanakamedala [1], Khalaf F. Alsharif [3], Maryam H. Mugri [4], Saranya Varadarajan [5], Ahmed Alamoudi [6], Ali Abdel-Halim Abdel-Azim Hassan [4], Mrim M. Alnfiai [7], Khalid J. Alzahrani [3], Maha A. Bahammam [8,9], Hosam Ali Baeshen [10], Thodur Madapusi Balaji [11] and Shilpa Bhandi [12,*]

[1] Department of Periodontics, Meenakshi Ammal Dental College and Hospital, Chennai 600095, Tamil Nadu, India
[2] Department of Periodontics, Maktoum Bin Hamdan Dental University, Dubai 122002, United Arab Emirates
[3] Department of Clinical Laboratory Sciences, College of Applied Medical Sciences, Taif University, P.O. Box 11099, Taif 21944, Saudi Arabia
[4] Department of Maxillofacial Surgery and Diagnostic Sciences, College of Dentistry, Jazan University, Jazan 45412, Saudi Arabia
[5] Department of Oral Pathology and Microbiology, Sri Venkateswara Dental College and Hospital, Chennai 600130, Tamil Nadu, India
[6] Department of Oral Biology, Faculty of Dentistry, King Abdulaziz University, Jeddah 21589, Saudi Arabia
[7] Department of Information Technology, College of Computers and Information Technology, Taif University, P.O. Box 11099, Taif 21944, Saudi Arabia
[8] Department of Periodontology, Faculty of Dentistry, King Abdulaziz University, Jeddah 80209, Saudi Arabia
[9] Executive Presidency of Academic Affairs, Saudi Commission for Health Specialties, Riyadh 11614, Saudi Arabia
[10] Department of Orthodontics, Faculty of Dentistry, King Abdulaziz University, Jeddah 21589, Saudi Arabia
[11] Department of Periodontology, Tagore Dental College and Hospital, Chennai 600127, Tamil Nadu, India
[12] College of Dental Medicine, Roseman University of Health Sciences, South Jordan, UT 84095, USA
* Correspondence: drjaideep.perio@madch.edu.in (J.M.); shilpa.bhandi@gmail.com (S.B.)

Abstract: Objectives: This study was conducted to evaluate the levels of salivary uric acid and arginase in patients with periodontitis, generalized gingivitis, and in healthy individuals. Then, the effects of non-surgical periodontal therapy on levels of salivary arginase and uric acid were also investigated. Methods: A total of 60 subjects were divided into three groups based on periodontal health: group I comprised 20 healthy individuals; group II comprised 20 subjects who had generalized gingivitis; group III comprised 20 subjects who had generalized periodontitis. On day 0, the clinical examination of periodontal status was recorded, following which saliva samples were collected. Group II and group III subjects underwent non-surgical periodontal therapy. These patients were re-called on day 30 to collect saliva samples. The periodontal parameters were reassessed on day 90, and saliva samples were collected for analysis of salivary arginase and uric acid levels. Results: Group II and group III showed improvement in clinical parameters following non-surgical periodontal therapy on the 90th day. The MGI score, PPD, and CAL showed improvement. On day 0, at baseline, salivary arginase levels in group III and group II were higher than those in healthy subjects, whereas on day 0, salivary uric acid levels in group III and group II were lower than those in healthy subjects. Both on day 0 and day 90, the salivary arginase level showed a positive correlation with the periodontal parameters, whereas the salivary uric acid level was positively correlated with the periodontal parameters on day 90. Conclusion: the level of salivary arginase was a pro-inflammatory marker and a raised level of salivary uric acid was an anti-inflammatory marker following periodontal therapy, suggesting their pivotal role in assessing periodontal status and evaluation of treatment outcome.

Keywords: salivary biomarkers; arginase; gingivitis; chronic periodontitis; root planing; scaling; uric acid

Citation: Priya, K.L.; Mahendra, J.; Mahendra, L.; Kanakamedala, A.; Alsharif, K.F.; Mugri, M.H.; Varadarajan, S.; Alamoudi, A.; Hassan, A.A.-H.A.-A.; Alnfiai, M.M.; et al. Salivary Biomarkers in Periodontitis Post Scaling and Root Planing. *J. Clin. Med.* **2022**, *11*, 7142. https://doi.org/10.3390/jcm11237142

Academic Editors: Francisco Mesa and Agostino Guida

Received: 8 October 2022
Accepted: 26 November 2022
Published: 1 December 2022

Publisher's Note: MDPI stays neutral with regard to jurisdictional claims in published maps and institutional affiliations.

Copyright: © 2022 by the authors. Licensee MDPI, Basel, Switzerland. This article is an open access article distributed under the terms and conditions of the Creative Commons Attribution (CC BY) license (https://creativecommons.org/licenses/by/4.0/).

1. Introduction

Periodontitis is an inflammatory disease of multifactorial origin, characterized by periods of exacerbation and remission [1]. The disease is initiated by the formation of plaque biofilm leading to a loss of equilibrium between microbial organisms and host response, resulting in disease progression. The inflammation of the surrounding periodontal tissues ultimately leads to alveolar bone and attachment loss [2]. The degree of tissue destruction has a log-linear relationship with the rise in microbial load. The main etiological factors for the disease include gram-negative anaerobic bacteria and a variety of facultative bacteria that reside in the subgingival biofilm [3].

Proper diagnosis and treatment modality has been recommended for periodontal and peri-implant diseases and conditions based on the recent classification reported by Caton et al. [4]. Various diagnostic methods are available for the early detection and diagnosis of periodontitis. They can be broadly divided into clinical and molecular methods. A biomarker or biologic marker is an objectively measured characteristic that provides an indicator of pharmacologic response, pathogenic processes, or normal biological processes after therapeutic intervention [5]. Analysis of biomarkers in fluids such as saliva, synovial fluid plasma, whole blood, cerebrospinal fluid, serum, semen, plasma, and urine have assisted in clinical diagnosis in medicine [6]. Among these sources, saliva is commonly used for early diagnosis and detection of biomarkers. Saliva collection is rapid, simple, and more importantly, painless, making it uncomplicated for screening purposes. Saliva contains systemically and locally derived markers related to periodontal disease, thus serving as a specific biomarker for the assessment of periodontitis [7].

Non-surgical periodontal therapy is the first recommended approach and gold standard to control periodontal infections. The primary objective of non-surgical therapy is to restore gingival health by removing the local factors that cause disease (plaque, calculus, and endotoxins). Hand and ultrasonic instruments are tools used in non-surgical therapy to drastically reduce the number of periodontopathogens in the oral environment, thus restoring gingival health [8]. The most relevant shortcoming of non-surgical therapy is the absence of a long-term effect due to an eventual bacterial recolonization after the therapy [8]. Accordingly, adjunctive treatments have been introduced in addition to SRP, e.g., the use of antibiotics, photodynamic therapy, administration of antioxidants, natural compounds, supplements (e.g., melatonin), and, in recent years, probiotic therapy to enhance the long-term effects of non-surgical therapy [9].

Salivary arginase and uric acid have been reported to play a significant role in periodontal disease [10,11]. Salivary arginase levels seem to be raised in chronic periodontitis, suggesting its role in the inflammatory process. Arginase is one of the five key enzymes of the urea cycle, which is essential for the metabolic conversion of ammonia into urea. Arginine, a semi-essential amino acid, mediates various physiologic processes, including urea and protein synthesis [10]. The increased levels of arginase reduce levels of nitric oxide, which is essential for destroying periodontal pathogens. This happens because both arginase and nitric oxide compete for the common substrate L-arginine. Through the urea cycle, arginase helps to produce polyamines, which are necessary for the survival of many oral bacteria. They provide nutritional support; hence, high arginase activity in saliva favors the growth of pathogens, leading to the progression of periodontal disease.

One of the major antioxidants present in saliva is uric acid, which is the most dominant antioxidant apart from glutathione, superoxide dismutase (SOD), albumin, and ascorbic acid. Uric acid is the end product of purine metabolism and it contributes to the antioxidant properties of saliva [11]. These biomarkers have both antioxidant and pro-oxidant properties in vitro by scavenging and producing reactive oxygen species and are known to have an impact during periodontal inflammation. Although studies in the past have shown the effects of these enzymes with regard to inflammation, very few studies have shown the effects of non-surgical therapy and periodontal status on levels of the above biomarkers. We hypothesized that decreased levels of salivary arginase and improved levels of uric acid post non-surgical therapy would have a positive impact on periodontal status. This study aims to quantify salivary arginase and uric acid levels in subjects with generalized gingivitis and periodontitis compared to those found in the healthy periodontium, and evaluate the effects of non-surgical periodontal therapy on salivary arginase and uric acid levels.

2. Materials and Methods

Sixty subjects (30 males and 30 females) were recruited from the outpatient section of the Department of Periodontology, Meenakshi Ammal Dental College and Hospital, Chennai, India. Ethical approval was obtained from Institutional Review Board of MAHER—Deemed to be University, Chennai (MADC/IRB-XXV/2018/393) before commencement of the study. The power of the study was calculated using G-power software. The power was calculated for 60 subjects, with a minimum of 20 subjects required in each group, which came out to be 95% based on the following calculation.

Calculation for power analysis:
t-tests—Means: Difference between two independent means (two groups)
Analysis: A priori: Compute required sample size
Input: Tail(s) = Two
Effect size d = 1.2041300
α err prob = 0.05
Power (1-β err prob) = 0.95
Allocation ratio N2/N1 = 1
Output: Noncentrality parameter δ = 3.7113779
Critical t = 2.0280940
Df = 36 Sample size group 1 = 19
Sample size group 2 = 19
Total sample size = 38
Actual power = 0.9506005

Written informed consent was obtained from all participants of the study. The subjects were divided into three groups of twenty subjects based on their periodontal health. Group I consisted of 20 periodontally and systemically healthy subjects (Controls). Group II included subjects with generalized chronic gingivitis. Group III comprised patients with chronic periodontitis according to the current classification of periodontal and peri-implant diseases, 2017 (Figure 1). The inclusion criteria included subjects willing to participate in the study, within 30–65 years of age, with ≥10 natural teeth.

Group I (control group) consisted of systemically healthy subjects with clinically healthy periodontium, probing pocket depth (PPD) ≤ 3 mm, without bone loss or attachment loss on radiographs [1].

Group II (experimental group) consisted of generalized chronic gingivitis subjects with PPD ≤ 3 mm having ≤ 10% bleeding on probing sites with clinical signs of gingival inflammation without signs of pseudo pockets, clinical attachment loss (CAL = 0), and radiographic evidence of bone loss.

Group III (experimental group) consisted of chronic periodontitis patients falling under Stage II/III, grade B category with interdental CAL detectable at ≥2 non-adjacent teeth or buccal or oral CAL ≥ 3 mm with pocketing > 3 mm and radiographic bone loss extending up to the middle third or apical third [1].

Individuals with a history of smoking, aggressive periodontitis, pregnant subjects, or subjects suffering from gout or systemic diseases that could affect periodontal status were excluded. Subjects with previous history of periodontal therapy in the last six months or were on medication affecting periodontal status were excluded from the study.

2.1. Non-Surgical Periodontal Therapy

On day 0, after periodontal examination and collection of saliva samples for molecular analysis, non-surgical periodontal therapy was performed, which consisted of complete scaling and root planing along with oral hygiene instructions, on subjects in group II and group III by a trained periodontist (J.M. and K.L.P.).

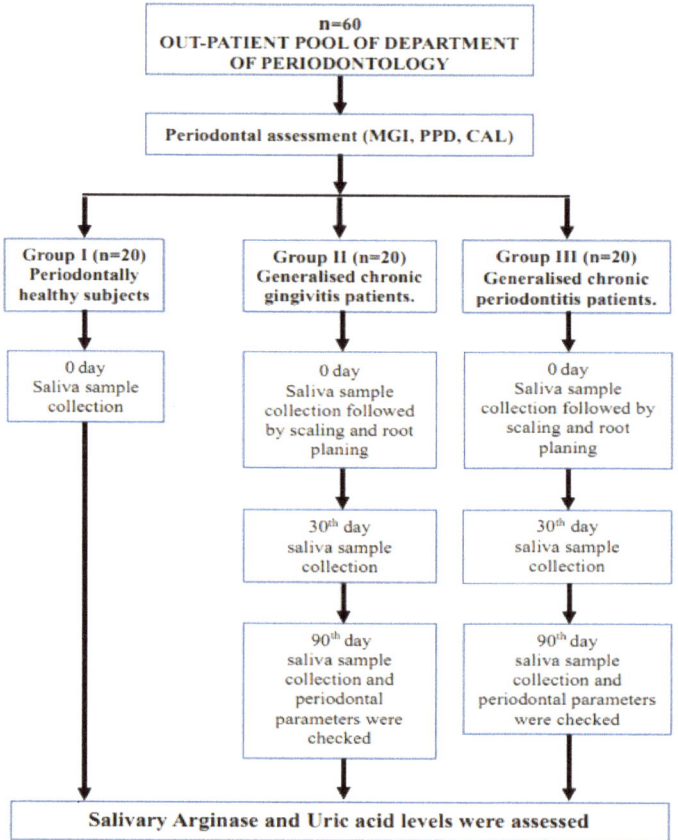

Figure 1. Flowchart of the study design.

2.2. Parameters Assessed

A detailed dental and medical history of the subjects was noted at the initial visit, followed by a periodontal examination that included: the modified gingival index (MGI) [10], clinical attachment level (CAL), and probing pocket depth (PPD), which were measured using a William's periodontal probe. Salivary arginase and uric acid levels were estimated at days 0, 30, and 90 (Figure 1). All parameters were assessed by calibrated investigators and taken as an average (K.L.P. and J.M.).

2.3. Collection of Unstimulated Saliva Samples

Saliva sample collection was standardized according to the circadian rhythm of the subjects. The individuals were requested to clean their mouths completely by rinsing with distilled water before the saliva samples were collected. The patients were instructed to swallow any leftover saliva in their mouth following the oral rinse. A 5 mL sample of unstimulated saliva was obtained in the morning between the hours of 10 am to 11 am, two hours after the last meal. The participants were asked to keep their mouths closed and not cough up mucus while their saliva was collected. They were instructed to let their saliva pool to its utmost extent on the floor of their mouths and then expectorate into the collection vessel until the necessary amount was gathered. The samples were taken to the laboratory using a standard gel coolant pack maintaining a temperature between 2 and 4 °C for immediate testing.

2.4. Estimation of Salivary Arginase and Uric Acid Levels

Saliva samples were centrifuged for 15 min and their supernatant was stored at minus 20 °C until the assay was performed. The salivary arginase level was estimated using an arginase activity assay kit ^. All reagents were brought to room temperature before the procedure. Both the urea reagent and substrate buffer were freshly prepared before the assay and used within 2 h. The substrate buffer was prepared for each well of the reaction by mixing 4 µL of arginine buffer and 2 µL of Mn solution provided in the kit. The urea reagent was created by mixing 105 µL of both reagents A and B provided in the kit. An aliquot of 40 µL of arginase was transferred to each individual well. Two wells were reserved as blank wells. A 5 µL test sample (saliva) was added to the remaining wells containing the arginase. The plate was incubated for 15 min at 25 °C. An aliquot of 5 µL of substrate was added to all wells, except the blank well. A volume of 5 µL of distilled water was added to the blank well and incubated for 30 min at 25 °C. Following incubation, 200 µL of urea reagent was added to all wells to stop the arginase reaction. The plate was incubated at room temperature (37 °C). An ELISA plate reader (LABSERV) was used to measure the optical density (O.D.) at 430 nm.

Uric acid analysis was performed using uric acid reagent (2 × 25 mL) and uric acid standard reagent (1.5 mL with a concentration of 8 mg/dL) **. The semi-auto analyzer was programmed to detect uric acid in the test samples at 510 nm. The kit contained ready-to-use components. The standard solution was pipetted and 0.5 µL was taken in Eppendorf tubes and incubated for 20 min at room temperature. The standard solution was aspirated through the analyzer and the concentration was measured to be 8 mg/dL, as provided by the uric acid estimation kit. An aliquot of 1.0 µL of uric acid reagent was taken in an Eppendorf tube and 0.5 µL of the test (saliva) sample was added. The contents were tapped, allowed to mix, and incubated for 10 min at room temperature. The working reagent along with the test sample was aspirated and the concentration of uric acid was estimated at 510 nm.

^ Sigma Aldrich—arginase activity assay kit (Sigma-Aldrich, St. Louis, MO, USA).

** Gen X uric acid estimation kit (Proton Biologicals India PVT LTD, Bangalore, Karnataka, India).

2.5. Statistical Analysis

Statistical analysis was performed using IBM SPSS software version 26.0 (IBM Corp., Armonk, NY, USA). The descriptive statistics were expressed using the mean and standard deviation. Shapiro-Wilk and Kolmogorov-Smirnov tests were used to assess the normality of the data. Based on the results obtained, the values followed a normal distribution. To compare mean values between groups, one-way ANOVA was applied, followed by Tukey's HSD post hoc test for multiple pairwise comparisons. Karl Pearson correlations were calculated to assess the linear relationship between biomarkers and clinical variables. The probability value <0.05 was considered significant.

3. Results

Intra- and intergroup comparisons revealed that mean changes in clinical attachment level (CAL), probing pocket depth (PPD), and modified gingival index (MGI) from day 0 to day 90 were statistically significant ($p = 0.000$) for group II and group III (Table 1).

All three groups showed a significant difference ($p = 0.000$) in salivary arginase levels on days 0, 30, and 90. Salivary arginase levels were found to be higher in group III at all time points compared to those in group II. Although the intragroup comparison of salivary arginase levels was reduced at different time points, they did not show any statistically significant difference in mean change (Table 2).

Table 1. Comparison of standard deviation, mean, and significant differences for periodontal parameters (MGI, PPD, CAL) within and between groups at different time intervals.

Periodontal Parameters	Time Interval (Days)	Group I (Mean ± SD)	Group II (Mean ± SD)	Group III (Mean ± SD)	p-Value
Modified gingival index	0	0.42 ± 0.20	1.17 ± 0.20	2.52 ± 0.21	0.000 *
	90	-	0.30 ± 0.13	1.66 ± 0.28	0.000 *
	Mean change 0 to 90	-	0.86 ± 0.20	0.86 ± 0.27	0.984 NS
	p-value	-	0.000 *	0.000 *	
Probing pocket depth (mm)	0	1.36 ± 0.27	1.48 ± 0.14	5.10 ± 0.26	0.000 *
	90	-	1.18 ± 0.07	2.29 ± 0.48	0.000 *
	Mean change 0 to 90	-	0.29 ± 0.15	2.80 ± 0.52	0.000 *
	p-value	-	0.000 *	0.000 *	
Clinical attachment level (mm)	0	1.35 ± 0.27	1.48 ± 0.14	5.47 ± 0.23	0.000 *
	90	-	1.18 ± 0.07	2.41 ± 0.62	0.000 *
	Mean change 0 to 90	-	0.29 ± 0.15	3.05 ± 0.60	0.000 *
	p-value	-	0.000 *	0.000 *	

*—Statistically significant; NS—Statistically not significant. Level of statistical significance $p < 0.05$.

Table 2. Comparison of mean, standard deviation, and significant differences for salivary arginase and uric acid levels within and between groups at different time intervals.

Salivary Parameters	Time Intervals (Days)	Group I	Group II	Group III	p-Value
Salivary arginase levels Units/L	0	3.21 ± 4.15	9.20 ± 5.93	14.31 ± 6.02	0.000 *
	30	-	7.74 ± 1.30	13.70 ± 1.37	0.003 *
	90	-	5.43 ± 1.17	11.18 ± 1.46	0.004 *
	p-value	-	0.076 NS	0.404 NS	-
	Mean change 0 to 30th day	-	1.46 ± 8.32	0.60 ± 7.23	0.731 NS
	p-value	-	1.000 NS	1.000 NS	
	Mean change 0 to 90th day	-	3.74 ± 6.75	3.13 ± 10.43	0.818 NS
	p-value	-	0.066 NS	0.586 NS	
	Mean change 30th to 90th day	-	2.31 ± 8.32	2.52 ± 8.71	0.938 NS
	p-value	-	0.687 NS	0.632 NS	
Salivary uric acid levels mg/dL	0	21.49 ± 10.01	9.73 ± 7.56	5.64 ± 4.32	0.000 *
	30	-	10.21 ± 11.19	16.30 ± 13.91	0.136 NS
	90	-	16.35 ± 12.10	18.54 ± 10.01	0.537 NS
	p-value	-	0.127 NS	0.000 *	-
	Mean change 0 to 30th day	-	0.48 ± 12.27	10.66 ± 13.68	0.018 *
	p-value	-	1.000 NS	0.007 *	
	Mean change 0 to 90th day	-	−6.62 ± 13.50	−12.90 ± 10.22	0.106 NS
	p-value	-	0.123 NS	0.000 *	
	Mean change 30th to 90th day	-	−6.13 ± 16.09	−2.23 ± 16.34	0.452 NS
	p-value	-	0.31 NS	1.000 NS	

*—Statistically significant; NS—Statistically not significant; Level of statistical significance $p < 0.05$.

Intergroup and intragroup assessments of salivary uric acid levels showed a statistically significant difference on day 0 among the groups. Intergroup comparisons of mean change in uric acid levels were statistically significant from day 0 to day 30. Similarly, intragroup comparisons also revealed statistically significant mean changes in uric acid levels from day 0 to day 30 and from day 0 to day 90 in group III (Table 2).

Karl Pearson correlation analysis was carried out to determine correlations between salivary arginase and uric acid levels with periodontal parameters on day 0 in all three groups. The results showed that both the levels of salivary arginase and uric acid were significantly correlated with MGI, PPD, and CAL on day 0 for all three groups ($p = 0.000$) (Table 3).

Table 3. Karl Pearson correlation analysis of salivary arginase and uric acid levels and all periodontal parameters on day 0 for all three groups (I, II, and III).

Periodontal Parameters		Salivary Arginase (units/L) (N = 60)	Salivary Uric Acid (mg/dL) (N = 60)
Modified gingival index	CORRELATION	0.625	−0.568
	p-value	0.000 *	0.000 *
Probing pocket depth (mm)	CORRELATION	0.556	−0.458
	p-value	0.000 *	0.000 *
Clinical attachment level (mm)	CORRELATION	0.555	−0.461
	p-value	0.000 *	0.000 *

*—Statistically significant; Level of statistical significance $p < 0.05$.

The salivary arginase levels were significantly correlated with the MGI, PPD, and CAL on day 90. However, the salivary uric acid level did not show any correlation with the clinical parameters on day 90 (Table 4).

Table 4. Karl Pearson correlation analysis of salivary arginase and uric acid levels and all periodontal parameters on the 90th day for groups II and III.

Periodontal Parameters		Salivary Arginase (units/L) (n = 40)	Salivary Uric Acid (mg/dL) (n = 40)
Modified gingival index	CORRELATION	0.426	0.124
	p-value	0.006 *	0.447 [NS]
Probing pocket depth (mm)	CORRELATION	0.343	0.100
	p-value	0.03 *	0.538 [NS]
Clinical attachment level (mm)	CORRELATION	0.316	0.090
	p-value	0.047 *	0.583 [NS]

*—Statistically significant; [NS]—Statistically not significant; Level of statistical significance $p < 0.05$.

4. Discussion

Periodontal disease is the sixth most prevalent disease globally, characterized by intermittent pain and destruction of tooth-supporting structures initiated by a complex microbial biofilm [12]. Saliva may prove to be an ideal diagnostic medium. Saliva contains a wide range of enzymes and molecules, including arginase, oxidized glutathione, uric acid, albumin, vitamin C, reduced glutathione, and SOD (superoxide dismutase), which work in concert to exert a defence against bacterial insult. Measuring the total enzyme status can reveal the severity of a disease, estimate the risk of diagnosing oral disease, and help monitor the host's response to various oral treatments. Quantifying these biomarkers can also help identify periodontal risk factors [13,14].

Salivary arginase is considered to be essential in inflammation. Arginase is found mainly in the liver and salivary glands. This enzyme catalyzes the hydrolysis of L-arginine to urea and ornithine and forms one of the five key enzymes in the urea cycle. Arginase helps in the synthesis of polyamines in saliva, which are nutritionally important to the oral microbiota. Raised levels of arginase may lead to a decrease in NO (nitric oxide) synthesis and increased susceptibility to bacterial infection [15].

Uric acid is a major non-enzymatic enzyme present in saliva in healthy and periodontitis conditions [16]. Salivary uric acid levels may relate to plasma uric acid levels and can be used to assess enzyme status. Gozalez-Hernadez et al. reported uric acid as a major enzyme present in saliva, contributing to 70% of the total enzyme capacity [17]. It acts as a pro-oxidant or as an enzyme depending on the environment [18]. In hydrophilic conditions, it acts as an enzyme combating ROS. In a hydrophobic environment, it acts as a pro-oxidant. Raised levels of uric acid can induce situations associated with oxidative stress, such as obesity, hypertension, and cardiovascular diseases. Hyperuricemia is a diseased state that could also indicate a protective response against oxidative damage [18].

This study quantified salivary arginase and uric acid levels in patients with periodontitis and generalized gingivitis compared to those in periodontally healthy subjects. We also examined the impact of non-surgical periodontal therapy on salivary arginase and uric acid levels in these patients.

Among the periodontal parameters assessed, the mean modified gingival index was reduced from day 0 to day 90 in group III and group II following scaling and root planing, which was statistically significant (Table 1, p = 0.000). These results are in accordance with earlier observations reported by Labao et al. and Kim et al. who found a reduction in inflammation following non-surgical therapy [19,20]. In intragroup and intergroup comparisons, we found the mean probing pocket depth (PPD) was significantly reduced from day 0 to 90 in group III and group II (p = 0.000). Van Der Weijden and Mesell et al. reported similar reductions in probing pocket depth following non-surgical therapy in chronic periodontitis subjects [21,22]. Similarly, in our study, there was an improvement in the mean clinical attachment level (CAL) from day 0 to 90 in group III and group II, which was also statistically significant (p = 0.000). These results corroborated the findings of Shah et al. and Schlagenhauf et al. who observed that non-surgical therapy resulted in a reduction of recession and clinical attachment gain [23,24]. Clinical attachment level is an important periodontal parameter that acts as an indicator of past tissue destruction, which helps to assess disease severity. Broadly consistent with previous research, we found that non-surgical therapy improved periodontal parameters in patients with gingivitis and periodontitis.

The levels of salivary arginase and uric acid were assessed before and after non-surgical periodontal therapy on day 0, day 30, and day 90. L-arginine is a common substrate that is used by NOS to synthesize nitric oxide, which has antimicrobial properties against periodontal pathogens and host inflammatory cells [24,25]. In the present study, intergroup comparisons of salivary arginase levels on days 0, 30, and 90 in group III and group II showed statistical significance (Table 2, p = 0.000). Similar results were obtained by Castro et al. who observed increased salivary levels of arginase in periodontitis subjects and concluded that the enzymes can be used as a marker for periodontal inflammation [25]. However, intragroup comparisons of the mean change in salivary arginase levels in group II and group III did not show any statistical significance (p = 0.07 and p = 0.404, respectively). A possible explanation could be that both groups had periodontal inflammation and hence had higher levels of arginase. These findings suggest that salivary arginase activity in periodontitis, along with the arginine-nitric oxide pathway, may be involved in the disease process using the common substrate L-arginine and inhibiting nitric oxide production. Periodontal therapy may result in an improvement in levels of salivary arginase [25]. Our results suggest that arginase is associated with the inflammatory processes of periodontal disease and its activity is decreased concurrently with progression in clinical parameters, making it a potential inflammatory biomarker [11].

Various salivary antioxidants, such as superoxide dismutase, albumin, and ascorbic acid, have been used as markers for the diagnosis of periodontitis. Due to their high sensitivity and specificity, salivary uric acid and arginase can be potent and reliable markers for evaluating periodontal status [10]. We observed a positive correlation between periodontal markers (MGI, PPD, and CAL) and salivary arginase in groups II and III on day 0 and day 90 (Tables 3 and 4). Similar results were obtained by Haririan et al. who found an improvement in clinical parameters with a reduction in salivary arginase levels following non-surgical periodontal treatment [26]. The subsequent reduction in levels of salivary arginase indicates that arginase levels are directly related to periodontal health status.

The intergroup comparison of salivary uric acid levels on day 0 in all three groups was statistically significant (Table 2, p = 0.000). These results are similar to those reported by Rizal and Vega, Pattanshetti et al., and Uppin et al. who found reduced levels of salivary uric acid in periodontitis patients compared to those in healthy subjects [11,27,28]. The difference in uric acid levels among the groups may be attributed to bacterial variability in gingivitis and periodontitis. We did not observe any significant difference in uric acid levels in group II and group III on day 30 and day 90 following non-surgical therapy.

The intragroup comparison of salivary uric acid levels in group II at different time points did not show any significant difference. However, in group III, the differences were statistically significant (Table 2, p = 0.000). These results are likely related to the inflammatory burden and oxidative stress in periodontitis being markedly higher than in gingivitis. Hence, non-surgical periodontal therapy that reduces inflammation could have a profound impact on salivary uric acid levels [29]. Uric acid levels tend to rise after non-surgical periodontal therapy, further facilitating healing of the tissues [28]. Nominal levels of oxidative stress trigger the action of protective enzymatic mechanisms, resulting in maintenance of the structural integrity of the periodontium. Non-surgical periodontal therapy results in a significant decrease in the bacterial load and oxidative stress in the periodontal tissues. The elimination of oxidative stress results in variations in the levels of uric acid, suggesting potential biomarkers for oral health [30]. Similar results were obtained by Sayar et al. and Baz et al. in gingivitis patients following non-surgical therapy [31,32]. An increase in salivary uric acid levels in periodontitis patients was attributed to a decrease in the abundance of free radicals following periodontal treatment [15].

Salivary uric acid levels showed a positive correlation with periodontal parameters (MGI, PPD, and CAL) on day 0, which was statistically significant (Table 3, p = 0.000). The improvement in periodontal status through non-surgical periodontal therapy increased salivary uric acid levels. Our result reflects those of Sayar et al. who observed a rise in uric acid levels with improvement in the periodontal status [31]. Bacterial invasion can cause a loss of balance between ROS and antioxidant defense, which contributes to the pathogenesis of periodontal disease. Similarly, Baz et al. found that the excessive amount of free radicals produced by periodontal inflammation exhausted the defensive capabilities of this enzyme, leading to tissue damage [32]. A decrease in free radical abundance can be achieved by eliminating inflammation through non-surgical therapy such as scaling and root planing, thereby neutralizing and restoring oxidative homeostasis and leading to improvement in the periodontal status. However, on the 90th day, salivary uric acid levels did not show any positive correlation with periodontal parameters (Table 4). The mouth is a heterogeneous environment for the resident microbiota but offers several distinct habitats for microbial colonization. These oral habitats form a highly heterogeneous ecological system and support the growth of significantly different microbial communities. The alternating warm and moist environment in the oral cavity suits the growth of many microorganisms and offers host-derived nutrients, such as saliva proteins, glycoproteins, and gingival crevicular fluid (GCF), among which the current study highlighted the effects of salivary uric acid and arginase on periodontal disease progression. In addition, an unbalanced oral microbiome could be detrimental not only to oral health but also have an effect on general health. Thus, balancing the host oral microbiota from a dysbiotic to a symbiotic environment is needed to achieve cessation of disease progression, which could be achieved by evolving adjunct pro- and prebiotic therapy [33].

The results of our study indicate the role and importance of salivary arginase in periodontal disease and highlight the relationship between periodontal inflammation and enzyme levels. Our results demonstrated that non-surgical periodontal therapy is capable of eliminating the inflammatory burden and producing a profound impact on levels of uric acid in groups II and III from day 0 to 90 after non-surgical periodontal treatment. Hence, salivary uric acid and arginase can be utilized as sensitive and specific biomarkers for the early detection of periodontal inflammation and tissue destruction, since they exert a definitive role in periodontal disease destruction and are widely distributed in saliva.

One limitation of our study was that only salivary enzymes were measured. In future, serum enzymatic levels can also be assessed and compared with salivary enzyme levels in order to authenticate the results. Further research can validate our findings by assessing the gene expression of arginase using RT-PCR. Another limitation of our study was the use of saliva as a diagnostic tool for the detection of biomarkers as it is prone to contamination and concentration variability of proteins and enzymes. GCF samples, as a more specific diagnostic tool, could be implemented for collecting oral samples. Further, future studies exploring the effects of non-surgical periodontal therapy on arginase and uric acid receptors and inhibitors in the gingival crevicular fluid would more specifically clarify the patho-immunogenic link between these biomarkers and periodontal disease.

5. Conclusions

The study showed decreased salivary arginase levels in patients with gingivitis and periodontitis following the non-surgical periodontal therapy (NSPT). Salivary arginase levels were also found to be positively correlated with periodontal parameters. On the other hand, salivary uric acid levels showed improvement following NSPT in these patients. Our findings indicate that levels of salivary arginase and uric acid can be used as potential biomarkers in the early detection of periodontal inflammation and indicators following periodontal therapy. In future, these biomarkers could help provide a non-invasive, chair-side diagnosis in the era of advancing diagnostic technology in order to provide point-of-care diagnosis, screening, and monitoring of treatment efficacy.

Author Contributions: Conceptualization, K.L.P., J.M., L.M. and K.F.A.; methodology, A.K., S.V. and S.B.; software, M.M.A., K.J.A. and M.A.B.; validation, A.A.-H.A.-A.H., H.A.B., A.A., T.M.B. and S.V.; formal analysis, K.L.P., L.M. and A.K..; investigation, K.F.A., K.L.P. and S.B.; resources, A.A.-H.A.-A.H., K.J.A. and M.A.B.; data curation, J.M., S.V. and M.H.M.; writing—original draft preparation, S.B., J.M., L.M., A.A., K.F.A., A.K. and M.A.B.; writing—review and editing, H.A.B., K.L.P., M.H.M., S.V., T.M.B., A.A.-H.A.-A.H., M.M.A. and K.J.A.; visualization, M.H.M., S.V. and S.B.; supervision, T.M.B., K.J.A. and L.M.; project administration, K.L.P., J.M. and A.K.; funding acquisition, M.M.A., K.F.A., L.M., S.B. and H.A.B. All authors have read and agreed to the published version of the manuscript.

Funding: This work was supported by Taif University Researchers Supporting Program (project number: TURSP-2020/153), Taif University, Saudi Arabia.

Institutional Review Board Statement: The study was conducted in accordance with the guidelines of Meenakshi Ammal Dental College and Hospital, Chennai, India. Ethical approval was obtained from the Institutional Review Board of MAHER—Deemed to be University, Chennai (MADC/IRB-XXV/2018/393).

Informed Consent Statement: Informed consent was obtained from all subjects involved in the study.

Data Availability Statement: Not applicable.

Conflicts of Interest: The authors declare no conflict of interest.

References

1. Papapanou, P.N.; Sanz, M.; Buduneli, N.; Dietrich, T.; Feres, M.; Fine, D.H.; Flemmig, T.F.; Garcia, R.; Giannobile, W.V.; Graziani, F.; et al. Periodontitis: Consensus report of workgroup 2 of the 2017 World Workshop on the Classification of Periodontal and Peri-Implant Diseases and Conditions. *J. Periodontol.* **2018**, *89*, S173–S182. [CrossRef] [PubMed]
2. Arigbede, A.; Babatope, B.; Bamidele, M. Periodontitis and systemic diseases: A literature review. *J. Indian Soc. Periodontol.* **2012**, *16*, 487. [CrossRef] [PubMed]
3. Bhusari, B.M.; Mahajan, R.; Rajbhoj, S.; Shah, S. Reactive Oxygen Species& Its Role in Periodontal Disease. *J. Dent. Sci.* **2014**, *13*, 52–59.
4. Caton, J.G.; Armitage, G.; Berglundh, T.; Chapple, I.L.; Jepsen, S.; Kornman, K.S.; Mealey, B.L.; Papapanou, P.N.; Sanz, M.; Tonetti, M.S. A new classification scheme for periodontal and peri-implant diseases and conditions–Introduction and key changes from the 1999 classification. *J. Periodontol.* **2018**, *89*, S1–S8. [CrossRef] [PubMed]
5. Ahamed, S.L.; Nalini, E.H.; Kumar, A.P.; Devi, R. Salivary biomarkers of periodontal disease-the ultimate diagnostic tool. *Int. J. Recent. Sci. Res.* **2018**, *9*, 25927–25932. [CrossRef]
6. Huang, L.; Shao, D.; Wang, Y.; Cui, X.; Li, Y.; Chen, Q.; Cui, J. Human body-fluid proteome: Quantitative profiling and computational prediction. *Brief. Bioinform.* **2021**, *22*, 315–333. [CrossRef]
7. Ji, S.; Choi, Y. Point-of-care diagnosis of periodontitis using saliva: Technically feasible but still a challenge. *Front. Cell. Infect. Microbiol.* **2015**, *5*, 65. [CrossRef]
8. Tanwar, J.; Hungund, S.; Dodani, K. Nonsurgical periodontal therapy: A review. *J. Oral Res. Rev.* **2016**, *8*, 39. [CrossRef]
9. Butera, A.; Gallo, S.; Pascadopoli, M.; Maiorani, C.; Milone, A.; Alovisi, M.; Scribante, A. Paraprobiotics in non-surgical periodontal therapy: Clinical and microbiological aspects in a 6-month follow-up domiciliary protocol for oral hygiene. *Microorganisms* **2022**, *10*, 337. [CrossRef]
10. Martí i Líndez, A.A.; Reith, W. Arginine-dependent immune responses. *Cell. Mol. Life Sci.* **2021**, *78*, 5303–5324. [CrossRef]
11. Rizal, M.I.; Vega, S. Level of Salivary Uric Acid in Gingivitis and Periodontitis Patients. *Sci. Dent. J.* **2017**, *1*, 7. [CrossRef]
12. Kajiya, M.; Kurihara, H. Molecular Mechanisms of Periodontal Disease. *Int. J. Mol. Sci.* **2021**, *22*, 930. [CrossRef] [PubMed]
13. Qasim, S.S.B.; Al-Otaibi, D.; Al-Jasser, R.; Gul, S.S.; Zafar, M.S. An Evidence-Based Update on the Molecular Mechanisms Underlying Periodontal Diseases. *Int. J. Mol. Sci.* **2020**, *21*, 3829. [CrossRef] [PubMed]
14. Ko, T.J.; Byrd, K.M.; Kim, S.A. The Chairside Periodontal Diagnostic Toolkit: Past, Present, and Future. *Diagnostics* **2021**, *11*, 932. [CrossRef]
15. Li, Z.; Wang, L.; Ren, Y.; Huang, Y.; Liu, W.; Lv, Z.; Qian, L.; Yu, Y.; Xiong, Y. Arginase shedding light on the mechanisms and opportunities in cardiovascular diseases. *Cell Death Discov.* **2022**, *8*, 413. [CrossRef]
16. Kalburgi, N.B.; Koregal, A.C.S.N. Arginase: An Emerging Key Player in Periodontal Disease and Diabetes Mellitus. *Int. J. Dent. Sci. Innov. Res.* **2019**, *2*, 153–159.
17. González-Hernández, J.M.; Franco, L.; Colomer-Poveda, D.; Martinez-Subiela, S.; Cugat, R.; Cerón, J.J.; Márquez, G.; Martínez-Aranda, L.M.; Jimenez-Reyes, P.; Tvarijonaviciute, A. Influence of sampling conditions, salivary flow, and total protein content in uric acid measurements in saliva. *Antioxidants* **2019**, *8*, 389. [CrossRef]
18. Schwartz MNeiers, F.; Feron, G.; Canon, F. The relationship between salivary redox, diet, and food flavo perception. *Front. Nutr.* **2021**, *7*, 612735. [CrossRef]
19. Lobao, W.; Carvalho, R.C.; Leite, S.A.; Rodrigues, V.P.; Batista, J.E.; Gomes-Filho, I.S.; Pereira, A.L. Relationship between periodontal outcomes and serum biomarkers changes after non-surgical periodontal therapy. *An. Da Acad. Bras. De Ciências* **2019**, *91*, e20170652. [CrossRef]
20. Kim, J.Y.; Kim, H.N. Changes in Inflammatory Cytokines in Saliva after Non-Surgical Periodontal Therapy: A Systematic Review and Meta-Analysis. *Int. J. Environ. Res. Public Health* **2021**, *18*, 194. [CrossRef]
21. Van der Wenden, G.A.; Dekkers, G.J.; Slot, D.E. Success of non-surgical periodontal therapy in adult periodontitis patients. A retrospective analysis. *Int. J. Dent. Hyg.* **2019**, *17*, 309–317. [CrossRef]
22. Mesell, S.E.; Bahar, K.U.; Leyla, K.U. Relationships between initial probing depth and changes in the clinical parameters following non-surgical periodontal treatment in chronic periodontitis. *J. Istanb. Univ. Fac. Dent.* **2017**, *51*, 11–17. [CrossRef]
23. Shah, H.K.; Sharma, S.; Goel, K.; Shrestha, S.; Niraula, S.R. Probing Pocket Depth and Clinical Attachment Level between Non-Surgical and Surgical Periodontal Therapy in Chronic Periodontitis Patients: A Randomised Controlled Clinical Trial. *J. Nepal. Soc. Periodontol. Oral Implantol.* **2018**, *2*, 40–44.22. [CrossRef]
24. Schlagenhauf, U.; Hess, J.V.; Stölzel, P.; Haubitz, I.; Jockel-Schneider, Y. Impact of a two-stage subgingival instrumentation scheme involving air polishing on attachment gain after active periodontal therapy. *J. Periodontol.* **2022**, *93*, 1500–1509. [CrossRef]
25. De Castro, M.V.M.; Cortelli, S.C.; Rodrigues, E.; de Moraes, A.; Costa, F.O.; de Maximo, P.M.; Cortelli, J.R. Salivary arginase activity after mechanical-chemical therapy. *Rev. Odontol. Da UNESP* **2018**, *47*, 261–266. [CrossRef]
26. Haririan, H.; Andrukhov, O.; Laky, M.; Rausch-Fan, X. Saliva as a Source of Biomarkers for Periodontitis and Periimplantitis. *Front. Dent. Med.* **2021**, *2*, 687638. [CrossRef]
27. Pattanshetti, J.; Kataria, N.; Kalburgi, N.B.; Athanasiadis, L.; Ioannidis, P.; Efrosini, K. Serum uric acid: Exploring the link between tobacco and periodontitis-Current Issue. *Int. J. Sci. Res.* **2017**, *6*, 420–423. [CrossRef]
28. Uppin, R.B.; Varghese, S.S. Estimation of serum, salivary, and gingival crevicular uric acid of individuals with and without periodontal disease: A systematic review and meta-analysis. *J. Int. Soc. Prev. Community Dent.* **2022**, *12*, 393. [CrossRef]

29. Fatima, G.; Uppin, R.B.; Kasagani, S.; Tapshetty, R.; Rao, A. Comparison of Salivary Uric Acid Level among Healthy Individuals without Periodontitis with that of Smokers and Non-smokers with Periodontitis. *J. Adv. Oral Res.* **2016**, *7*, 24–28. [CrossRef]
30. Ghezzi, P.; Jaquet, V.; Marcucci, F.; Schmidt, H.H.H.W. The oxidative stress theory of disease: Levels of evidence and epistemological aspects. *Br. J. Pharmacol.* **2017**, *174*, 1784–1796. [CrossRef]
31. Sayar, F.; Ahmadi, R.S.; Montazeri, M. Effect of nonsurgical periodontal therapy on the level of salivary antioxidants in patients with generalized moderate-to-severe chronic periodontitis. *J. Adv. Periodontol. Implant. Dent.* **2019**, *11*, 21–27. [CrossRef]
32. Baz, E.L.; Mohamed, K.; Abd El Gwad, A.; Awadallah, H.I.; Mahallawy, O.S. The use of antioxidants in treatment of patients with gingivitis & chronic periodontitis-intervention study. *J. Environ. Sci. Ain Shams* **2021**, *50*, 217–237. [CrossRef]
33. Deo, P.N.; Deshmukh, R. Oral microbiome: Unveiling the fundamentals. *J. Oral Maxillofac. Pathol. JOMFP* **2019**, *23*, 122. [CrossRef]

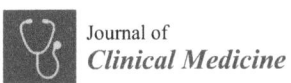

Article

METTL3-Mediated lncSNHG7 m⁶A Modification in the Osteogenic/Odontogenic Differentiation of Human Dental Stem Cells

Yeqing Yang [1,2,3,†], Junkai Zeng [1,3,†], Chong Jiang [4,†], Jiawen Chen [1,3], Ci Song [1], Ming Chen [2,*] and Buling Wu [1,3,5,*]

1. Nanfang Hospital, Southern Medical University, 1838 Guangzhou Avenue North, Guangzhou 510515, China
2. Stomatological Hospital, Southern Medical University, No. 366 Jiangnan Avenue South, Haizhu District, Guangzhou 510280, China
3. School of Stomatology, Southern Medical University, Guangzhou Avenue North, Guangzhou 510515, China
4. Guangdong Provincial People's Hospital, Guangdong Academy of Medical Sciences, Guangzhou 510080, China
5. Shenzhen Stomatology Hospital (Pingshan), Southern Medical University, 143 Dongzong Road, Pingshan District, Shenzhen 518118, China
* Correspondence: kumiming@smu.edu.cn (M.C.); bulingwu@smu.edu.cn (B.W.); Tel.: +86-020-84403983 (M.C.); +86-755-82929331 (B.W.)
† These authors contributed equally to this work.

Abstract: Background: Human dental pulp stem cells (hDPSCs) play an important role in endodontic regeneration. N6-methyladenosine (m⁶A) is the most common RNA modification, and noncoding RNAs have also been demonstrated to have regulatory roles in the expression of m⁶A regulatory proteins. However, the study on m⁶A modification in hDPSCs has not yet been conducted. **Methods**: Single base site PCR (MazF) was used to detect the m⁶A modification site of lncSNHG7 before and after mineralization of hDPSCs to screen the target m⁶A modification protein, and bioinformatics analysis was used to analyze the related pathways rich in lncSNHG7. After knockdown and overexpression of lncSNHG7 and METTL3, the osteogenic/odontogenic ability was detected. After METTL3 knockdown, the m⁶A modification level and its expression of lncSNHG7 were detected by MazF, and their binding was confirmed. Finally, the effects of lncSNHG7 and METTL3 on the Wnt/β-catenin pathway were detected. **Results**: MazF experiments revealed that lncSNHG7 had a m⁶A modification before and after mineralization of hDPSCs, and the occurrence site was 2081. METTL3 was most significantly upregulated after mineralization of hDPSCs. Knockdown/ overexpression of lncSNHG7 and METTL3 inhibited/promoted the osteogenic/odontogenic differentiation of hDPSCs. The m⁶A modification and expression of lncSNHG7 were both regulated by METTL3. Subsequently, lncSNHG7 and METTL3 were found to regulate the Wnt/β-catenin signaling pathway. **Conclusion**: These results revealed that METTL3 can activate the Wnt/β-catenin signaling pathway by regulating the m⁶A modification and expression of lncSNHG7 in hDPSCs to enhance the osteogenic/odontogenic differentiation of hDPSCs. Our study provides new insight into stem cell-based tissue engineering.

Keywords: human dental pulp stem cells; N6-methyladenosine; osteogenic/odontogenic differentiation; RNA epigenetics; long noncoding RNA

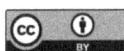

1. Introduction

Bone tissue engineering is based on the concepts of stem cells, growth factors and scaffold materials [1,2]. Many situations, such as trauma, tumor and necrosis, lead to bone defects, which may, eventually, lead to extensive dysfunction [3]. For example, if bacterial invasion and other factors exceed the resistance of the pulp tissue itself, it will further develop into pulpitis and periapical periodontitis [4]. Clinically regenerative endodontic treatment is considered the ideal treatment for necrotic permanent teeth [5]. Therefore, the introduction of effective new strategies to achieve functional and physiological bone reconstruction is urgently required to improve the potential of pulp tissue repair. Human dental pulp stem cells (hDPSCs), initially identified by Gronthos [6], have lower immunogenicity, and higher proliferation rates and cloning potential compared with mesenchymal stem cells [7,8]; moreover, hDPSCs from different species can form regenerative tissue after implantation in animals. In addition, hDPSCs come from a wide range of sources, in sufficient quantity and as a convenient material, showing great potential in regenerative medicine for the treatment of various human diseases; as a consequence, they present good potential for clinical transformation. However, the exact mechanism of osteogenic/odontogenic differentiation is still unclear and requires investigation to achieve the best clinical bone enhancement results.

N6 methyladenosine (m^6A) is the most common modification method in mRNA and was implicated in all aspects of posttranscriptional RNA metabolism [9]. The widespread presence of m^6A in the human transcriptome has aroused great interest among researchers. Exploration of methylation patterns in cells can not only reveal the specific distribution of the m^6A modification in many transcripts, but also the differences in m^6A status under different physiological conditions [10]. The biological function of m^6A modification mainly depends on methyltransferases, demethylases and methylated reading proteins. Among them, methyltransferases such as methyltransferase 3 (METTL3) were most extensively studied: their main role is to catalyze the m^6A modification of adenosine on RNA [11]. It was demonstrated that m^6A modification plays an important role in cancer, metabolism, embryonic stem cell processes and tissue development [12–14]. Studies have shown that the m^6A modification mediated by METTL3 can promote the osteogenic differentiation of bone marrow mesenchymal stem cells through different pathways and help to inhibit the progression of osteoporosis [15]. In addition, the m^6A modification of METTL3 can also promote osteogenic differentiation in human adipose-derived stem cells induced by NEL-like 1 protein [16]. For hDPSCs, it was shown that the m^6A modification of METTL3 has a regulatory role in the cell cycle [17] and METTL3 might affect the LPS-induced inflammatory response by regulating the alternative splicing of MyD88 [18]. However, research on the osteogenic/odontogenic differentiation of hDPSCs is still lacking; improving the osteogenic/odontogenic differentiation ability of hDPSCs is a key issue to be solved before their clinical application and transformation. Therefore, the effects and mechanisms of m^6A modification on the osteogenic/odontogenic differentiation of hDPSCs require further exploration.

Many factors are involved in regulating osteogenic/odontogenic differentiation of mesenchymal stem cells. Among them, long noncoding RNAs (lncRNAs), as a large class of regulatory molecules, have attracted much attention in recent years. A type of noncoding RNA (ncRNA) with a length of more than 200 nucleotides, lncRNAs cannot be translated into protein. Studies have shown that lncRNAs are involved in a variety of biological processes and disease pathogenesis, and they play a significant role in the osteogenic/odontogenic differentiation of stem cells [19,20]. An increasing number of studies have also shown that lncRNAs can affect the osteogenic/odontogenic differentiation of hDPSCs by regulating the expression of downstream target genes in combination with microRNAs (miRNAs) [21–23]. However, current research on whether lncRNAs can play a regulatory role in this process is still in the preliminary stage, and the functions and mechanisms of a large number of lncRNAs are still unclear. In addition, because hDPSCs are ideal seed cells for regenerative tissue engineering, it is of clinical significance to improve their osteogenic/odontogenic differentiation ability through in vitro editing technology before implantation in vivo. Thus far, there has been no research on the regulation of lncRNA m^6A modification in the process of hDPSC osteogenic/odontogenic differentiation, so further research is required.

In this study, and for the first time, m^6A modification of lncRNAs was combined with the hDPSC osteogenic/odontogenic differentiation pathway: it confirmed the promoting effect of METTL3 in the osteogenic/odontogenic differentiation of hDPSCs; it also confirmed the regulatory effect of METTL3 on the m^6A modification of lncRNA SNHG7 and its relationship with the Wnt/β-catenin signaling pathway. The aim was to provide a new concept and method for bone tissue engineering.

2. Methods

2.1. hDPSCs Culture and Characterization

The hDPSCs used in this study were obtained from healthy third molar teeth (without caries and intact after extraction) from 15 patients (6 males and 9 females) aged 18–25 years; the teeth were indicated for extraction at the Department of Stomatology in Nanfang Hospital, Southern Medical University, Guangzhou, Guangdong, China. All experimental protocols were approved by the Ethical Committee, Southern Medical University (NFEC-2022-173). As previously described in [24], the hDPSCs were cultured in Dulbecco's modified Eagle's medium (DMEM) with 10% fetal bovine serum (FBS; GIBCO, Life Technologies, NSW, Australia), 100 U/mL penicillin and 100 μg/mL streptomycin (Sigma, St. Louis, MO, USA) added, at a temperature of 37 °C, and air containing 5% CO_2. The medium was changed every 3 days, and hDPSCs at passages 3–5 were used for the subsequent experiments [25,26]. We divided the samples into two groups: the undifferentiated hDPSC group, in which cells were cultured in 10% FBS in DMEM with no supplements, and the differentiated hDPSC group, in which cells were cultured in 50 mg/mL ascorbic acid, 100 nmol/l dexamethasone and 10 mmol/l β-glycerophosphate (Sigma, St Louis, MO, USA) in DMEM for 14 days. Flow cytometry was performed to identify the phenotypes of the hDPSCs by screening the surface markers against CD29, CD44, CD90, CD45 and CD34.

2.2. Single Base Site PCR (MazF)

The conserved motif region (m^6A ACA site) of the core ACA sequence on lncSNHG7 was verified. The m^6A modification levels in the hDPSC undifferentiated group, differentiated group and after METTL3 knockdown were detected. The RNA endonuclease MazF recognized the RNA single strand and cleaved at the 5' end of the unmethylated ACA site but could not cleave the methylated m^6A ACA site. The extracted total RNA samples were divided into two parts, one without MazF treatment and the other after MazF treatment. The m^6A methylation level of specific ACA sites in the samples was then detected by real-time quantitative polymerase chain reaction (qRT-PCR) [27,28].

2.3. Alkaline Phosphatase (ALP) and Alizarin Red Staining (ARS)

Samples were first washed three times with phosphate-buffered saline and were fixed in 4% paraformaldehyde for 15 min. After washing, the hDPSCs were stained with the NBT/BCIP Staining Kit and Alizarin red. The results for each group were photographed under an inverted microscope.

2.4. Real-Time Polymerase Chain Reaction

The total RNAs were isolated from the undifferentiated hDPSC and differentiated hDPSC groups, obtained by culturing, as described above. A quantity of 1 μg of RNA per sample was reverse-transcribed into cDNA using a cDNA Reverse Transcription Kit (Takara, Tokyo, Japan). qRT-PCR was performed in a 20 μL reaction system. Finally, the relative expression of RNAs was calculated using the $2^{-\Delta\Delta Ct}$ method with glyceraldehyde-3-phosphate dehydrogenase (GAPDH) as the reference gene. Each sample was taken in triplicate, and the results were obtained from the independent experiments. The primer sequences used in the real-time PCR are summarized in Table 1.

Table 1. The sequences of the primers used in PCR.

Gene		Sequence 5′–3′
GAPDH	Forward:	TCAACAGCGACACCCACTC
	Reverse:	GCTGTAGCCAAATTCGTTGTC
ALP	Forward:	CCAAAGGCTTCTTCTTGCTG
	Reverse:	CCACCAAATGTGAAGACGTG
Runx2	Forward:	TCGCCAGGCTTCATAGCAAA
	Reverse:	GGCCTTGGGTAAGGCAGATT
DSPP	Forward:	CAGCAGCGACAGCAGTGATAGC
	Reverse:	TGTCACTGTCACTGTCACTTCCATTG
DMP1	Forward:	CTCCGAGTTGGACGATGAGG
	Reverse:	TCATGCCTGCACTGTTCATTC
METTL3	Forward:	GAGGAGTGCATGAAAGCCAG
	Reverse:	GGCCTCAGAATCCATGCAAG
METTL14	Forward:	GACGGGGACTTCATTCATGC
	Reverse:	CCAGCCTGGTCGAATTGTAC
IGF2BP1	Forward:	TGAAGCTGGAGACCCACATA
	Reverse:	GGGTCTGGTCTCTTGGTACT
IGF2BP2	Forward:	AGTGGAATTGCATGGGAAAATCA
	Reverse:	CAACGGCGGTTTCTGTGTC
IGF2BP3	Forward:	TATATCGGAAACCTCAGCGAGA
	Reverse:	GGACCGAGTGCTCAACTTCT
ALKBH5	Forward:	ACCCCATCCACATCTTCGAG
	Reverse:	CTTGATGTCCTGAGGCCGTA
HNRNPA2B1	Forward:	CAGTTCTCACTACAGCGCCA
	Reverse:	TTCCTCTCCAAAGGAACAGTTT
FTO	Forward:	AGACACCTGGTTTGGCGATA
	Reverse:	CCAAGGTTCCTGTTGAGCAC
YTHDC1	Forward:	CTTCTGATGAGCAAGGGAACAA
	Reverse:	GGCCTCACTTCGAGTGTCATAA
YTHDF1	Forward:	ACCTGTCCAGCTATTACCCG
	Reverse:	TGGTGAGGTATGGAATCGGAG
FMR1	Forward:	TATGCAGCATGTGATGCAACT
	Reverse:	TTGTGGCAGGTTTGTTGGGAT
HNRNPC	Forward:	GTTACCAACAAGACAGATCCTCG
	Reverse:	AGGCAAAGCCCTTATGAACAG
WTAP	Forward:	ACGCAGGGAGAACATTCTTG
	Reverse:	CACACTCGGCTGCTGAACT
lncSNHG7	Forward:	TTGCTGGCGTCTCGGTTAAT
	Reverse:	GGAAGTCCATCACAGGCGAA

2.5. Western Blot Analysis

The hDPSC protein was lysed by radioimmunoprecipitation assay buffer (Pierce, Rockford, IL, USA). The lysate containing loading buffer (2% SDS and 1% 2-mercaptoethanol) was prepared at 99 °C for 5 min. The samples were separated on 10% SDS polyacrylamide gel and transferred to 0.22 µm polyvinylidene fluoride membranes using a semidry transfer apparatus. Afterward, the membranes were blocked with skim milk powder solution at room temperature for 1 h. The transferred proteins were reacted with the primary antibody overnight at 4 °C and then labeled with the secondary antibody for 1 h at room temperature. Primary antibodies in this study included METTL3, GAPDH, dentin sialophosphoprotein (DSPP), dentin matrix acidic phosphoprotein 1 (DMP1), runt-related transcription factor 2 (Runx2) and ALP, phosphorylation-GSK-3β, and GSK-3β and β-catenin. Immunoreactive proteins were detected by using the ECL Kit (Beyotime Biotech, Shanghai, China), and the band densities were quantified using Image J software (National Institutes of Health, MD, USA) (v1.8.0).

2.6. Gene Knockdown and Overexpression

The undifferentiated hDPSC group and differentiated hDPSC group were cultured as described above and seeded into six-well plates at a density of 2×10^5 cells per well.

Transfection was performed when cells had grown to 60–80% confluency according to the instruction manual. For METTL3 and lncSNHG7 knockdown, the small interfering RNAs (siRNAs) for METTL3, lncSNHG7 and negative control siRNA were synthesized by Genechem (Shanghai, China). The overexpression lentivirus of METTL3 and lncSNHG7 were also synthesized by Genechem (Shanghai, China). The transfection procedure followed the manufacturer's instructions.

2.7. Bioinformatic Analysis

The m^6A modification position of lncSNHG7 was predicted by the SRAMP website tool. The binding site of lncSNHG7 to METTL3 was predicted using the catRAPID website, and the interaction probability of lncSNHG7 to METTL3 was predicted using the RPISeq website. Differentially expressed lncRNAs during the osteogenic differentiation of hDPSCs were analyzed using GEO2R in GSE138179 [29] and SRP214747 [30]. m^6Avar, WHISTLE software was used to predict the ACA sites where m^6A modification may occur in lncSNHG7. The Starbase database was used to predict related m^6A-modifying enzymes that may bind to lncSNHG7. Both Gene Ontology (GO) analysis and analysis using the Kyoto Encyclopedia of Genes and Genomes (KEGG) were carried out. GO (http://geneontology.org/, Accessed on 21 September 2021) enrichment analysis was used to define gene attributes in organisms from three fields: biological processes (BP), cellular components (CC) and molecular functions (MF) ($p < 0.05$ was used). David software was used to test the statistical enrichment of the target gene candidates in the KEGG pathway database (KEGG; https://david.ncifcrf.gov/, Accessed on 21 September 2021).

2.8. RNA-Binding Protein Immunoprecipitation (RIP) Assay

Based on the manufacturer's instructions, the RIP assay was removed with an RNA-Binding Protein Immunoprecipitation Kit. Cells were dissolved with RIP lysis buffer. Cell lysates (100 µL) were treated with the RIP buffer and cultured with Proteinase K and magnetic beads conjugated with anti-METTL3 antibody or control (anti-IgG) (Millipore, Burlington, MA, USA). The RNA bound to the beads was purified and then reverse-transcribed into cDNA for qRT-PCR.

2.9. Statistical Analysis

All experiments were performed three times. The data were processed by SPSS 25.0 software (SPSS, Chicago, IL, USA). Analysis of variance and Student's *t*-test were used to evaluate statistical differences in different groups. All results were summarized and shown as means ± standard deviation. Results were treated with statistical significance at $p < 0.05$. One-way analysis of variance (ANOVA) followed by Dunnett's post hoc test was used for multiple group comparisons. Prism software (Graphpad Prism Software, CA, USA) (v8.2.1.441) was used to create the figures.

3. Results

3.1. Characteristics of hDPSCs

hDPSCs were extracted from the third molars of healthy people. Primary cultured hDPSCs grew around the tissue blocks (Figure 1A). Morphological observation showed that the cells had a fibroblast-like appearance (Figure 1B). To further identify the multidirectional differentiation potential of hDPSCs, the isolated hDPSCs were induced to differentiate into osteoblasts and adipocytes. Lipid droplets were observed in the cytoplasm using Oil Red O staining, and the matrix mineralization increased significantly in the process of osteogenic induction compared with the undifferentiated group (Figure 1C–F). In addition, hDPSCs exhibited a high expression of CD29 (99.88%), CD44 (97.87%) and CD90 (99.37%), but were negative for CD34 (0.39%) and CD45 (0.53%) (Figure 1G). The qRT–PCR results suggest that the expression levels of DSPP, DMP1, RUNX2, ALP were upregulated (Figure 1H).

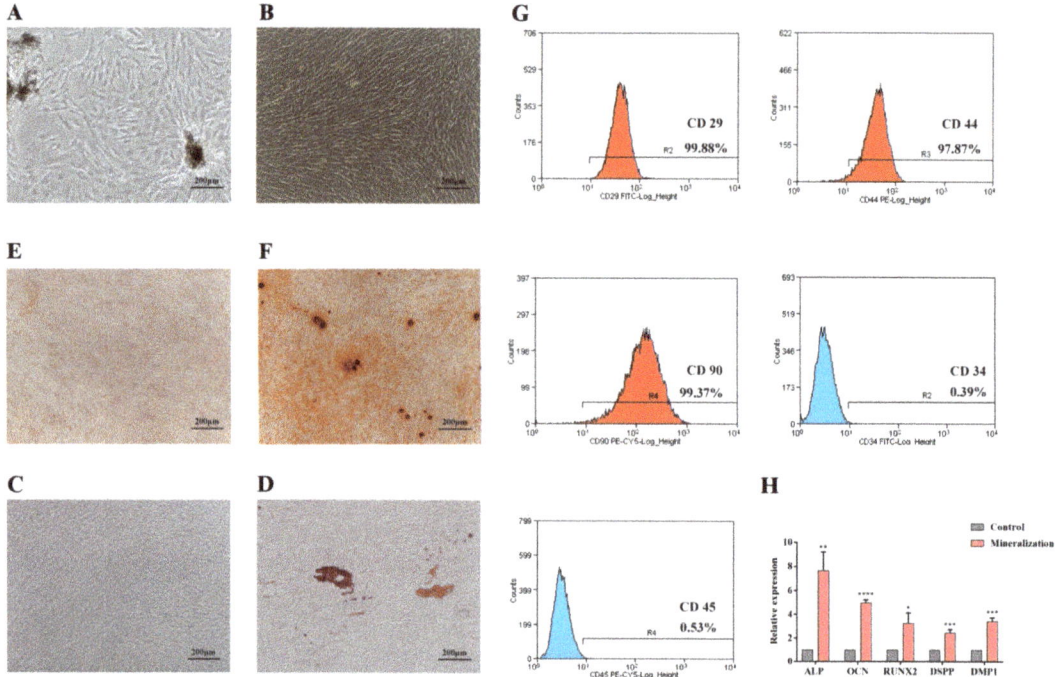

Figure 1. Culture and identification of hDPSCs. (**A,B**) Primary cultured and passage hDPSCs. (**C,D**) Oil red O staining of hDPSCs showed that no lipid droplet was observed in the undifferentiated hDPSCs group but a few lipid droplets were found in the differentiated hDPSCs group. (**E,F**) Alizarin Red S staining of hDPSCs showed that no obvious nodules in the undifferentiated hDPSCs but obviously more nodules and mineralized matrix were formed in the differentiated hDPSCs group. (**G**) The flow cytometric analysis revealed that hDPSCs were positive for mesenchymal stem cell marker (CD29, CD44, CD90) but were negative for hematopoietic stem cell marker (CD34, CD45). (**H**) mRNA expressions of osteogenic/odontogenic genes ALP, OCN, RUNX2, DSPP and DMP1 were detected by qRT-PCR. All samples were performed in triplicate. The data are represented as means ± SD. * $p < 0.05$, ** $p < 0.01$, *** $p < 0.001$, **** $p < 0.0001$.

3.2. lncSNHG7 m^6A Modification in hDPSCs

By analyzing the GSE138179 and SRP214747 datasets, we found that the expression of lncSNHG7 was enhanced after osteogenic/odontogenic differentiation of hDPSCs. Through m^6Avar, the WHISTLE database predicted that lncSNHG7 might have 19 m^6A modification sites (Supplementary Table S1 and Figure 2A), among which there were three ACA modification sites with very high confidence. The m^6A single base site PCR (MazF) verified that lncSNHG7 had an m^6A modification on the 2081 ACA site (Figure 2B). Thus, according to the results of the StarBase database, m^6A-related modifying enzymes that might bind to lncSNHG7 include METTL3/14, IGF2BP1/2/3, ALKBH5, HNRNPA2B1, FTO, YTHDC1, YTHDF1, FMR1, HNRNPC and WTAP (Supplementary Table S2). The expression of all m^6A-related enzymes was detected in hDPSCs, and it was found that the expression levels of most of them increased in hDPSCs after osteogenic/odontogenic differentiation ($p < 0.05$). METTL3 exhibited the highest expression (Figure 2C).

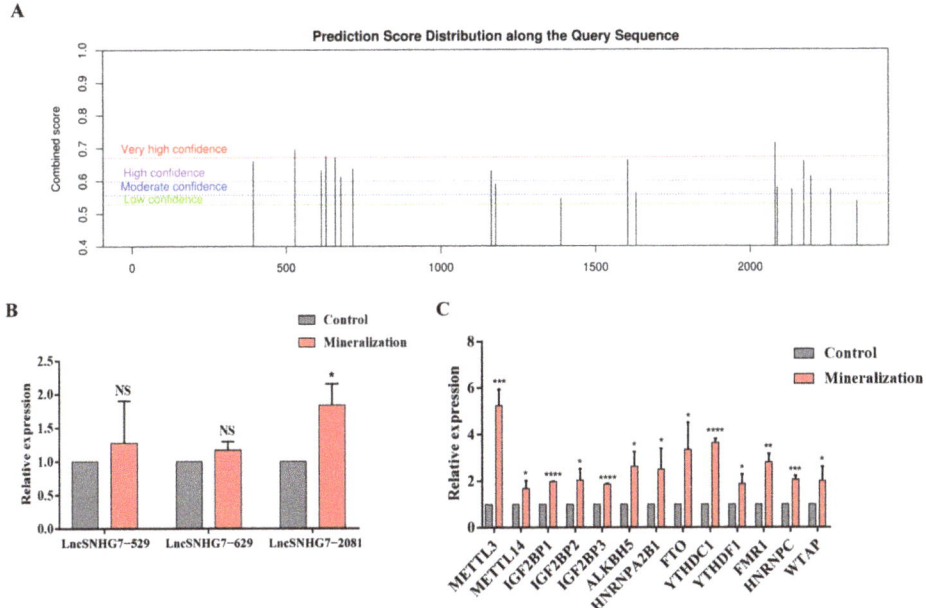

Figure 2. The m⁶A modification on lncSNHG7. (**A**) The m⁶A prediction score distribution of lncSNHG7 predicted by SRAMP website tools. (**B**) Single base site PCR (MazF) analysis was used to confirm the m⁶A modification site of lncSNHG7 after mineralization. (**C**) mRNA expressions of m⁶A modification-related enzymes detected by qRT-PCR. The data were represented as means ± SD for each group: * $p < 0.05$, ** $p < 0.01$, *** $p < 0.001$, **** $p < 0.0001$. NS: Not Statistically Significant.

3.3. METTL3 Promoted Osteogenic/Odontogenic Differentiation of hDPSCs

After mineralization of the hDPSCs, the protein level of METTL3 increased (Figure 3A,B). We speculated that METTL3 might be involved in the regulation of the osteogenic/odontogenic differentiation of hDPSCs. We then knocked down METTL3 using siRNA and the efficiency of the knockdown was verified by qRT–PCR (Figure 3C). After the knockdown of METTL3, decreased mRNA expression levels of the osteogenic/odontogenic genes DSPP, DMP1, RUNX2 and ALP were observed (Figure 3D). The expression of osteogenic/odontogenic differentiation-related proteins was detected by Western Blotting, and the data were consistent with the qRT–PCR results (Figure 3G,H). Similarly, as shown in Figure 3I, after the knockdown of METTL3, both ALP activity and mineralized nodules decreased in the siMETTL3 group compared with the control groups (Figure 3I). In contrast, METTL3 overexpression resulted in reverse impacts on the expression levels of these osteogenic/odontogenic differentiation-related genes (Figure 3E–G). The ALP activity and mineralized nodules also increased after the overexpression of METTL3 (Figure 3I).

3.4. lncSNHG7 Promoted Osteogenic/Odontogenic Differentiation of hDPSCs

The ability of lncSNHG7 to regulate hDPSC osteogenic /odontogenic differentiation was further validated in vitro. siRNA-SNHG7 was constructed and transduced into hDPSCs and was confirmed by qRT–PCR (Figure 4A). As shown in Figure 4B,E,F, lnc-SNHG7 silencing decreased the mRNA and protein expression levels of DSPP, DMP1, RUNX2 and ALP after induction for 14 days. The ALP activity and mineralized nodules also decreased in the si-SNHG7 group compared with the control group (Figure 4G). However, when lncSNHG7 was overexpressed, the phenotypic changes were reversed (Figure 4C–G). The results above demonstrate that lncSNHG7 is an important regulator that could promote osteogenic/odontogenic differentiation of hDPSCs.

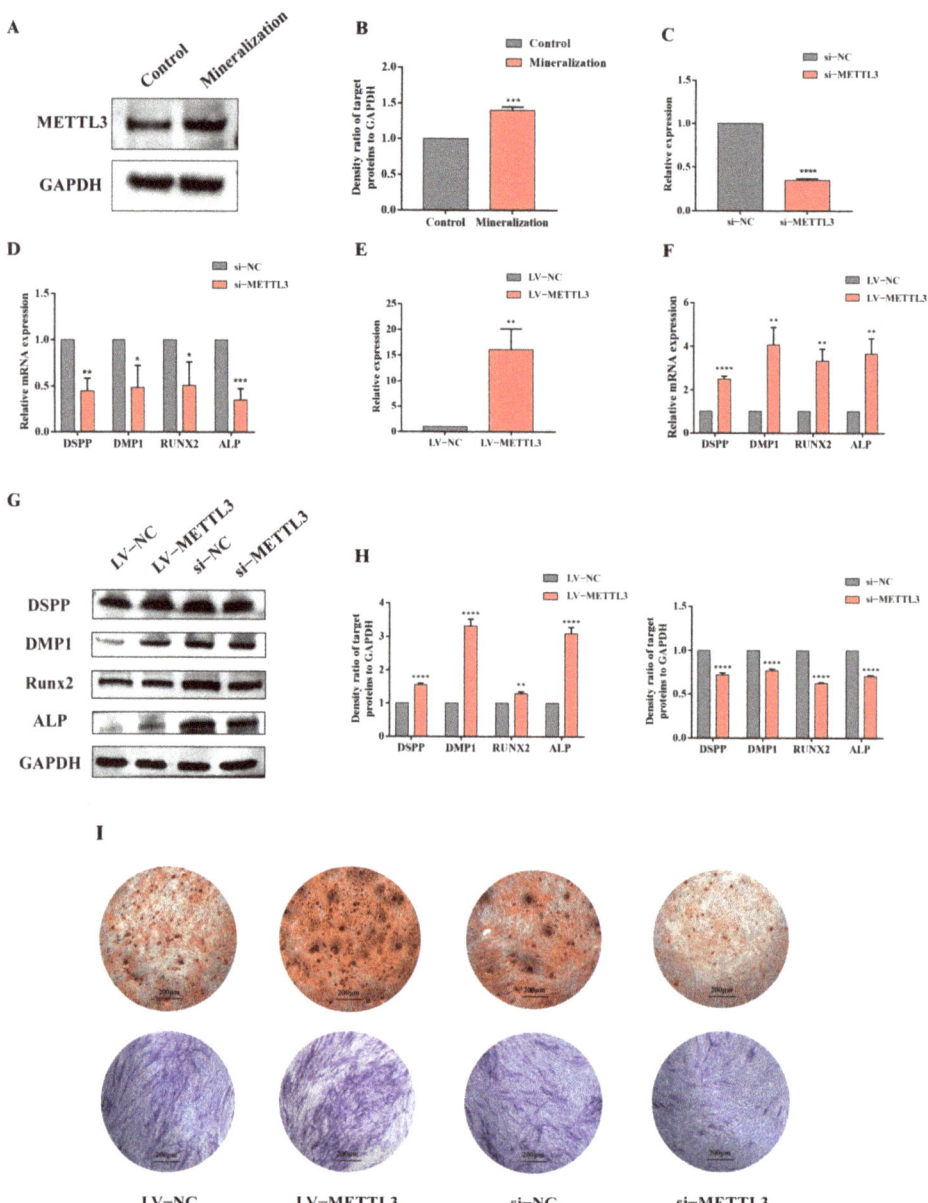

Figure 3. METTL3 promoted osteogenic/odontogenic differentiation of hDPSCs. (**A**) The protein expression of METTL3 detected by Western blot. (**B**) The density ratio of target proteins to GAPDH. (**C**,**E**) The knockdown and overexpression effect of si-METTL3 and LV-METTL3 detected by qRT-PCR. (**D**,**F**) mRNA expressions of osteogenic/odontogenic genes detected by qRT-PCR after the knockdown and overexpression of METTL3. (**G**) Western blot results showed the expression level of osteogenic/odontogenic proteins decreased in the si-METTL3 group and increased in the LV-METTL3 after mineralization. (**H**) The density ratio of target proteins to GAPDH. (**I**) ARS and ALP staining after the knockdown and overexpression of METTL3. The data were represented as means ± SD for each group: * $p < 0.05$, ** $p < 0.01$, *** $p < 0.001$, **** $p < 0.0001$.

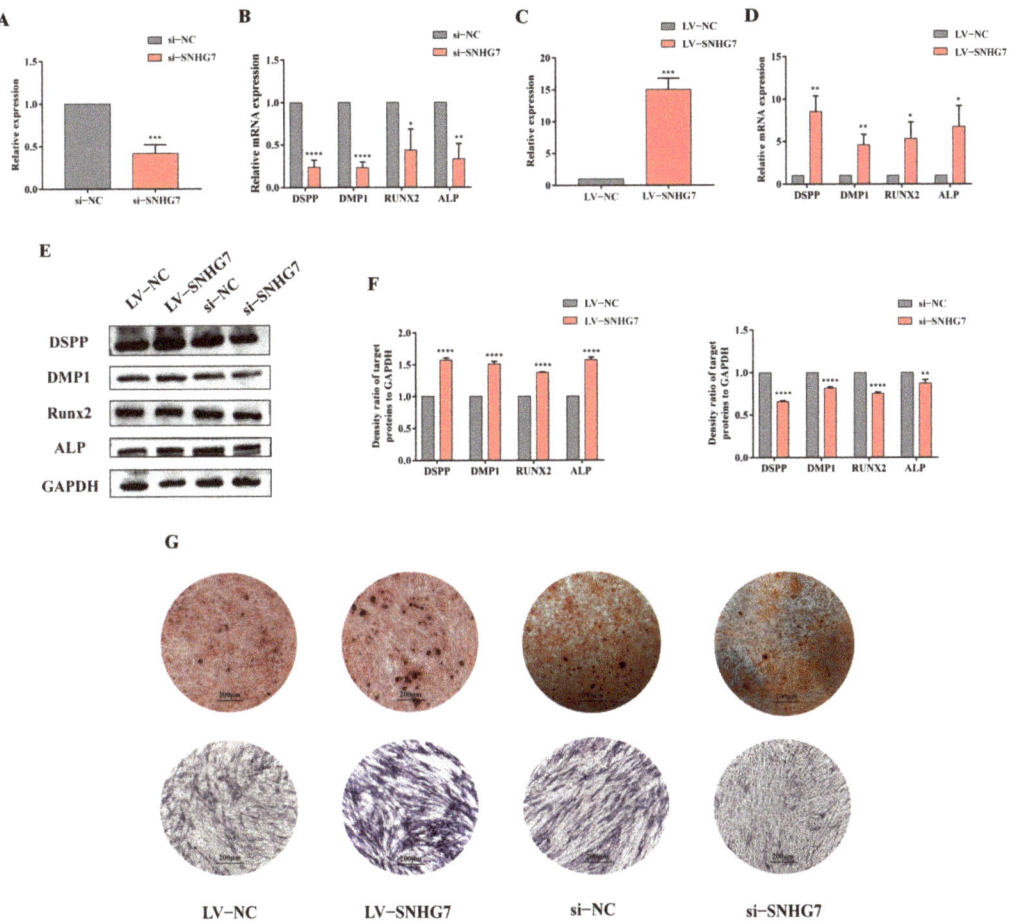

Figure 4. lncSNHG7 promoted osteogenic/odontogenic differentiation of hDPSCs. (**A**,**C**) The knockdown and overexpression effect of si-lncSNHG7 and LV- lncSNHG7 detected by qRT-PCR. (**B**,**D**) mRNA expressions of osteogenic/odontogenic genes detected by qRT-PCR after the knockdown and overexpression of lncSNHG7. (**E**) Western blot results showed the expression level of osteogenic/odontogenic proteins decreased in the si-lncSNHG7 group and increased in the LV- lncSNHG7 group after mineralization. (**F**) The density ratio of target proteins to GAPDH. (**G**) ARS and ALP staining after the knockdown and overexpression of lncSNHG7. The data were represented as means ± SD for each group: * $p < 0.05$, ** $p < 0.01$, *** $p < 0.001$, **** $p < 0.0001$.

To further understand the possible roles of lncSNHG7 in functional regulation, GO analysis and KEGG pathway analysis were performed, using the predicted target mRNAs of the lncRNAs based on the StarBase database. The enriched functions in the three GO categories (BP, MF and CC) are shown in Figure 5A. The enriched GO terms for the biological process category are the regulation of transcription from the RNA polymerase II promoter, signal transduction and protein phosphorylation, etc. The molecular-function-structured networks indicate protein binding, transcription factor activity and sequence-specific DNA binding. Through cellular component analysis, the target genes were found to be widely involved in the cytoplasm, nucleus and plasma membrane, etc. The results of the KEGG pathway analysis show that the target mRNAs of lncSNHG7 were enriched in many pathways, including cancer, cytokine–cytokine receptor interactions and transcriptional misregulation in cancer. Four enriched pathways were closely related to osteogenic/odontogenic differentiation, such as MAPK, NF-kappa B, Wnt and TGF-beta (Figure 5B). Figure 5C shows a map of the Wnt signaling pathway.

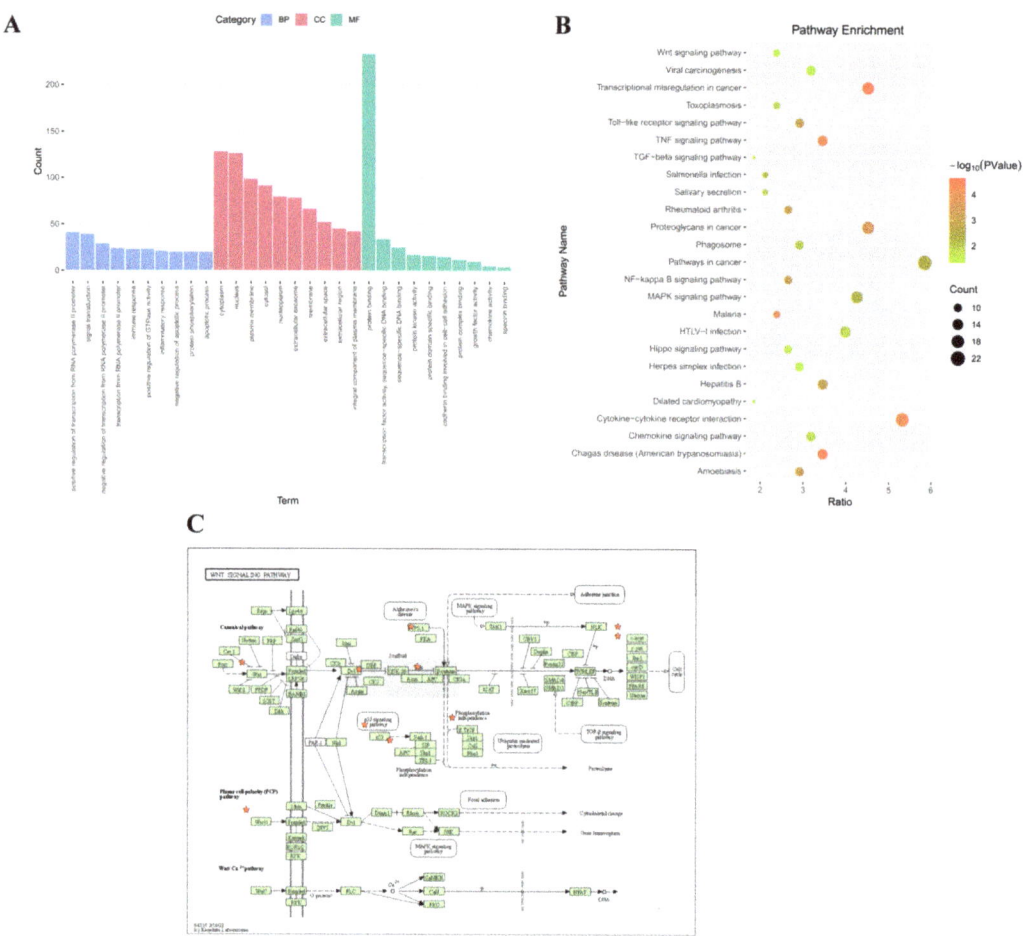

Figure 5. Bioinformatics analysis of lncSNHG7. (**A**,**B**) GO and KEGG pathway analysis of lncSNHG7. (**C**) Wnt signaling pathway map. Red Stars: The potential target gene of lncSNHG7 involved in Wnt signaling pathway.

3.5. METTL3 Regulated the m^6A Modification of lncSNHG7

METTL3 was shown to be an m^6A methyltransferase involved in regulating a variety of physiological processes [31]. Because lncSNHG7 has three ACA modification sites with very high confidence, we speculated that METTL3 could target and regulate the m^6A modification of lncSNHG7. First, after knocking down METTL3, it was found that the m^6A modification level of lncSNHG7 was reduced (Figure 6A), and the expression level of lncSNHG7 was also reduced, indicating that METTL3 not only regulated the m^6A modification of lncSNHG7, but also affected its expression (Figure 6B). The overexpression of lncSNHG7 could rescue the reduced expression levels of DSPP, DMP1, RUNX2 and ALP caused by the knockdown of METTL3 (Figure 6C–E). In addition, we analyzed the nucleotide sequence of lncSNHG7 by catRAPID and found that nucleotides at 70–121 and 495–546 had a high potential to bind with proteins (Figure 6F). The possibility of the combination of lncSNHG7 and METTL3 is shown in Figure 6G and the binding between METTL3 and lncSNHG7 was confirmed by RIP-qPCR (Figure 6H).

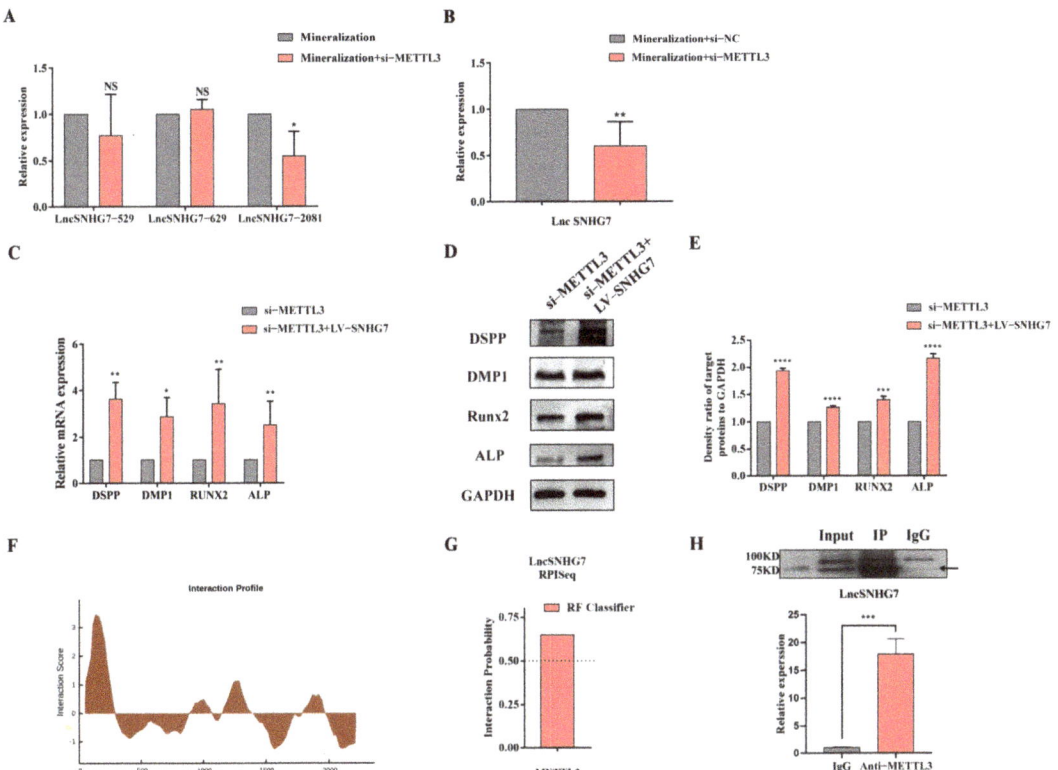

Figure 6. METTL3 regulated the m^{6}A modification of lncSNHG7. (**A**) Single base site PCR (MazF) analysis was used to confirm the m^{6}A modification site of lncSNHG7 after the knockdown of METTL3. (**B**) The expression level of lncSNHG7 after the knockdown of METTL3. (**C,D**) The mRNA and protein expression of osteogenic/ odontogenic genes (DSPP, DMP1, RUNX2 and ALP) under METTL3 knockdown and co-transfection of LV-lncSNHG7. (**E**) The density ratio of target proteins to GAPDH. (**F**) The binding sites between METTL3 and lncSNHG7 were predicted online. (**G**) RPISeq assay showed that METTL3 could bind to lncSNHG7 (The value greater than 0.50 indicates high binding possibility). (**H**) RIP-qPCR confirmed the interaction between METTL3 and lncSNHG7. The data were represented as means ±SD for each group: * $p < 0.05$, ** $p < 0.01$, *** $p < 0.001$, **** $p < 0.0001$. NS: Not Statistically Significant.

3.6. The METTL3/lncSNHG7 Axis Regulated the Wnt/β-Catenin Signaling Pathway

Bioinformatics analysis predicted that the lncSNHG7 target gene was enriched in the Wnt/β-catenin signaling pathway. We speculated that METTL3 could affect the Wnt/β-catenin signaling pathway by regulating the m^{6}A modification of lncSNHG7 to ultimately promote the osteogenic/odontogenic differentiation of hDPSCs. First, lncSNHG7 knockdown resulted in decreased phosphorylation of the key protein GSK-3β in the Wnt/β-catenin signaling pathway and the expression of β-catenin also decreased (Figure 7A,B), indicating that lncSNHG7 activated the Wnt/β-catenin signaling pathway. After METTL3 was knocked down, a decreased expression of phosphorylation of GSK-3β and β-catenin were then observed (Figure 7C,D). These results confirm the presence of the METTL3/lncSNHG7 axis, which could regulate the Wnt/β-catenin signaling pathway and affect the osteogenic/odontogenic differentiation of hDPSCs.

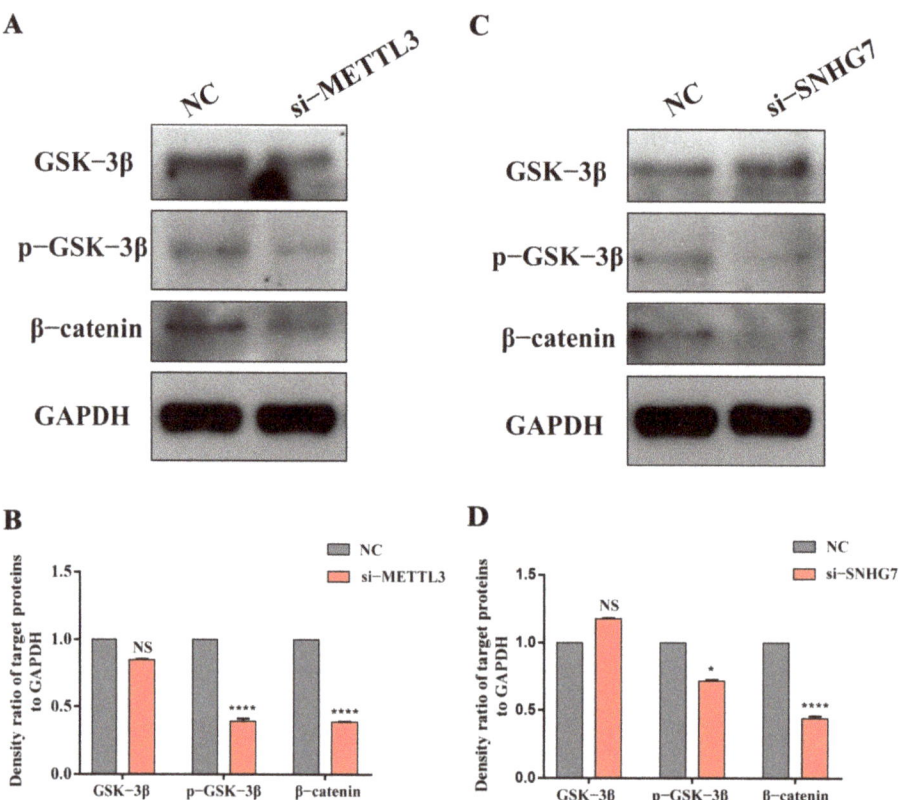

Figure 7. Demonstration of the METTL3/lncSNHG7axis and its regulatory analysis of Wnt/β-catenin signaling pathway. (**A**,**C**) The protein expression levels of β-catenin and GSK-3β phosphorylation under lncSNHG7 and METTL3 knockdown. (**B**,**D**) The density ratio of target proteins to GAPDH. The data were represented as means ± SD for each group: * $p < 0.05$, **** $p < 0.0001$, NS: Not Statistically Significant.

4. Discussion

The m^6A modification is the most common modification in post-transcriptional RNA. It can also regulate noncoding RNAs, such as miRNAs, lncRNAs and circRNAs. The change in its level may be closely related to the metabolism and function of RNA. It has been reported that m^6A modification is involved in the biological processes of a variety of stem cells and plays an important role in bone metabolism. For example, the demethylase ALKBH5 can promote the expression of osteogenic genes [32]. METTL14 plays a regulatory role in osteoporosis. METTL14 can promote osteoclast activity by inhibiting miRNA expression [33]. The importance of METTL3-mediated m^6A methylation of XIST in OPLL provides new insights into therapeutic strategies for OPLL [34]. However, few studies have been conducted to examine m^6A modification of hDPSCs. Luo et al. demonstrated that METTL3 plays a regulatory role in the cell cycle [17]. In addition, METTL3 was found to be involved in the development of tooth roots, the deletion of which led to the reduction in odontogenic differentiation, shortening of molar roots and thinning of dentin by weakening the translation efficiency of nuclear factor IC (NFIC) (a key regulator of tooth roots) [35]. METTL3 can also directly interact with ATP citrate lyase (ACLY) and mitochondrial citrate transporter (SLC25A1) to then further affect the glycolysis pathway and glucose metabolism during the osteogenesis of hDPSCs [36]. However, based on the literature, the mechanism underlying the m^6A modification involved in bone metabolism of hDPSCs has not been fully clarified. It is still controversial and requires further exploration. Recent studies have shown that m^{6}A modification can also affect the stability and metabolism of lncRNAs [37–39]. However, to the best of our knowledge, there has been no research on the regulation of bone homeostasis and bone tissue engineering by m^{6}A of lncRNA in hDPSCs. Therefore, this study is expected to provide a new theoretical basis for the study of the mechanism of osteogenic/odontogenic differentiation in hDPSCs.

In this study, we first identified the m^{6}A modification of lncSNHG7 in hDPSCs by a MazF experiment. Its occurrence region was the 2081 site of the conserved motif region containing the core ACA sequence, but whether the m^{6}A modification of lncSNHG7 still occurs at other sites requires further study. The potential regulatory mechanism of METTL3 in the osteogenic/odontogenic differentiation of hDPSCs was then discussed. Knockdown and overexpression of METTL3, respectively, reduced and increased expression levels of DSPP, DMP1, RUNX2 and ALP, ALP activity and the level of mineralized nodules, which supported the positive regulatory role of METTL3 in the mineralization of hDPSCs, consistent with other studies [40,41]. However, other studies have revealed that METTL3 can inhibit osteogenesis through m^{6}A modification [42,43]. Altogether, these results confirm that METTL3 may be an important regulator of osteogenic/odontogenic differentiation, but the specific regulation of different stem cells requires further study.

lncRNAs can regulate gene expression at the level of chromatin modification, transcription and post-transcriptional processing, and are very important in almost all biological processes, including pluripotency, cell development, the immune response and differentiation. Many studies have shown that lncRNAs play an important role in the osteogenic/odontogenic differentiation of hDPSCs [29,44]. However, there has been no research on the regulation of lncRNA m^{6}A modification in hDPSC osteogenic/odontogenic differentiation. In our study, METTL3 increased m^{6}A methylation and the expression levels of lncSNHG7, leading to promotion of the osteogenic/odontogenic differentiation of hDPSCs. These findings reveal a new role of METTL3 in hDPSCs, showing that METTL3 could promote osteogenic/odontogenic differentiation of hDPSCs through the upregulation of lncSNHG7.

Osteogenic/odontogenic differentiation is regulated by a variety of signaling pathways, including the Wnt/β-catenin signaling pathway. The expression of β-catenin is very important for tooth formation, and β-catenin may play an important role in BMP-9-induced osteogenic and odontogenic signal transduction [45]. Recent data suggested that the treated dentin matrix directly targeted GSK-3β and activated the typical Wnt/β-catenin signaling pathway to promote odontogenic differentiation of hDPSCs [46]. These reports strongly suggested that Wnt/β-catenin signaling regulated osteogenic/odontogenic differentiation. In the present study, through bioinformatics analysis of lncSNHG7, we found that osteogenic/odontogenic differentiation was enriched in the Wnt/β-catenin signaling pathway. We, therefore, speculate that METTL3 can affect the Wnt/β-catenin signaling pathway and that it ultimately promoted the osteogenic/odontogenic differentiation of hDPSCs by regulating the m^{6}A modification of lncSNHG7. Our results show that knockdown of lncSNHG7 and METTL3 led to decreased expression levels of p-GSK-3β and β-catenin in the Wnt/β-catenin signaling pathway.

Improving the differentiation ability of stem cells before clinical application is necessary. Studies demonstrated that Alx3-Wnt3a promoted angiogenesis and newly formed dentin with a structural–mechanical equivalency suggesting that conceptualizing recombinant human Wnt3a delivery in disinfected root canals is one of the possible methods in tooth regeneration [47]. The present study revealed that METTL3-mediated lncSNHG7 m^{6}A modification is involved in the Wnt/β-catenin signaling pathway and could promote osteogenic/odontogenic differentiation of hDPSCs. Similarly, hDPSCs stably transfected with METTL3-lncSNHG7 and synthetic scaffolds (such as collagen, hydrogel, decellularized bioscaffold and nanofibrous spongy microspheres) might be constructed and injected into the disinfected root canal to replace the original root-filling materials for regeneration. Until then, however, the specific underlying mechanisms on the correlation of m^{6}A modification, lncSNHG7 and the Wnt/β-catenin signaling pathway in the process of osteogenic/odontogenic differentiation require further exploration and will be a focus of our future studies.

5. Conclusions

To conclude, the present study revealed that lncSNHG7, mediated by METTL3 through m^6A modification, could activate the Wnt/β-catenin signaling pathway to promote the osteogenic/odontogenic differentiation of hDPSCs (Figure 8). As the activation of molecular pathways is a pivotal characteristic in tissue regeneration, our study might provide a key clue for the future application of hDPSCs in clinically regenerative endodontic treatment. The function of METTL3-mediated lncSNHG7 in vivo will be investigated in our future studies.

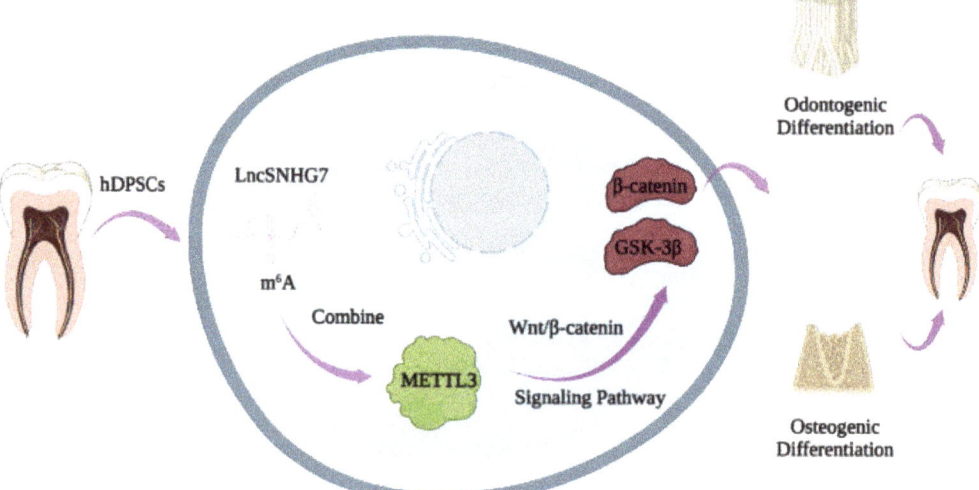

Figure 8. A schematic illustration of the molecular mechanism of lncSNHG7 promoting osteogenic/odontogenic differentiation of hDPSCs. This schematic illustration created in BioRender.com (Accessed on 20 September 2022).

Supplementary Materials: The following supporting information can be downloaded at: https://www.mdpi.com/article/10.3390/jcm12010113/s1, Table S1. Prediction of m6A modification sites of lncSNHG7. Table S2 Prediction of m6A modifying enzymes possibly bound to lncSNHG7.

Author Contributions: Conceptualization, Y.Y., J.Z., C.J., M.C. and B.W.; Data curation, Y.Y. and J.C.; Formal analysis, J.Z.; Funding acquisition, Y.Y., M.C. and B.W.; Resources, B.W.; Supervision, B.W.; Validation, J.Z.; Writing—original draft, Y.Y.; Writing—review and editing, C.J. and C.S. All authors have read and agreed to the published version of the manuscript.

Funding: This work was supported by the General Program of National Natural Scientific Foundation of China (No.81870755); Medical Scientific Research Foundation of Guangdong Province of China (No. A2022199); Science Research Cultivation Program of Stomatological Hospital, Southern Medical University (PY2020018 and PY2021021).

Institutional Review Board Statement: This study was approved by the Ethics Committee of Nanfang Hospital, Southern Medical University (NFEC-2022-173). All subjects were informed and performed under the supervision of the Nanfang Hospital, Southern Medical University Medical Ethics Committee.

Informed Consent Statement: Not applicable.

Data Availability Statement: Not applicable.

Conflicts of Interest: The authors declare no conflict of interest.

Abbreviations

(hDPSCs) Human dental pulp stem cells, (m⁶A) N6 methyladenosine, (METTL3) methyltransferase 3, (lncRNAs) Long noncoding RNAs, (ncRNA) oncoding RNA, (miRNA) microRNA, (DMEM) Dulbecco's modified Eagle's medium, (FBS) Fetal bovine serum, (qRT-PCR) real-time quantitative polymerase chain reaction, (ALP) Alkaline Phosphatase, (ARS) Alizarin Red Staining, (GAPDH) glyceraldehyde-3-phosphate dehydrogenase, (siRNAs) small interfering RNAs, (GO) Gene Ontology, (KEGG) Kyoto Encyclopedia of Genes and Genomes, (BP) biological processes, (CC) cellular components, (MF) molecular functions, (RIP) RNA-binding protein immunoprecipitation, (DSPP) dentin sialophosphoprotein, (DMP1) dentin matrix acidic phosphoprotein 1, (Runx2) runt-related transcription factor 2.

References

1. Zhang, Z. Bone regeneration by stem cell and tissue engineering in oral and maxillofacial region. *Front. Med.* **2011**, *5*, 401–413. [CrossRef] [PubMed]
2. de Souza Lucena, E.E.; Guzen, F.P.; de Paiva Cavalcanti JR, L.; Barboza CA, G.; do Nascimento Júnior, E.S.; de Sousa Cavalcante, J. Experimental considerations concerning the use of stem cells and tissue engineering for facial nerve regeneration: A systematic review. *J. Oral Maxillofac. Surg.* **2014**, *72*, 1001–1012. [CrossRef] [PubMed]
3. Ercal, P.; Pekozer, G.G.; Kose, G.T. Dental stem cells in bone tissue engineering: Current overview and challenges. In *Cell Biology and Translational Medicine*; Springer International Publishing: Cham, Switzerland, 2018; Volume 3, pp. 113–127.
4. Brodzikowska, A.; Ciechanowska, M.; Kopka, M.; Stachura, A.; Włodarski, P.K. Role of Lipopolysaccharide, Derived from Various Bacterial Species, in Pulpitis—A Systematic Review. *Biomolecules* **2022**, *12*, 138. [CrossRef] [PubMed]
5. Elnawam, H.; Abdelmougod, M.; Mobarak, A.; Hussein, M.; Aboualmakarem, H.; Girgis, M.; El Backly, R. Regenerative Endodontics and Minimally Invasive Dentistry: Intertwining Paths Crossing over into Clinical Translation. *Front. Bioeng. Biotechnol.* **2022**, *10*, 837639. [CrossRef]
6. Gronthos, S.; Mankani, M.; Brahim, J.; Robey, P.G.; Shi, S. Postnatal human dental pulp stem cells (DPSCs) in vitro and in vivo. *Proc. Natl. Acad. Sci. USA* **2000**, *97*, 13625–13630. [CrossRef] [PubMed]
7. Yamada, Y.; Nakamura-Yamada, S.; Kusano, K.; Baba, S. Clinical Potential and Current Progress of Dental Pulp Stem Cells for Various Systemic Diseases in Regenerative Medicine: A Concise Review. *Int. J. Mol. Sci.* **2019**, *20*, 1132. [CrossRef] [PubMed]
8. Ching, H.; Luddin, N.; Rahman, I.; Ponnuraj, K. Expression of Odontogenic and Osteogenic Markers in DPSCs and SHED: A Review. *Curr. Stem Cell Res. Ther.* **2016**, *12*, 71–79. [CrossRef] [PubMed]
9. Fazi, F.; Fatica, A. Interplay between N6-Methyladenosine (m6A) and Non-coding RNAs in Cell Development and Cancer. *Front. Cell Dev. Biol.* **2019**, *7*, 116. [CrossRef]
10. Zhou, C.; Molinie, B.; Daneshvar, K.; Pondick, J.V.; Wang, J.; Van Wittenberghe, N.; Xing, Y.; Giallourakis, C.C.; Mullen, A.C. Genome-Wide Maps of m6A circRNAs Identify Widespread and Cell-Type-Specific Methylation Patterns that Are Distinct from mRNAs. *Cell Rep.* **2017**, *20*, 2262–2276. [CrossRef]
11. Wang, P.; Doxtader, K.A.; Nam, Y. Structural Basis for Cooperative Function of Mettl3 and Mettl14 Methyltransferases. *Mol. Cell* **2016**, *63*, 306–317. [CrossRef]
12. Lin, S.; Zhu, Y.; Ji, C.; Yu, W.; Zhang, C.; Tan, L.; Long, M.; Luo, D.; Peng, X. METTL3-Induced miR-222-3p Upregulation Inhibits STK4 and Promotes the Malignant Behaviors of Thyroid Carcinoma Cells. *J. Clin. Endocrinol. Metab.* **2021**, *107*, 474–490. [CrossRef] [PubMed]
13. Xia, C.; Wang, J.; Wu, Z.; Miao, Y.; Chen, C.; Li, R.; Li, J.; Xing, H. METTL3-mediated M6A methylation modification is involved in colistin-induced nephrotoxicity through apoptosis mediated by Keap1/Nrf2 signaling pathway. *Toxicology* **2021**, *462*, 152961. [CrossRef] [PubMed]
14. Bhattarai, P.Y.; Kim, G.; Poudel, M.; Lim, S.-C.; Choi, H.S. METTL3 induces PLX4032 resistance in melanoma by promoting m6A-dependent EGFR translation. *Cancer Lett.* **2021**, *522*, 44–56. [CrossRef] [PubMed]
15. Yan, G.; Yuan, Y.; He, M.; Gong, R.; Lei, H.; Zhou, H.; Wang, W.; Du, W.; Ma, T.; Liu, S.; et al. m6A Methylation of Precursor-miR-320/RUNX2 Controls Osteogenic Potential of Bone Marrow-Derived Mesenchymal Stem Cells. *Mol. Ther.—Nucleic Acids* **2020**, *19*, 421–436. [CrossRef] [PubMed]
16. Song, Y.; Pan, Y.; Wu, M.; Sun, W.; Luo, L.; Zhao, Z.; Liu, J. METTL3-Mediated lncRNA m6A Modification in the Osteogenic Differentiation of Human Adipose-Derived Stem Cells Induced by NEL-Like 1 Protein. *Stem Cell Rev. Rep.* **2021**, *17*, 2276–2290. [CrossRef]
17. Luo, H.; Liu, W.; Zhang, Y.; Yang, Y.; Jiang, X.; Wu, S.; Shao, L. METTL3-mediated m6A modification regulates cell cycle progression of dental pulp stem cells. *Stem Cell Res. Ther.* **2021**, *12*, 159. [CrossRef]

18. Feng, Z.; Li, Q.; Meng, R.; Yi, B.; Xu, Q. METTL 3 regulates alternative splicing of MyD88 upon the lipopolysaccharide-induced inflammatory response in human dental pulp cells. *J. Cell. Mol. Med.* **2018**, *22*, 2558–2568. [CrossRef]
19. Liu, H.; Hu, L.; Yu, G.; Yang, H.; Cao, Y.; Wang, S.; Fan, Z. LncRNA, PLXDC2-OT promoted the osteogenesis potentials of MSCs by inhibiting the deacetylation function of RBM6/SIRT7 complex and OSX specific isoform. *Stem Cells* **2021**, *39*, 1049–1066. [CrossRef]
20. Zhou, Z.; Hossain, M.S.; Da Liu, D. Involvement of the long noncoding RNA H19 in osteogenic differentiation and bone regeneration. *Stem Cell Res. Ther.* **2021**, *12*, 1–9. [CrossRef]
21. Wang, J.; Liu, X.; Wang, Y.; Xin, B.; Wang, W. The role of long noncoding RNA THAP9-AS1 in the osteogenic differentiation of dental pulp stem cells via the miR-652-3p/VEGFA axis. *Eur. J. Oral Sci.* **2021**, *129*, e12790. [CrossRef]
22. Liao, C.; Zhou, Y.; Li, M.; Xia, Y.; Peng, W. LINC00968 promotes osteogenic differentiation in vitro and bone formation in vivo via regulation of miR-3658/RUNX2. *Differentiation* **2020**, *116*, 1–8. [CrossRef] [PubMed]
23. Wu, Y.; Lian, K.; Sun, C. LncRNA LEF1-AS1 promotes osteogenic differentiation of dental pulp stem cells via sponging miR-24-3p. *Mol. Cell. Biochem.* **2020**, *475*, 161–169. [CrossRef] [PubMed]
24. Chen, M.; Yang, Y.; Zeng, J.; Deng, Z.; Wu, B. circRNA Expression Profile in Dental Pulp Stem Cells during Odontogenic Differentiation. *Stem Cells Int.* **2020**, *2020*, 1–19. [CrossRef] [PubMed]
25. Jiang, W.; Lv, H.; Wang, H.; Wang, D.; Sun, S.; Jia, Q.; Wang, P.; Song, B.; Ni, L. Activation of the NLRP3/caspase-1 inflammasome in human dental pulp tissue and human dental pulp fibroblasts. *Cell Tissue Res.* **2015**, *361*, 541–555. [CrossRef] [PubMed]
26. Wei, X.; Ling, J.; Wu, L.; Liu, L.; Xiao, Y. Expression of Mineralization Markers in Dental Pulp Cells. *J. Endod.* **2007**, *33*, 703–708. [CrossRef]
27. Garcia-Campos, M.A.; Edelheit, S.; Toth, U.; Safra, M.; Shachar, R.; Viukov, S.; Winkler, R.; Nir, R.; Lasman, L.; Brandis, A.; et al. Deciphering the "m6A Code" via Antibody-Independent Quantitative Profiling. *Cell* **2019**, *178*, 731–747.e16. [CrossRef]
28. Zhang, Z.; Chen, L.-Q.; Zhao, Y.-L.; Yang, C.-G.; Roundtree, I.A.; Zhang, Z.; Ren, J.; Xie, W.; He, C.; Luo, G.-Z. Single-base mapping of m^{6}A by an antibody-independent method. *Sci. Adv.* **2019**, *5*, eaax0250. [CrossRef]
29. Chen, Z.; Zhang, K.; Qiu, W.; Luo, Y.; Pan, Y.; Li, J.; Yang, Y.; Wu, B.; Fang, F. Genome-wide identification of long noncoding RNAs and their competing endogenous RNA networks involved in the odontogenic differentiation of human dental pulp stem cells. *Stem Cell Res. Ther.* **2020**, *11*, 114. [CrossRef]
30. Liu, Z.; Xu, S.; Dao, J.; Gan, Z.; Zeng, X. Differential expression of lncRNA/miRNA/mRNA and their related functional networks during the osteogenic/odontogenic differentiation of dental pulp stem cells. *J. Cell. Physiol.* **2019**, *235*, 3350–3361. [CrossRef]
31. Xin, Y.; He, Q.; Liang, H.; Zhang, K.; Guo, J.; Zhong, Q.; Chen, D.; Li, J.; Liu, Y.; Chen, S. m6A epitranscriptomic modification regulates neural progenitor-to-glial cell transition in the retina. *Elife* **2022**, *11*, e79994. [CrossRef]
32. Feng, L.; Fan, Y.; Zhou, J.; Li, S.; Zhang, X. The RNA demethylase ALKBH5 promotes osteoblast differentiation by modulating Runx2 mRNA stability. *FEBS Lett.* **2021**, *595*, 2007–2014. [CrossRef] [PubMed]
33. Sun, Z.; Wang, H.; Wang, Y.; Yuan, G.; Yu, X.; Jiang, H.; Wu, Q.; Yang, B.; Hu, Z.; Shi, F.; et al. MiR-103-3p targets the m^{6}A methyltransferase METTL14 to inhibit osteoblastic bone formation. *Aging Cell* **2021**, *20*, e13298. [CrossRef] [PubMed]
34. Yuan, X.; Shi, L.; Guo, Y.; Sun, J.; Miao, J.; Shi, J.; Chen, Y. METTL3 Regulates Ossification of the Posterior Longitudinal Ligament via the lncRNA XIST/miR-302a-3p/USP8 Axis. *Front. Cell Dev. Biol.* **2021**, *9*, 629895. [CrossRef] [PubMed]
35. Sheng, R.; Wang, Y.; Wu, Y.; Wang, J.; Zhang, S.; Li, Q.; Zhang, D.; Qi, X.; Xiao, Q.; Jiang, S.; et al. METTL3-Mediated m^{6}A mRNA Methylation Modulates Tooth Root Formation by Affecting NFIC Translation. *J. Bone Miner. Res.* **2021**, *36*, 412–423. [CrossRef] [PubMed]
36. Cai, W.; Ji, Y.; Han, L.; Zhang, J.; Ni, Y.; Cheng, Y.; Zhang, Y. METTL3-Dependent Glycolysis Regulates Dental Pulp Stem Cell Differentiation. *J. Dent. Res.* **2021**, *101*, 580–589. [CrossRef] [PubMed]
37. Liu, H.; Xu, Y.; Yao, B.; Sui, T.; Lai, L.; Li, Z. A novel N6-methyladenosine (m6A)-dependent fate decision for the lncRNA THOR. *Cell Death Dis.* **2020**, *11*, 613. [CrossRef]
38. Wu, Y.; Yang, X.; Chen, Z.; Tian, L.; Jiang, G.; Chen, F.; Li, J.; An, P.; Lu, L.; Luo, N.; et al. m6A-induced lncRNA RP11 triggers the dissemination of colorectal cancer cells via upregulation of Zeb1. *Mol. Cancer* **2019**, *18*, 87. [CrossRef]
39. Ni, W.; Yao, S.; Zhou, Y.; Liu, Y.; Huang, P.; Zhou, A.; Liu, J.; Che, L.; Li, J. Long noncoding RNA GAS5 inhibits progression of colorectal cancer by interacting with and triggering YAP phosphorylation and degradation and is negatively regulated by the m6A reader YTHDF3. *Mol. Cancer* **2019**, *18*, 143. [CrossRef]
40. Wu, Y.; Xie, L.; Wang, M.; Xiong, Q.; Guo, Y.; Liang, Y.; Li, J.; Sheng, R.; Deng, P.; Wang, Y.; et al. Mettl3-mediated m^{6}A RNA methylation regulates the fate of bone marrow mesenchymal stem cells and osteoporosis. *Nat. Commun.* **2018**, *9*, 4772. [CrossRef]
41. Tian, C.; Huang, Y.; Li, Q.; Feng, Z.; Xu, Q. Mettl3 Regulates Osteogenic Differentiation and Alternative Splicing of Vegfa in Bone Marrow Mesenchymal Stem Cells. *Int. J. Mol. Sci.* **2019**, *20*, 551. [CrossRef]
42. Li, D.; Cai, L.; Meng, R.; Feng, Z.; Xu, Q. METTL3 Modulates Osteoclast Differentiation and Function by Controlling RNA Stability and Nuclear Export. *Int. J. Mol. Sci.* **2020**, *21*, 1660. [CrossRef] [PubMed]
43. Yu, J.; Shen, L.; Liu, Y.; Ming, H.; Zhu, X.; Chu, M.; Lin, J. The m6A methyltransferase METTL3 cooperates with demethylase ALKBH5 to regulate osteogenic differentiation through NF-κB signaling. *Mol. Cell. Biochem.* **2020**, *463*, 203–210. [CrossRef]
44. Zhong, J.; Tu, X.; Kong, Y.; Guo, L.; Li, B.; Zhong, W.; Cheng, Y.; Jiang, Y.; Jiang, Q. LncRNA H19 promotes odontoblastic differentiation of human dental pulp stem cells by regulating miR-140-5p and BMP-2/FGF9. *Stem Cell Res. Ther.* **2020**, *11*, 202. [CrossRef] [PubMed]

45. Luo, W.; Zhang, L.; Huang, B.; Zhang, H.; Zhang, Y.; Zhang, F.; Liang, P.; Chen, Q.; Cheng, Q.; Tan, D.; et al. BMP9-initiated osteogenic/odontogenic differentiation of mouse tooth germ mesenchymal cells (TGMCS) requires Wnt/β-catenin signalling activity. *J. Cell. Mol. Med.* **2021**, *25*, 2666–2678. [CrossRef] [PubMed]
46. Lim, H.-M.; Nam, M.-H.; Kim, Y.-M.; Seo, Y.-K. Increasing Odontoblast-like Differentiation from Dental Pulp Stem Cells through Increase of β-Catenin/p-GSK-3β Expression by Low-Frequency Electromagnetic Field. *Biomedicines* **2021**, *9*, 1049. [CrossRef] [PubMed]
47. He, L.; Zhou, J.; Chen, M.; Lin, C.-S.; Kim, S.G.; Zhou, Y.; Xiang, L.; Xie, M.; Bai, H.; Yao, H.; et al. Parenchymal and stromal tissue regeneration of tooth organ by pivotal signals reinstated in decellularized matrix. *Nat. Mater.* **2019**, *18*, 627–637. [CrossRef] [PubMed]

Disclaimer/Publisher's Note: The statements, opinions and data contained in all publications are solely those of the individual author(s) and contributor(s) and not of MDPI and/or the editor(s). MDPI and/or the editor(s) disclaim responsibility for any injury to people or property resulting from any ideas, methods, instructions or products referred to in the content.

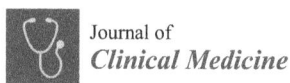 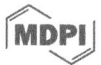

Systematic Review

Comparative Efficacy and Safety of Interventions for the Treatment of Oral Lichen Planus: A Systematic Review and Network Meta-Analysis

Xin Yi Leong [1], Divya Gopinath [2], Sakil M. Syeed [3], Sajesh K. Veettil [3], Naresh Yedthare Shetty [4] and Rohit Kunnath Menon [4,*]

[1] School of Dentistry, International Medical University, Kuala Lumpur 57000, Malaysia
[2] Department of Basic Medical and Dental Sciences, College of Dentistry, Ajman University, Ajman P.O. Box 346, United Arab Emirates
[3] Department of Pharmacotherapy, College of Pharmacy, University of Utah, Salt Lake City, UT 84112, USA
[4] Department of Clinical Sciences, College of Dentistry, Ajman University, Ajman P.O. Box 346, United Arab Emirates
* Correspondence: r.menon@ajman.ac.ae

Abstract: Background: This systematic review and network meta-analysis aimed to assess comparative efficacy and safety of interventions to treat symptomatic, biopsy-proven oral lichen planus (OLP). Methods: Search was conducted for trials published in Medline, Embase and Cochrane Central Register of Controlled Trials. Network meta-analysis was performed on data from randomized controlled trials that assessed efficacy and safety of interventions used in the treatment of OLP. Agents were ranked according to their effectiveness in treatment of OLP based on outcomes using surface under the cumulative ranking [SUCRA]. Results: In total, 37 articles were included in the quantitative analysis. Purslane was clinically significant and ranked first in improving clinical symptoms [RR = 4.53; 95% CI: 1.45, 14.11], followed by aloe vera [RR = 1.53; 95% CI: 1.05, 2.24], topical calcineurin [RR = 1.38; 95% CI: 1.06, 1.81] and topical corticosteroid [RR = 1.35 95% CI: 1.05, 1.73]. Topical calcineurin demonstrated the highest incidence of adverse effects [RR, 3.25 [95% CI: 1.19, 8.86. Topical corticosteroids were significant in achieving clinical improvement of OLP with RR1.37 [95% CI: 1.03, 1.81]. PDT [MD = −5.91 [95% CI: −8.15, −3.68] and showed statistically significant improvement in the clinical score for OLP. Conclusions: Purslane, aloe vera and photodynamic therapy appear promising in treatment of OLP. More high-quality trials are recommended for strengthening the evidence. Although topical calcineurin is significantly efficacious in the treatment of OLP, significant adverse effects are a concern for clinical use. Based on the current evidence, topical corticosteroids are recommended for treatment of OLP owing to their predictable safety and efficacy.

Keywords: systematic review; network meta-analysis; oral lichen planus; management; OLP

Citation: Leong, X.Y.; Gopinath, D.; Syeed, S.M.; Veettil, S.K.; Shetty, N.Y.; Menon, R.K. Comparative Efficacy and Safety of Interventions for the Treatment of Oral Lichen Planus: A Systematic Review and Network Meta-Analysis. *J. Clin. Med.* **2023**, *12*, 2763. https://doi.org/10.3390/jcm12082763

Academic Editor: Agostino Guida

Received: 7 February 2023
Revised: 18 March 2023
Accepted: 20 March 2023
Published: 7 April 2023

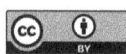

Copyright: © 2023 by the authors. Licensee MDPI, Basel, Switzerland. This article is an open access article distributed under the terms and conditions of the Creative Commons Attribution (CC BY) license (https://creativecommons.org/licenses/by/4.0/).

1. Introduction

Lichen Planus [LP] is a common chronic inflammatory disease involving both the skin and the mucous membranes of the body, including the oral cavity [1,2]. LP involving the oral mucosa is known as oral lichen planus [OLP]. It is a common autoimmune chronic inflammatory oral mucosal disorder affecting the stratified squamous epithelium by a cell-mediated immunological dysfunction [3]. OLP is more common in females between 30–60 years. The prevalence of OLP is reported to be at 1.27% [4]. Traditionally, several forms of OLP were described, such as reticular, papular, plaque, atrophic and ulcerative [erosive] form [5]. Atrophic and erosive forms of OLP usually present with burning sensation to intense pain, requiring treatment and hence are associated with difficulty in eating, swallowing and burning sensation with hot and spicy food [2,6–8]. However, currently, OLP is a dynamic disease, fluctuating often in distribution and extent of the lesions, clinical types, and their severity [9]. Hence, remission is rarely achieved in OLP and relapse is often seen even after treatment [6,7].

Numerous drugs have been used to treat OLP and proposed therapies given are typically symptomatic. However, evidence is inadequate to support the effectiveness of any specific treatment as being more superior than the other [10]. Although a wide range of systemic and topical therapies have been used to treat OLP, a majority of these therapies have not been evaluated in randomized controlled clinical trials [RCTs] [11]. Previous systematic reviews [12–14] on treatment of OLP demonstrated beneficial effects of using topical corticosteroids [TopCORT] or topical calcineurin inhibitors [TopCALN] in treatment settings. Other interventions such as aloe vera [AV] and photochemotherapy [PDT] were also tested in clinical trials. Most of the reported previous systematic reviews [12,13] have focused only on pairwise comparison of interventions. Comprehensive evidence comparing the relative efficacy and safety of all the available interventions has not been previously investigated. A network meta-analysis [NMA] allows for assessing the comparative efficacy and safety across a network of RCTs of all interventions to date through the enablement of investigations to combine both direct and indirect evidence [15]. NMA makes it possible to identify the most effective intervention for a given issue for which there are several potential solutions. Therefore, we aimed to perform a NMA to assess the comparative efficacy and safety of interventions used to treat symptomatic biopsy-proven OLP.

2. Materials and Methodology

This systematic review was performed with a priori published protocol [PROSPERO CRD42021256151] and was reported according to the Preferred Reporting Items for Systematic Reviews and Meta-Analysis [PRISMA] extension statement for incorporating network meta-analysis [NMA] for healthcare interventions [15].

2.1. Search Strategy and Study Selection

We identified relevant studies through a systematic search of Medline, Embase and Cochrane Central Register of Controlled Trials from the inception of databases to August 2022. To identify studies not captured by database searches, we manually checked the reference lists of published systematic reviews and identified articles.

Studies included were RCTs that met the following inclusion criteria.

(i) Population was patients with clinically- and histologically-proven lichen planus.
(ii) Intervention includes any form of local or systemic treatment for OLP.
(iii) Comparison is placebo, any other antifungal agent or no treatment.
(iv) Outcome.

Split mouth studies, in vitro studies, letter to editors, conference abstracts and non-English articles were excluded.

Two reviewers [L.X.Y. and RKM] independently screened titles and abstracts for eligible studies, followed by full text reading. Ineligible studies were excluded from the full text review, and the reasons for exclusion were documented. Any disagreements were resolved by consensus.

2.2. Outcomes of Interest

The primary outcome of interest was a clinical improvement (Thongprasom scale) of the disease. Secondary outcomes were clinical resolution, reduction in pain score (Thongprasom scale), clinical score and adverse effects.

2.3. Data Extraction and Quality Assessment

Data were extracted independently and in duplicates by the two reviewers into a data extraction form created following the Cochrane Handbook of Systematic Reviews of Interventions guidelines, by a consensus of all the reviewers. If multiple publications of the same trial were retrieved, only the most recent information or relevant data was included from these publications. The data from the RCTs were separated into the following sections:

study characteristics, population characteristics, intervention characteristics, outcome definitions and measures. For all outcomes, we used the initial number of participants randomized to each trial arm and performed the analyses irrespective of how the authors of the original trials had analysed the data [intention-to-treat principle] [14]. The risk of bias [ROB] within each study was independently assessed by two reviewers [LYC, RKM] by using the revised Cochrane risk of bias tool [RoB 2.0] [16,17]. Disagreements were resolved by reviewers over discussion.

2.4. Data Synthesis and Statistical Analysis

The treatment effect was evaluated and calculated as the risk ratio [RR], along with a 95% confidence interval [CI]. A random-effects network meta-analysis [NMA] using a consistency model within a frequentist approach was applied to incorporate indirect with direct comparisons [18]. Network inconsistency assumption, which refers to a disagreement between the direct and indirect estimates, was evaluated using a global inconsistency test by fitting design-by-treatment in the inconsistency model [19,20]. For the missing data, we have followed the Cochrane assumption that data are assumed missing at random and that missing values were assumed to have a particular value, such as a poor outcome [21]. Heterogeneity was assessed by I^2 statistics. The percentages indicate low (25%), medium (50%) and high (75%) heterogeneity [22,23]. Surface under the cumulative ranking [SUCRA] curves were estimated to rank the intervention hierarchy in the network meta-analysis [24]. Higher SUCRA scores [ranging from 0 to 1] correspond to higher ranking for clinical effectiveness [i.e., clinical resolution, clinical improvement] of OLP treatment. A comparison-adjusted funnel plot was used to examine the publication bias [24]. Stata version 15.0 [StataCorp, College Station, TX, USA] was used for statistical analysis and graph generation. To assess the robustness of primary efficacy outcome, a sensitivity analysis was performed by restricting studies with low risk of bias.

3. Results

3.1. Study Selection

Our search yielded a total of 975 articles. A total of 88 articles were retained for full-text review following titles and abstracts screening and duplicate references removal. Finally, 37 articles were selected to be included in the meta-analysis. Figure 1 depicts the flow of the study selection process. The list of the excluded is provided in Supplementary Table S1.

3.2. Study Characteristics

Supplementary Table S2 shows the characteristics of included RCTs. The interventions assessed included amlexanox paste [AML], aloe vera [AV], curcumin gel [CUR], photodynamic therapy [PDT], placebo [PLA], purslane [PUR], systemic corticosteroid [SysCORT], topical corticosteroid [TopCORT], topical calcineurin [TopCALN] and topical calcineurin and systemic corticosteroid combined [TopCALNcoSysCORT]. Of thirty-seven included studies, five compared TopCORT and PLA [25–29], fifteen compared TopCORT and TopCALN [1,11,26,30–41], two compared corticosteroids with each other [39,42], six compared corticosteroids with other treatments such as PDT, AML, CUR and HA [43–48], four compared other treatments with PLA, including AV, PUR and HA [49–52], four compared TopCALN and PLA [53–56] and one compared other treatments, including aloe vera with photodynamic therapy [57].

3.3. Quality of RCTs

Quality assessment of each study using the ROB assessment tool is provided in Figure 2. Among the RCTs, 13 trials were evaluated to be at high ROB, 6 were evaluated to be at low ROB, whereas the remaining studies were of unclear ROB.

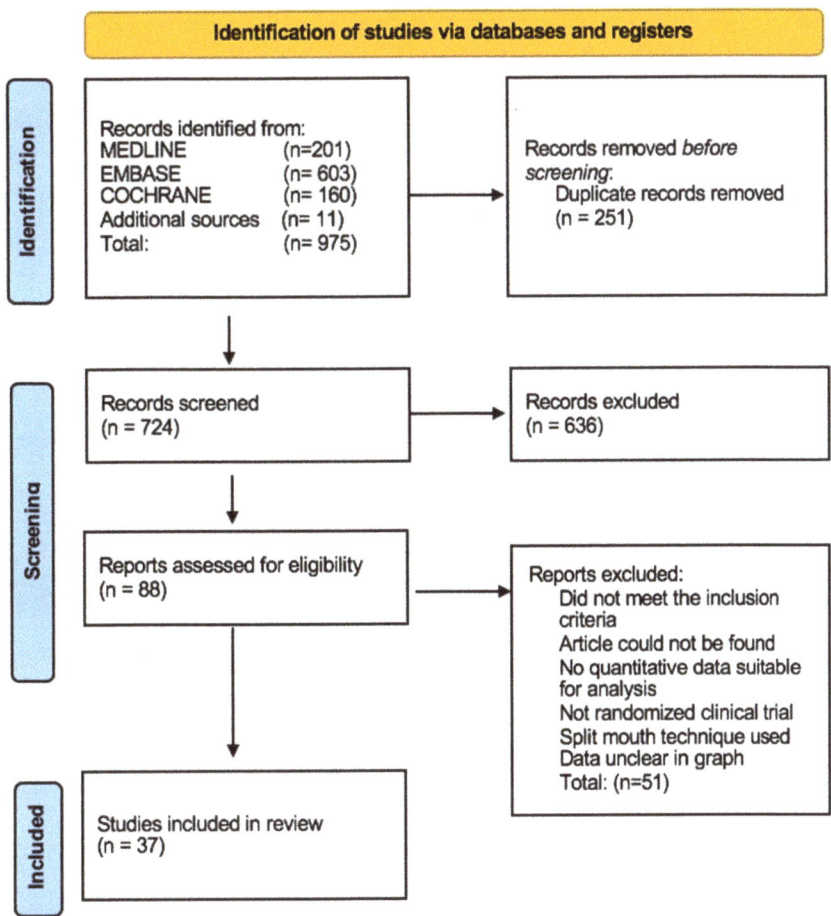

Figure 1. Prisma flow chart.

3.4. NMA Results

3.4.1. Clinical Symptoms Improvement

A total of 37 RCTs comparing 9 interventions were included for this outcome measuring improvement in clinical symptoms. The network plot is provided in Figure 3. Network meta-analysis suggested that, compared with placebo, PUR ranked first in improving clinical symptoms [RR = 4.53; 95% CI: 1.45, 14.11, SUCRA 96.5], followed by AV [RR = 1.53; 95% CI: 1.05, 2.24, SUCRA 57.2], TopCALN [RR = 1.38; 95% CI: 1.06, 1.81, SUCRA 47.3] and TopCORT [RR = 1.35; 95% CI: 1.05, 1.73, SUCRA 40.5]. Other interventions were not statistically significant. Detailed results of SUCRA ranks and curves are presented in Supplementary Table S3 and Supplementary Figure S1, respectively. The league table showing the comparative efficacies shown as the risk ratio [RR] along with a 95% confidence interval [CI] is provided in Figure 4.

Figure 2. Risk of Bias [1,11,25–57].

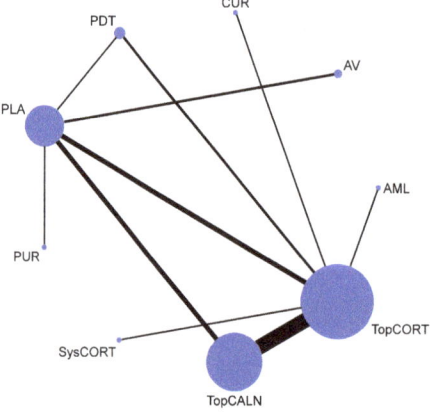

Figure 3. Network plot: Clinical Improvement of Oral Lichen Planus. Abbreviations: AML, amlexanox paste; AV, aloe vera; CUR, curcumin gel; PDT, photodynamic therapy; PLA, placebo; PUR, purslane; SysCORT, systemic corticosteroid; TopCALN, topical calcineurin; TopCALNcoSysCORT, topical calcineurin combined with systemic corticosteroid; TopCORT, topical corticosteroid.

TopCORT								
0.97 (0.84,1.13)	TopCALN							
0.98 (0.55,1.75)	1.01 (0.55,1.83)	SysCORT						
0.30 (0.09,0.95)	0.31 (0.10,0.98)	0.30 (0.08,1.12)	PUR					
0.86 (0.58,1.26)	0.88 (0.59,1.32)	0.87 (0.43,1.76)	2.87 (0.85,9.73)	PDT				
0.79 (0.44,1.41)	0.81 (0.45,1.48)	0.81 (0.35,1.83)	2.65 (0.72,9.70)	0.92 (0.46,1.85)	CUR			
0.88 (0.56,1.38)	0.91 (0.57,1.44)	0.90 (0.43,1.88)	2.96 (0.89,9.79)	1.03 (0.58,1.84)	1.12 (0.54,2.33)	AV		
1.11 (0.69,1.80)	1.14 (0.69,1.89)	1.13 (0.53,2.41)	3.73 (1.06,13.11)	1.30 (0.70,2.40)	1.41 (0.66,2.99)	1.26 (0.65,2.44)	AML	
1.35 (1.06,1.73)	1.39 (1.06,1.81)	1.38 (0.73,2.59)	4.53 (1.46,14.11)	1.58 (1.01,2.46)	1.71 (0.91,3.22)	1.53 (1.05,2.24)	1.22 (0.71,2.09)	PLA

Figure 4. League table for the Clinical Improvement of OLP. Abbreviations: AML, amlexanox paste; AV, aloe vera; CUR, curcumin gel; PDT, photodynamic therapy; PLA, placebo; PUR, purslane; SysCORT, systemic corticosteroid; TopCALN, topical calcineurin; TopCALNcoSysCORT, topical calcineurin combined with systemic corticosteroid; TopCORT, topical corticosteroid. The green gihlights indicate the interventions and the dark highlights indicate the significant results.

3.4.2. Adverse Effects

In the case of adverse effects, there are 20 RCTs that reported those data. The network plot is provided in Figure 5. Network meta-analysis suggested that there was a significant adverse effect compared with placebo only for topical calcineurin [RR, 3.25 [95% CI: 1.19, 8.86]. When ranked, purslane was the best [SUCRA 63] and topical calcineurin was the worst [SUCRA 26.1], indicating the probability of the most adverse effects. Detailed results for SUCRA ranks and curves are presented in Supplementary Table S4 and Supplementary Figure S2, respectively. The league table showing the comparative safety shown as the risk ratio [RR] along with a 95% confidence interval [CI] is provided in Figure 6.

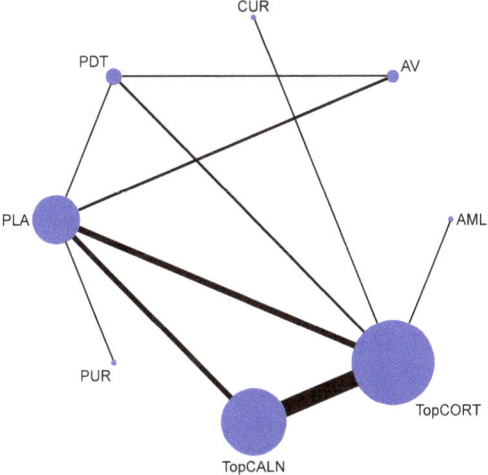

Figure 5. Network plot: Clinical Improvement of Oral Lichen Planus. Abbreviations: AML, amlexanox paste; AV, aloe vera; CUR, curcumin gel; PDT, photodynamic therapy; PLA, placebo; PUR, purslane; SysCORT, systemic corticosteroid; TopCALN, topical calcineurin; TopCALNcoSysCORT, topical calcineurin combined with systemic corticosteroid; TopCORT, topical corticosteroid.

TopCORT							
0.60 (0.31,1.16)	TopCALN						
2.27 (0.03,173.08)	3.79 (0.05,291.97)	PUR					
0.80 (0.12,5.54)	1.34 (0.18,9.91)	0.35 (0.00,36.95)	PDT				
1.00 (0.01,69.36)	1.67 (0.02,121.79)	0.44 (0.00,189.32)	1.25 (0.01,132.10)	CUR			
0.77 (0.07,9.13)	1.29 (0.11,15.69)	0.34 (0.00,42.58)	0.97 (0.07,13.80)	0.77 (0.01,104.53)	AV		
1.48 (0.17,13.06)	2.47 (0.25,24.02)	0.65 (0.01,83.41)	1.85 (0.10,34.09)	1.48 (0.01,173.87)	1.91 (0.07,51.32)	AML	
1.94 (0.75,5.06)	3.25 (1.19,8.86)	0.86 (0.01,58.75)	2.43 (0.35,16.96)	1.94 (0.03,150.07)	2.51 (0.24,25.76)	1.31 (0.12,14.15)	PLA

Figure 6. League table for adverse effects. Abbreviations: AML, amlexanox paste; AV, aloe vera; CUR, curcumin gel; PDT, photodynamic therapy; PLA, placebo; PUR, purslane; SysCORT, systemic corticosteroid; TopCALN, topical calcineurin; TopCALNcoSysCORT, topical calcineurin combined with systemic corticosteroid; TopCORT, topical corticosteroid. The green gihlights indicate the interventions and the dark highlights indicate the significant results.

3.4.3. SUCRA Value for Safety and Efficacy

Figure 7 shows an overall analysis of the safety and efficacy of the interventions that were statistically significant. PUR was the safest and the most efficacious in treatment of OLP. TopCALN caused statistically significant adverse effects, therefore, it is ranked the lowest in safety. TopCORT was considered safe and effective in the treatment of OLP.

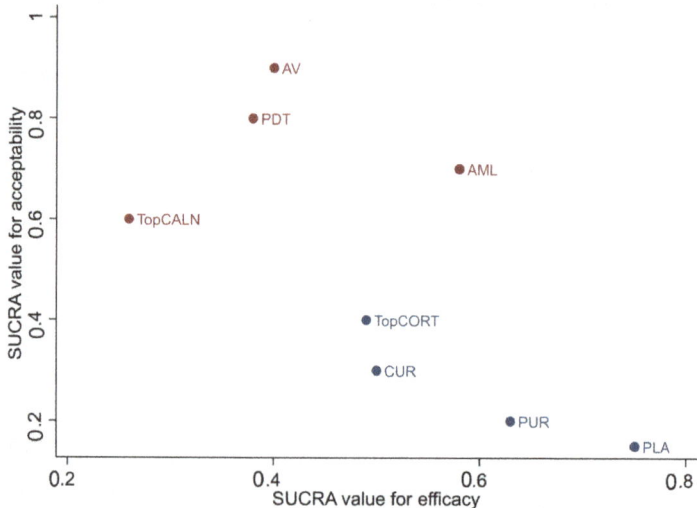

Figure 7. SUCRA Value for Safety and Efficacy of Interventions Used for Treatment of Oral Lichen Planus. Abbreviations: AV, aloe vera; PDT, photodynamic therapy; PUR, purslane; TopCALN, topical calcineurin; TopCORT, topical corticosteroid.

3.4.4. Clinical Resolution

Clinical resolution of OLP was considered as only when the lesion was completely healed. The network plot is provided in Figure 8. Network meta-analysis suggested that only TopCALN [RR = 3.07; 95% CI: 1.20, 7.83] was statistically significant in showing clinical resolution of OLP compared to placebo. Accordingly, on SUCRA ranking, TopCALN was ranked highest [SUCRA 72] for clinical resolution of OLP and TopCORT was the lowest [SUCRA 47.7] compared to placebo. Detailed results of SUCRA ranks and curves are presented in Supplementary Table S5 and Supplementary Figure S3. The league table showing the comparative efficacies shown as the risk ratio [RR] along with a 95% confidence interval [CI] is provided in Figure 9.

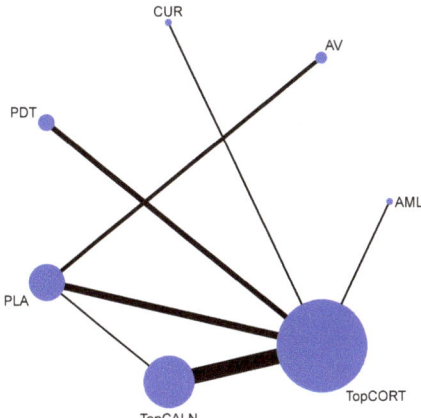

Figure 8. Network Plot: Clinical Resolution of Oral Lichen Planus. Abbreviations: AML, amlexanox paste; AV, aloe vera; CUR, curcumin gel; PDT, photodynamic therapy; PLA, placebo; TopCALN, topical calcineurin; TopCORT, topical corticosteroid.

TopCORT							
0.71 (0.42,1.22)	TopCALN						
0.73 (0.28,1.85)	1.02 (0.35,2.96)	PDT					
1.00 (0.05,19.79)	1.40 (0.07,29.07)	1.38 (0.06,31.48)	CUR				
1.00 (0.19,5.10)	1.40 (0.26,7.51)	1.37 (0.21,9.01)	1.00 (0.03,29.94)	AV			
1.11 (0.25,4.94)	1.56 (0.32,7.60)	1.53 (0.26,8.92)	1.11 (0.04,31.27)	1.11 (0.12,10.18)	AML		
2.19 (0.95,5.04)	3.07 (1.20,7.83)	3.02 (0.85,10.66)	2.19 (0.10,48.56)	2.19 (0.54,8.99)	1.97 (0.36,10.89)	PLA	

Figure 9. League table for adverse effects. Abbreviations: AML, amlexanox paste; AV, aloe vera; CUR, curcumin gel; PDT, photodynamic therapy; PLA, placebo; TopCALN, topical calcineurin; TopCORT, topical corticosteroid. The green highlights indicate the interventions and the dark highlights indicate the significant results.

3.4.5. Clinical Score

Improvement of clinical score for OLP was measured based on Thongprasom scale scoring. It is a scoring system for OLP based on the surface area involved and the severity of the lesion. The output results for clinical score were calculated using mean difference, and the network plot is presented in Figure 10. Based on the NMA findings, PDT [MD = −5.91 [95% CI: −8.15, −3.68] and TopCORT [MD = −1.02 [95% CI: −1.98, −0.06] showed statistically significant improvement in clinical score for OLP. When ranked, PDT demonstrated the highest score in improvement of clinical score for OLP [SUCRA 0] and SysCORT was ranked last [SUCRA 70.8]. Detailed SUCRA ranks and curves are presented in Supplementary Table S6 and Supplementary Figure S4. The league table showing the comparative efficacies shown as the risk ratio [RR] along with a 95% confidence interval [CI] is provided in Figure 11.

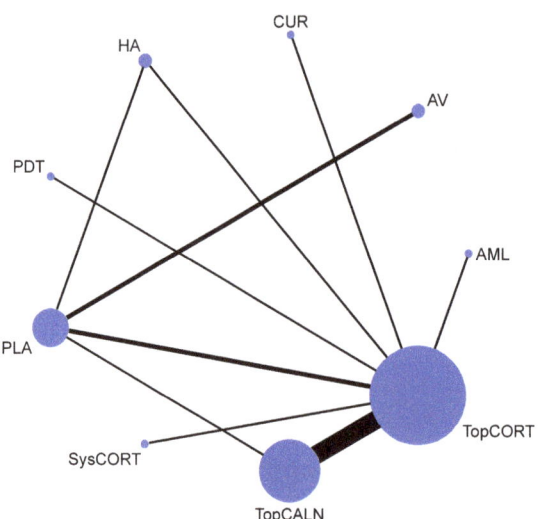

Figure 10. Network Plot: Clinical Score. Abbreviations: AML, amlexanox paste; AV, aloe vera; CUR, curcumin gel; PDT, photodynamic therapy; PLA, placebo; PUR, purslane; SysCORT, systemic corticosteroid; TopCALN, topical calcineurin; TopCORT, topical corticosteroid; HA, hyaluronic acid.

TopCORT								
0.01 (-0.57,0.59)	**TopCALN**							
-0.60 (-2.28,1.08)	-0.61 (-2.38,1.17)	**SysCORT**						
4.90 (2.88,6.92)	4.89 (2.79,7.00)	5.50 (2.88,8.13)	**PDT**					
-0.26 (-1.53,1.01)	-0.27 (-1.64,1.10)	0.34 (-1.77,2.44)	-5.16 (-7.55,-2.78)	**HA**				
0.34 (-1.33,2.01)	0.33 (-1.44,2.10)	0.94 (-1.43,3.31)	-4.56 (-7.18,-1.94)	0.60 (-1.50,2.70)	**CUR**			
0.05 (-1.47,1.58)	0.04 (-1.54,1.63)	0.65 (-1.61,2.92)	-4.85 (-7.38,-2.32)	0.32 (-1.41,2.05)	-0.29 (-2.55,1.98)	**AV**		
-0.13 (-1.83,1.57)	-0.14 (-1.93,1.66)	0.47 (-1.92,2.86)	-5.03 (-7.67,-2.39)	0.13 (-1.99,2.26)	-0.47 (-2.85,1.91)	-0.18 (-2.47,2.10)	**AML**	
-1.02 (-1.97,-0.06)	-1.02 (-2.07,0.02)	-0.42 (-2.35,1.51)	-5.92 (-8.15,-3.68)	-0.75 (-2.01,0.50)	-1.36 (-3.28,0.57)	-1.07 (-2.26,0.12)	-0.89 (-2.83,1.06)	**PLA**

Figure 11. League table for clinical score. Abbreviations: AML, amlexanox paste; AV, aloe vera; CUR, curcumin gel; PDT, photodynamic therapy; PLA, placebo; PUR, purslane; SysCORT, systemic corticosteroid; TopCALN, topical calcineurin; TopCORT, topical corticosteroid; HA, hyaluronic acid. The green highlights indicate the interventions and the dark highlights indicate the significant results.

3.4.6. Pain Score

Pain score was measured with visual analog scale [VAS] scoring. Based on the NMA (Figure 12), PDT showed statistically significant improvement in the pain score [MD −1.63, 95%CI: −2.73, −0.53]. In SUCRA ranks and curves, PDT was ranked the best in improving pain score [SUCRA 94.0], and AV ranked the worst [SUCRA 23.2]. Detailed SUCRA ranks and curves are presented in Supplementary Table S7 and Supplementary Figure S5. The league table showing the comparative efficacies shown as the mean deviation [MD] along with a 95% confidence interval [CI] is provided in Figure 13.

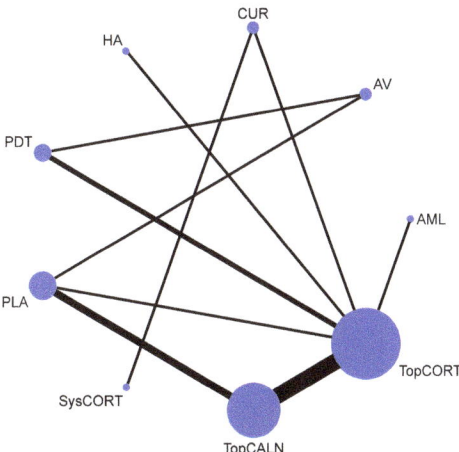

Figure 12. Network Plot: Pain Score. Abbreviations: AML, amlexanox paste; AV, aloe vera; CUR, curcumin gel; PDT, photodynamic therapy; PLA, placebo; PUR, purslane; SysCORT, systemic corticosteroid; TopCALN, topical calcineurin; TopCORT, topical corticosteroid; HA, hyaluronic acid.

TopCORT								
0.18 (-0.32,0.67)	TopCALN							
-0.16 (-2.09,1.77)	-0.34 (-2.33,1.65)	SysCORT						
1.04 (0.12,1.95)	0.86 (-0.15,1.87)	1.20 (-0.93,3.33)	PDT					
-0.11 (-1.51,1.29)	-0.29 (-1.77,1.20)	0.05 (-2.33,2.43)	-1.15 (-2.82,0.52)	HA				
-0.32 (-1.69,1.05)	-0.50 (-1.95,0.96)	-0.16 (-1.51,1.20)	-1.36 (-3.01,0.29)	-0.21 (-2.17,1.75)	CUR			
-0.79 (-1.97,0.39)	-0.96 (-2.17,0.24)	-0.63 (-2.89,1.63)	-1.83 (-2.96,-0.69)	-0.68 (-2.51,1.15)	-0.47 (-2.28,1.34)	AV		
0.08 (-1.33,1.48)	-0.10 (-1.59,1.39)	0.24 (-2.15,2.62)	-0.96 (-2.64,0.71)	0.18 (-1.80,2.17)	0.39 (-1.57,2.36)	0.86 (-0.97,2.70)	AML	
-0.59 (-1.40,0.21)	-0.77 (-1.54,-0.00)	-0.43 (-2.52,1.66)	-1.63 (-2.73,-0.53)	-0.48 (-2.10,1.13)	-0.27 (-1.86,1.32)	0.19 (-0.92,1.30)	-0.67 (-2.29,0.95)	PLA

Figure 13. League table for pain score. Abbreviations: AML, amlexanox paste; AV, aloe vera; CUR, curcumin gel; PDT, photodynamic therapy; PLA, placebo; PUR, purslane; SysCORT, systemic corticosteroid; TopCALN, topical calcineurin; TopCORT, topical corticosteroid; HA, hyaluronic acid. The green highlights indicate the interventions and the dark highlights indicate the significant results.

3.5. Subgroup Analysis of Individual Agents

3.5.1. Clinical Improvement

The network plot for this subgroup analysis with individual agents for clinical outcome is presented in Figure 14. Network meta-analysis suggested that PUR [RR = 4.53; 95% CI: 1.49, 13.79], AV [RR = 1.53, 95% CI: 1.08, 2.15], TAC [RR = 1.43; 95% CI: 1.06, 1.95], and CLO [RR = 1.34; 95% CI: 1.02, 1.78] are statistically significant in clinical improvement of OLP. According to SUCRA ranking, PUR was ranked the first [SUCRA 98.1], followed by AV [SUCRA 68.5] and TAC [SUCRA 64.7]. Detailed SUCRA ranks of individual interventions and SUCRA curves are presented in Supplementary Table S8 and Supplementary Figure S6, respectively. The league table showing the comparative efficacies shown as the risk ratio [RR] along with a 95% confidence interval [CI] is provided in Figure 15.

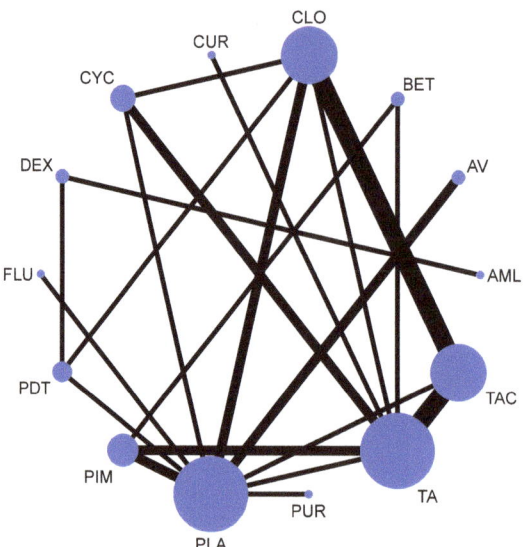

Figure 14. Network plot: Clinical Improvement (subgroup analysis). Abbreviations: AML, amlexanox paste; AV, aloe vera; CUR, curcumin gel; PDT, photodynamic therapy; PLA, placebo; PUR, purslane; TAC, tacrolimus; FLU, flucinonide acetonide; CLO, clobetasol propionate; PIM, pimecrolimus; BET, betamethasone; TA, triamcinolone acetonide; DEX, dexamethasone; CYC, cyclosporine.

TAC													
1.20 (0.95,1.50)	TA												
0.32 (0.10,1.01)	0.27 (0.08,0.84)	PUR											
1.13 (0.81,1.58)	0.95 (0.73,1.23)	3.57 (1.11,11.54)	PIM										
0.98 (0.66,1.46)	0.82 (0.54,1.24)	3.08 (0.93,10.19)	0.86 (0.54,1.39)	PDT									
0.96 (0.52,1.77)	0.80 (0.44,1.48)	3.02 (0.88,10.39)	0.85 (0.44,1.62)	0.98 (0.49,1.95)	FLU								
1.96 (0.53,7.20)	1.64 (0.44,6.05)	6.16 (1.30,34.48)	1.72 (0.46,6.51)	2.00 (0.58,6.91)	2.04 (0.49,8.42)	DEX							
1.55 (1.06,2.26)	1.30 (0.92,1.83)	4.88 (1.49,16.03)	1.37 (0.89,2.09)	1.58 (0.97,2.59)	1.62 (0.82,3.18)	0.79 (0.21,3.01)	CY						
0.94 (0.53,1.69)	0.79 (0.46,1.35)	2.98 (0.84,10.60)	0.83 (0.46,1.51)	0.96 (0.49,1.90)	0.98 (0.44,2.22)	0.48 (0.12,1.99)	0.61 (0.32,1.15)	CUR					
1.07 (0.86,1.32)	0.89 (0.70,1.14)	3.36 (1.07,10.60)	0.94 (0.67,1.32)	1.09 (0.77,1.55)	1.11 (0.61,2.04)	0.55 (0.15,1.98)	0.69 (0.48,0.98)	1.13 (0.63,2.04)	CLO				
1.15 (0.76,1.74)	0.96 (0.67,1.37)	3.61 (1.09,12.01)	1.01 (0.73,1.40)	1.17 (0.68,2.01)	1.20 (0.59,2.40)	0.59 (0.15,2.27)	0.74 (0.45,1.21)	1.21 (0.64,2.31)	1.07 (0.70,1.64)	BET			
0.94 (0.60,1.48)	0.79 (0.50,1.24)	2.97 (0.93,9.52)	0.83 (0.50,1.37)	0.96 (0.56,1.67)	0.98 (0.52,1.86)	0.48 (0.12,1.87)	0.61 (0.36,1.04)	1.00 (0.50,2.01)	0.88 (0.57,1.37)	0.82 (0.47,1.44)	AV		
2.17 (0.55,8.56)	1.82 (0.46,7.19)	6.85 (1.16,40.35)	1.92 (0.48,7.73)	2.22 (0.60,8.24)	2.27 (0.52,9.96)	1.11 (0.72,1.70)	1.40 (0.35,5.68)	2.30 (0.53,10.08)	2.04 (0.52,7.91)	1.89 (0.46,7.83)	2.30 (0.56,9.55)	AML	
1.64 (1.06,1.95)	1.20 (0.89,1.62)	4.53 (1.49,13.80)	1.27 (0.88,1.84)	1.47 (0.95,2.27)	1.50 (0.88,2.56)	0.74 (0.20,2.74)	0.93 (0.61,1.41)	1.52 (0.83,2.81)	1.35 (1.02,1.78)	1.25 (0.80,1.97)	1.53 (1.08,2.15)	0.66 (0.17,2.64)	PLA

Figure 15. League table for clinical Improvement (subgroup analysis). Abbreviations: AML, amlexanox paste; AV, aloe vera; CUR, curcumin gel; PDT, photodynamic therapy; PLA, placebo; PUR, purslane; TAC, tacrolimus; FLU, flucinonide acetonide; CLO, clobetasol propionate; PIM, pimecrolimus; BET, betamethasone; TA, triamcinolone acetonide; DEX, dexamethasone; CYC, cyclosporine. The green highlights indicate the interventions and the dark highlights indicate the significant results.

3.5.2. Adverse Effects

Network meta-analysis suggested that CYC [RR = 4.96; 95% CI: 1.21, 20.34], DEX [RR = 9.01; 95% CI: 1.29, 62.67] and CLO [RR = 6.25; 95% CI: 2.04, 19.09] were statistically significant for adverse effects. According to SUCRA ranking, TA is the one with the least adverse effects, followed by CUR. Detailed SUCRA ranks of individual interventions and SUCRA curves are presented in Supplementary Table S9 and Supplementary Figure S7, respectively. The network plot is presented in Figure 16 and the league table showing the comparative efficacies is provided in Figure 17.

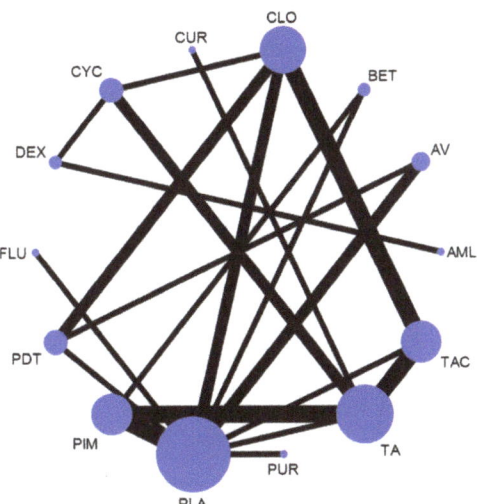

Figure 16. Network plot: Adverse Effects (subgroup analysis). Abbreviations: AML, amlexanox paste; AV, aloe vera; CUR, curcumin gel; PDT, photodynamic therapy; PLA, placebo; PUR, purslane; TAC, tacrolimus; FLU, flucinonide acetonide; CLO, clobetasol propionate; PIM, pimecrolimus; BET, betamethasone; TA, triamcinolone acetonide; DEX, dexamethasone; CYC, cyclosporine.

TAC													
2.60 (1.10,6.13)	TA												
3.37 (0.06,199.49)	1.30 (0.02,75.73)	PUR											
1.21 (0.34,4.30)	0.47 (0.13,1.67)	0.36 (0.01,21.11)	PIM										
0.64 (0.09,4.31)	0.25 (0.04,1.67)	0.19 (0.00,14.01)	0.53 (0.07,4.03)	PDT									
2.89 (0.05,171.63)	1.11 (0.02,65.15)	0.86 (0.00,221.20)	2.39 (0.04,141.26)	4.53 (0.06,337.35)	FLU								
0.32 (0.05,2.16)	0.12 (0.02,0.70)	0.10 (0.00,7.58)	0.27 (0.03,2.22)	0.50 (0.04,6.04)	0.11 (0.00,8.87)	DEX							
0.58 (0.15,2.27)	0.22 (0.07,0.67)	0.17 (0.00,11.17)	0.48 (0.09,2.52)	0.91 (0.11,7.44)	0.20 (0.00,13.08)	1.81 (0.48,6.88)	CYC						
2.60 (0.05,146.27)	1.00 (0.02,51.29)	0.77 (0.00,221.49)	2.15 (0.03,135.05)	4.08 (0.05,325.75)	0.90 (0.00,259.11)	8.10 (0.13,597.71)	4.47 (0.07,266.67)	CUR					
0.46 (0.17,1.27)	0.18 (0.06,0.54)	0.14 (0.00,8.11)	0.38 (0.09,1.58)	0.73 (0.12,4.23)	0.16 (0.00,9.50)	1.44 (0.22,9.63)	0.79 (0.21,3.08)	0.18 (0.00,10.62)	CLO				
3.96 (1.17,13.40)	1.52 (0.42,5.46)	1.17 (0.02,66.19)	3.27 (1.18,9.08)	6.21 (0.87,44.49)	1.37 (0.02,77.52)	12.33 (1.49,101.95)	6.80 (1.32,35.01)	1.52 (0.02,95.56)	8.56 (3.25,33.20)	BET			
0.95 (0.09,10.01)	0.36 (0.04,3.78)	0.28 (0.00,24.26)	0.78 (0.07,8.45)	1.48 (0.13,16.89)	0.33 (0.00,28.40)	2.95 (0.17,50.37)	1.63 (0.13,19.92)	0.36 (0.00,35.50)	2.05 (0.20,20.89)	0.24 (0.02,2.41)	AV		
0.48 (0.04,5.40)	0.18 (0.02,1.81)	0.14 (0.00,14.44)	0.39 (0.03,5.31)	0.75 (0.04,13.64)	0.16 (0.00,16.91)	1.48 (0.33,6.68)	0.82 (0.11,6.10)	0.18 (0.00,17.42)	1.03 (0.09,11.61)	0.12 (0.01,1.61)	0.50 (0.02,12.48)	AML	
2.89 (0.95,8.81)	1.11 (0.38,3.23)	0.86 (0.02,43.41)	2.39 (0.80,7.17)	4.53 (0.77,26.65)	1.00 (0.02,50.84)	9.01 (1.30,62.67)	4.97 (1.21,20.34)	1.11 (0.02,65.72)	6.25 (2.05,19.09)	0.73 (0.29,1.85)	3.05 (0.37,25.40)	8.08 (0.52,70.89)	PLA

Figure 17. League table for adverse effects (subgroup analysis). Abbreviations: AML, amlexanox paste; AV, aloe vera; CUR, curcumin gel; PDT, photodynamic therapy; PLA, placebo; PUR, purslane; TAC, tacrolimus; FLU, flucinonide acetonide; CLO, clobetasol propionate; PIM, pimecrolimus; BET, betamethasone; TA, triamcinolone acetonide; DEX, dexamethasone; CYC, cyclosporine. The green highlights indicate the interventions and the dark highlights indicate the significant results.

3.5.3. Clinical Resolution

Based on the NMA findings, only TAC was significant in clinical resolution of OLP [RR = 5.40; 95% CI: 1.48, 19.67]. SUCRA ranks reported that TAC scored the highest [SUCRA 83], and CYC [SUCRA score: 17.8] scored the worst. Detailed SUCRA ranks of individual interventions and SUCRA curves are presented in Supplementary Table S10 and Supplementary Figure S8, respectively. The network plot is presented in Figure 18 and the league table showing the comparative efficacies is provided in Figure 19.

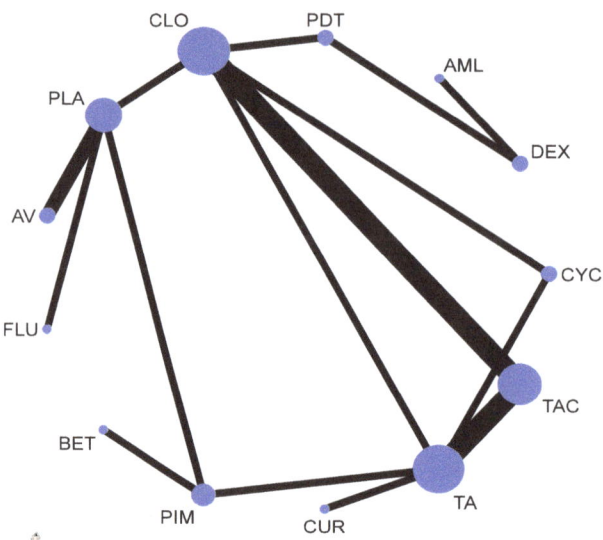

Figure 18. Network plot: Clinical Resolution (subgroup analysis). Abbreviations: AML, amlexanox paste; AV, aloe vera; CUR, curcumin gel; PDT, photodynamic therapy; PLA, placebo; PUR, purslane; TAC, tacrolimus; FLU, flucinonide acetonide; CLO, clobetasol propionate; PIM, pimecrolimus; BET, betamethasone; TA, triamcinolone acetonide; DEX, dexamethasone; CYC, cyclosporine.

TAC												
1.99 (0.85,4.63)	TA											
1.97 (0.56,7.02)	0.99 (0.34,2.91)	PIM										
1.52 (0.43,5.34)	0.77 (0.21,2.76)	0.77 (0.17,3.53)	PDT									
0.60 (0.02,17.19)	0.30 (0.01,8.38)	0.30 (0.01,8.17)	0.39 (0.01,11.97)	FLU								
4.57 (0.13,161.99)	2.30 (0.06,82.29)	2.31 (0.06,90.81)	3.00 (0.11,84.72)	7.62 (0.06,902.95)	DEX							
7.47 (1.42,39.13)	3.76 (0.76,18.64)	3.78 (0.60,23.63)	4.90 (0.86,27.93)	12.44 (0.35,445.62)	1.63 (0.04,70.57)	CYC						
1.99 (0.09,43.34)	1.00 (0.05,19.39)	1.01 (0.04,23.55)	1.30 (0.05,32.93)	3.31 (0.04,284.08)	0.43 (0.00,45.24)	0.27 (0.01,7.73)	CUR					
1.96 (0.83,4.63)	0.99 (0.41,2.37)	0.99 (0.30,3.31)	1.29 (0.51,3.28)	3.27 (0.12,87.15)	0.43 (0.01,13.78)	0.26 (0.06,1.14)	0.99 (0.04,21.74)	CLO				
4.04 (0.87,18.89)	2.04 (0.49,8.51)	2.05 (0.62,6.72)	2.66 (0.48,14.61)	6.74 (0.25,182.47)	0.88 (0.02,37.61)	0.54 (0.07,4.02)	2.04 (0.08,54.76)	2.06 (0.49,8.59)	BET			
2.48 (0.38,16.13)	1.25 (0.20,7.77)	1.25 (0.21,7.37)	1.63 (0.22,11.89)	4.13 (0.14,122.31)	0.54 (0.01,26.43)	0.33 (0.03,3.20)	1.25 (0.04,40.62)	1.26 (0.22,7.34)	0.61 (0.10,3.66)	AV		
5.08 (0.11,238.95)	2.56 (0.05,121.30)	2.57 (0.05,132.97)	3.33 (0.09,127.21)	8.46 (0.06,1244.23)	1.11 (0.26,4.74)	0.68 (0.01,38.49)	2.56 (0.02,332.14)	2.59 (0.06,111.14)	1.26 (0.02,69.97)	2.05 (0.03,129.97)	AML	
5.40 (1.48,19.67)	2.72 (0.82,9.07)	2.74 (0.89,8.37)	3.55 (0.84,14.94)	9.00 (0.41,198.97)	1.18 (0.03,44.83)	0.72 (0.12,4.36)	2.72 (0.11,66.74)	2.75 (0.92,8.22)	1.34 (0.43,4.17)	2.18 (0.55,8.67)	1.06 (0.02,53.30)	PLA

Figure 19. League table: Clinical Resolution (subgroup analysis). Abbreviations: AML, amlexanox paste; AV, aloe vera; CUR, curcumin gel; PDT, photodynamic therapy; PLA, placebo; PUR, purslane; TAC, tacrolimus; FLU, flucinonide acetonide; CLO, clobetasol propionate; PIM, pimecrolimus; BET, betamethasone; TA, triamcinolone acetonide; DEX, dexamethasone; CYC, cyclosporine. The green highlights indicate the interventions and the dark highlights indicate the significant results.

3.5.4. Clinical Score

None of the interventions were statistically significant in improving clinical score except PDT MD = −5.92; 95% CI: −8.76, 3.09]. When ranked, PDT scored the highest and BET scored the worst. Detailed SUCRA ranks of individual interventions and SUCRA curves are presented in Supplementary Table S11 and Supplementary Figure S9, respectively. The network plot is presented in Figure 20 and the league table showing the comparative efficacies with a 95% confidence interval [CI] is provided in Figure 21.

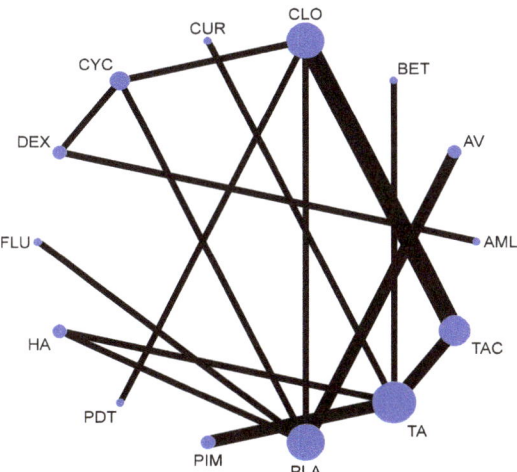

Figure 20. Network plot: Clinical Score (subgroup analysis). Abbreviations: AML, amelexanox paste; AV, aloe vera; CUR, curcumin gel; PDT, photodynamic therapy; PLA, placebo; PUR, purslane; TAC, tacrolimus; FLU, flucinonide acetonide; CLO, Clobetasol propionate; PIM, pimecrolimus; BET, betamethasone; TA, triamcinolone acetonide; DEX, dexamethasone; CYC, cyclosporine.

TAC													
-0.13 (-1.49,1.24)	TA												
-0.39 (-2.41,1.63)	0.77 (0.17,3.43)	PIM											
4.68 (2.05,7.31)	122.24 (6.79,2200.24)	5.07 (1.81,8.32)	PDT										
-0.44 (-2.37,1.49)	0.73 (0.13,4.26)	.05 (-2.36,2.26)	-5.12 (-8.18,-2.06)	HA									
-0.14 (-2.90,2.62)	0.99 (0.06,17.22)	0.25 (-2.97,3.47)	-4.82 (-8.35,-1.29)	0.30 (-2.42,3.03)	FLU								
-1.18 (-63.22,60.86)	0.35 (0.00,3.09e+26)	-0.79 (-62.85,61.27)	-5.86 (-67.93,56.22)	-0.73 (-62.77,61.30)	-1.04 (-63.09,61.01)	DEX							
-0.36 (-2.36,1.63)	0.79 (0.08,7.45)	0.03 (-2.66,2.72)	-5.04 (-7.96,-2.12)	0.08 (-2.21,2.37)	-0.22 (-2.98,2.53)	0.82 (-61.22,62.86)	CYC						
0.21 (-2.27,2.69)	1.40 (0.18,11.15)	0.60 (-1.96,3.16)	-4.47 (-8.02,-0.91)	0.65 (-2.07,3.37)	0.35 (-3.18,3.88)	1.39 (-60.69,63.47)	0.57 (-2.48,3.62)	CUR					
-0.22 (-1.38,0.93)	0.91 (0.17,4.80)	0.17 (-2.07,2.40)	-4.90 (-7.26,-2.54)	0.22 (-1.73,2.17)	-0.08 (-2.71,2.54)	0.95 (-61.08,62.99)	0.14 (-1.57,1.85)	-0.43 (-3.09,2.22)	CLO				
-0.73 (-3.21,1.76)	0.55 (0.07,4.38)	-0.34 (-2.90,2.22)	-5.41 (-8.96,-1.85)	-0.28 (-3.01,2.44)	-0.59 (-4.12,2.94)	0.45 (-61.63,62.53)	-0.37 (-3.42,2.69)	-0.94 (-3.87,2.00)	-0.51 (-3.17,2.16)	BET			
-0.16 (-2.47,2.15)	0.97 (0.09,10.95)	0.23 (-2.62,3.08)	-4.84 (-8.03,-1.65)	0.28 (-1.99,2.55)	-0.02 (-2.59,2.55)	1.01 (-61.02,63.05)	0.20 (-2.11,2.51)	-0.37 (-3.57,2.82)	0.06 (-2.09,2.21)	0.57 (-2.63,3.76)	AV		
-1.31 (-63.35,60.73)	0.31 (0.00,2.71e+26)	-0.92 (-62.98,61.14)	-5.98 (-68.06,56.09)	-0.86 (-62.90,61.17)	-1.17 (-63.22,60.88)	-0.13 (-2.23,1.97)	-0.95 (-62.99,61.09)	-1.52 (-63.60,60.56)	-1.08 (-63.12,60.95)	-0.58 (-62.66,61.50)	-1.14 (-63.17,60.89)	AML	
-1.25 (-3.03,0.53)	0.33 (0.05,2.25)	-0.86 (-3.30,1.58)	-5.92 (-8.76,-3.09)	-0.80 (-2.53,0.93)	-1.11 (-3.21,1.00)	-0.07 (-62.08,61.95)	-0.89 (-2.66,0.89)	-1.46 (-4.29,1.38)	-1.02 (-2.59,0.54)	-0.52 (-3.35,2.32)	-1.08 (-2.56,0.39)	0.06 (-61.95,62.07)	PLA

Figure 21. Network plot: Clinical Score (subgroup analysis). Abbreviations: AML, amelexanox paste; AV, aloe vera; CUR, curcumin gel; PDT, photodynamic therapy; PLA, placebo; PUR, purslane; TAC, tacrolimus; FLU, flucinonide acetonide; CLO, Clobetasol propionate; PIM, pimecrolimus; BET, betamethasone; TA, triamcinolone acetonide; DEX, dexamethasone; CYC, cyclosporine. The green highlights indicate the interventions and the dark highlights indicate the significant results.

3.5.5. Pain Score

Network meta-analysis suggested that TAC [MD = −1.67; 95% CI: −2.78, −48, SUCRA 86.3] and PDT [MD = −1.90 [95% CI: −3.06, −0.76, SUCRA 92.1] are statistically significant compared to placebo in improving the pain score. Detailed SUCRA ranks of individual interventions and curves are presented in Supplementary Table S12 and Supplementary Figure S10, respectively. The network plot is presented in Figure 22. The league table showing the comparative efficacies with a 95% confidence interval [CI] is provided in Figure 23.

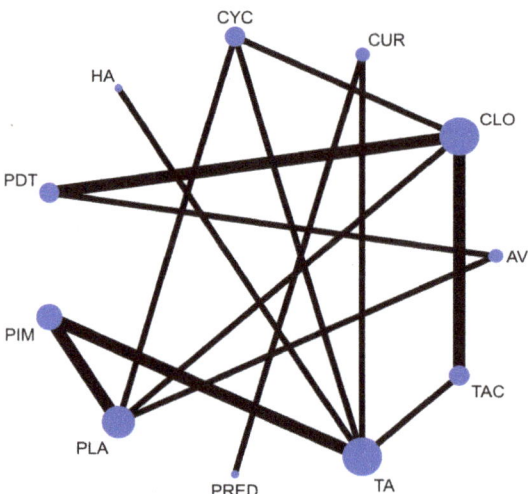

Figure 22. Network plot: Pain Score (subgroup analysis). Abbreviations: AML, amlexanox paste; AV, aloe vera; CUR, curcumin gel; PDT, photodynamic therapy; PLA, placebo; TAC, tacrolimus; FLU, flucinonide acetonide; CLO, clobetasol propionate; PIM, pimecrolimus; TA, triamcinolone acetonide; CYC, cyclosporine; PRED, prednisolone; HA, hyaluronic acid.

TAC										
-0.86 (-1.92,0.19)	TA									
-1.03 (-3.21,1.16)	-0.16 (-2.08,1.75)	PRED								
-1.19 (-2.42,0.04)	-0.33 (-1.21,0.56)	-0.17 (-2.27,1.94)	PIM							
0.28 (-0.96,1.53)	1.15 (-0.17,2.47)	1.31 (-1.02,3.64)	1.48 (0.11,2.84)	PDT						
-0.97 (-2.72,0.77)	-0.11 (-1.50,1.28)	0.05 (-2.31,2.42)	0.22 (-1.43,1.86)	-1.26 (-3.17,0.66)	HA					
-0.74 (-1.92,0.44)	0.12 (-0.87,1.12)	0.28 (-1.88,2.44)	0.45 (-0.71,1.61)	-1.03 (-2.33,0.27)	0.23 (-1.48,1.94)	CYC				
-1.18 (-2.90,0.54)	-0.32 (-1.68,1.04)	-0.16 (-1.50,1.19)	0.01 (-1.61,1.63)	-1.47 (-3.36,0.43)	-0.21 (-2.15,1.73)	-0.44 (-2.13,1.25)	CUR			
-0.68 (-1.57,0.20)	0.18 (-0.87,1.23)	0.34 (-1.84,2.53)	0.51 (-0.64,1.65)	-0.97 (-1.88,-0.05)	0.29 (-1.45,2.03)	0.06 (-0.95,1.07)	0.50 (-1.22,2.22)	CLO		
-1.68 (-3.12,-0.25)	-0.82 (-2.23,0.60)	-0.66 (-3.04,1.72)	-0.49 (-1.89,0.91)	-1.97 (-3.11,-0.82)	-0.71 (-2.69,1.27)	-0.94 (-2.35,0.47)	-0.50 (-2.46,1.47)	-1.00 (-2.21,0.22)	AV	
-1.61 (-2.78,-0.45)	-0.75 (-1.79,0.29)	-0.59 (-2.77,1.59)	-0.42 (-1.37,0.53)	-1.90 (-3.07,-0.73)	-0.64 (-2.38,1.10)	-0.87 (-1.93,0.18)	-0.43 (-2.15,1.28)	-0.93 (-1.88,0.02)	0.07 (-1.05,1.18)	PLA

Figure 23. League table: Pain Score (subgroup analysis). Abbreviations: AML, amlexanox paste; AV, aloe vera; CUR, curcumin gel; PDT, photodynamic therapy; PLA, placebo; TAC, tacrolimus; FLU, flucinonide acetonide; CLO, clobetasol propionate; PIM, pimecrolimus; TA, triamcinolone acetonide; CYC, cyclosporine; PRED, prednisolone; HA, hyaluronic acid. The green highlights indicate the interventions and the dark highlights indicate the significant results.

3.6. Network Consistency and Small Study Effects and GRADE Quality

For all outcomes, the test of global inconsistency showed no evidence of inconsistency within any network comparisons. We did not find any evidence of publication bias on any outcome assessed based on the comparison-adjusted funnel plots, as all plots were symmetrical (Supplementary Figures S11–S20). The GRADE analysis of quality of evidence is provided in Supplementary Table S13. The evidence generated was classified as moderate quality evidence for all outcomes.

4. Discussion

Defining the most appropriate intervention used for treating OLP is challenging due to the wide variety of interventions that has been used to treat OLP, giving a wide range of beneficial results in various aspects. The majority of previous systematic reviews only conducted a pairwise comparison of interventions in clinical trials. The Cochrane Database of Systematic Reviews have also reported two reviews [12,13]. However, there is a lack of comprehensive evidence that compares the relative efficacy and safety of all interventions combined [1,11,25,30–32,42,49–56,58–70]. NMA enables the combination of both direct and indirect evidence to establish comparative efficacy and acceptability across a network of randomized controlled trials of all compounds [15]. A recent NMA has investigated the efficacy of topical administration for treatment of OLP [14]. The scope of the aforementioned review was restricted to topical agents only, whereas our review comprehensively evaluates all the available agents for the management of OLP. Further, our review has also included additional trials published in the recent couple of years. Therefore, our NMA presents the most recent cumulative evidence of comparative effectiveness of agents on symptomatic, biopsy-proven OLP on five major outcomes including clinical improvement, clinical resolution, adverse effects, clinical score and pain score. Further, the RCTs included in the present study included participants with clinically- and histologically-proven symptomatic forms of OLP, thus improving the reliability of the results. According to our results, purslane is the most effective agent, followed by aloe vera and topical calcineurin inhibitors in bringing clinical improvement. Topical calcineurin inhibitors are the best agents in terms of clinical resolution, however, they were the least safe. Photodynamic therapy was the most effective agent in terms of reduction in clinical score and pain score.

Purslane, a type of green leafy vegetable in which plant extract was granulated with lactose and other inert substances, has the highest SUCRA ranking for clinical improvement of OLP and has the least adverse effects according to our analysis. However, this information was obtained from one study that was identified to have a high risk of bias [49]. It is prescribed to the patients in capsule form. The antioxidant activity of purslane is well established. This helps mitigate the oxidative stress brought about by inflammatory-cell-associated free radicals and reactive oxygen species [71–73]. Imbalance in antioxidant activity is reported in vulvar and skin LP [71,72]. Keratinocytes can also release ROS subsequent to stimulation by pro-inflammatory cytokines and endotoxins as well [71]. Both of the aforementioned can be reduced by the antioxidant activity of purslane. However, since the antioxidant activity of purslane has been demonstrated by only one study with a high risk of bias, more trials are required before a recommendation for routine use may be made.

Aloe vera (AV) has been previously reported with only mild side effects restricted to mild itching and stinging sensation [50]. OLP is a T-cell-mediated disease and an autoimmune disease [51]. OLP upregulates adhesion through activated keratinocytes and lymphocytes which release interleukin [IL]-2, IL-4, IL-10 and tumour necrosis factor [TNF-alpha] [14,73,74]. AV acts by interfering with the arachidonic acid pathway via cyclooxygenase and by reducing TNF-alpha levels and leukocyte adhesion, thus contributing to the treatment of OLP [75–78]. However, more high-quality trials are recommended to be performed on AV for evidence synthesis, as there were only two trials with unclear risk of bias which were included in this review [50,51].

Calcineurin inhibitors impair transcription of interleukin [IL]-2 and several other cytokines in T lymphocytes [79]. TopCALN was found to be statistically significant in clinical improvement and clinical resolution of OLP. Clinical resolution is measured by the complete resolution of the lesion intraorally. TopCALN is usually recommended as the second line of therapy after the failure of TopCORT [10,55,80,81]. However, it has the highest incidence of adverse effects. The most common adverse effects caused by calcineurin inhibitors are transient burning or stinging sensation at the site of application [10,11,25,31,33,55,56,82]. Others include dysgeusia [82], mucosal paraesthesia [57] and gastrointestinal upsets [10,32]. However, a definitive conclusion on the long-term resolution cannot be made at this stage as most of the trials have a short follow-up period [10]. Moreover, systemic use of calcineurin has been linked to malignancy due to promotion of metastasis, tumour growth and angiogenesis [83]. A better understanding of adverse effects caused by calcineurin inhibitors is imperative before a recommendation for routine use may be made [10].

Corticosteroids have remained the treatment of choice for symptomatic OLP in many studies that had been conducted previously [34,84–86]. After balancing out all the outcomes from the results of the current study, our study also confirms that TopCORT is the most effective treatment option for OLP. It is statistically significant in causing clinical improvement of OLP and also in improving the clinical score. Clinical score is measured with Thongprasom scale scoring. Moreover, TopCORT is associated with adverse effects with lesser impact, including slight burning sensation [33,35,43,67], gastrointestinal upsets [43], xerostomia [44], candidiasis [58,65] and general discomfort [69]. This finding is in accordance with previous research which implicates corticosteroids as the most successful and predictable interventions in the treatment of OLP with minimal potential for systemic side effects [32,85,87–90]. Anti-inflammatory and immunosuppressive actions of corticosteroids contribute to its efficacy in the treatment of OLP [34,85,87]. Therefore, continued use of TopCORT for the treatment of OLP is recommended since it is implemented in current practice.

After considering TopCORT, TopCALN, PUR and AV as clinically significant interventions that can be used for effective treatment of OLP, a subgroup analysis was performed for a more specific understanding of the interventions for treatment of OLP. TopCORT evaluated in this review were BET, CLO, DEX, FLU and TA. For TopCALN, PIM, CYC and TAC were included. It is observed that PUR, AV and TAC are statistically significant in the clinical improvement of OLP. They are also ranked top three in the SUCRA ranking. Based on the adverse effects, CLO and CYC can be seen being statistically significant in adverse effects.

The current review has several strengths. In this review, different interventions were compared as a group as well as individually with a range of outcome measures. Efficacy and safety of a large number of interventions have been included in this review of both topical and systemic agents. Another strength of this NMA is that the comparison-adjusted funnel plot for clinical improvements of OLP and adverse effects were symmetrical, suggesting that results are not influenced by the sample size of literature and publication bias.

Our study is not without limitations. A limitation of the current NMA is that it remains unclear in which concentration or dosage regimen represents "standard of care" for the recommended intervention. Dosages reported in individual trials varied. Outcomes were reported in different measurements when comparing the effectiveness and safety of interventions, which makes pooling the data challenging. Further the timing of the outcome measurements and of follow-up length varied between the studies. For meaningful comparison of data, there is a need to standardise parameters for the outcome measurement and the length of treatment OLP for intervention trials. International associations can keep standardised guidelines for the conduct of trials. In addition, future trials should focus on long-term follow up, particularly in terms of relapses. Cost-effectiveness and economic utility could also be considered as an area of research in in future trials to improve the clinical usefulness.

5. Conclusions

After performing the NMA with 37 studies, the available evidence suggests that purslane and aloe vera are the most effective drugs in the management for OLP, but only a small number of studies were performed on these interventions. There is also evidence that TopCALN is effective in treatment of OLP; however, the safety is a concern. The newer PDT is shown to be efficacious for pain and reduction in clinical scores and safe as well. Nevertheless, further RCTs are warranted to confirm and improve the accuracy of the findings from the present review.

Supplementary Materials: The following supporting information can be downloaded at: https://www.mdpi.com/article/10.3390/jcm12082763/s1. Table S1: Articles excluded and reasons for exclusion. Table S2: Characteristics of included RCTs.

Author Contributions: Conceptualization, R.K.M. and X.Y.L.; methodology, R.K.M., S.M.S. and S.K.V.; software, S.M.S. and S.K.V.; validation, R.K.M. and D.G.; formal analysis, X.Y.L. and S.M.S.; investigation, X.Y.L., R.K.M. and D.G.; resources, R.K.M.; data curation, X.Y.L., R.K.M. and D.G.; writing—original draft preparation, X.Y.L. and D.G.; writing—review and editing, R.K.M., D.G. and N.Y.S.; visualization, X.Y.L. and S.M.S.; supervision, R.K.M. and N.Y.S.; project administration, R.K.M. All authors have read and agreed to the published version of the manuscript.

Funding: This research received no external funding.

Institutional Review Board Statement: Not applicable.

Informed Consent Statement: Not applicable.

Data Availability Statement: Supporting data is provided in the Supplementary Materials.

Conflicts of Interest: The authors declare no conflict of interest.

References

1. Conrotto, D.; Carbone, M.; Carrozzo, M.; Arduino, P.; Broccoletti, R.; Pentenero, M.; Gandolfo, S. Ciclosporin vs. clobetasol in the topical management of atrophic and erosive oral lichen planus: A double-blind, randomized controlled trial. *Br. J. Dermatol.* **2006**, *154*, 139–145. [CrossRef] [PubMed]
2. Scully, C.; Eisen, D.; Carrozzo, M. Management of oral lichen planus. *Am. J. Clin. Dermatol.* **2000**, *1*, 287–306. [CrossRef] [PubMed]
3. Thornhill, M.H. Immune mechanisms in oral lichen planus. *Acta Odontol. Scand.* **2001**, *59*, 174–177. [CrossRef] [PubMed]
4. McCartan, B.E.; Healy, C.M. The reported prevalence of oral lichen planus: A review and critique. *J. Oral Pathol. Med.* **2008**, *37*, 447–453. [CrossRef] [PubMed]
5. Lodi, G.; Scully, C.; Carrozzo, M.; Griffiths, M.; Sugerman, P.B.; Thongprasom, K. Current controversies in oral lichen planus: Report of an international consensus meeting. Part Viral infections and etiopathogenesis. *Oral Surg. Oral Med. Oral Pathol. Oral Radiol. Endod.* **2005**, *100*, 40–51. [CrossRef]
6. Carrozzo, M.; Gandolfo, S. The management of oral lichen planus. *Oral Dis.* **1999**, *5*, 196–205. [CrossRef]
7. Eisen, D. The clinical features, malignant potential, and systemic associations of oral lichen planus: A study of 723 patients. *J. Am. Acad. Dermatol.* **2002**, *46*, 207–214. [CrossRef]
8. Adamo, D.; Calabria, E.; Coppola, N.; Lo Muzio, L.; Giuliani, M.; Bizzoca, M.E.; Azzi, L.; Croveri, F.; Colella, G.; Boschetti, C.E.; et al. Psychological profile and unexpected pain in oral lichen planus: A case-control multicenter SIPMO study. *Oral Dis.* **2021**, *28*, 398–414. [CrossRef]
9. Kaplan, I.; Ventura-Sharabi, Y.; Gal, G.; Calderon, S.; Anavi, Y. The Dynamics of Oral Lichen Planus: A Retrospective Clinicopathological Study. *Head Neck Pathol.* **2011**, *6*, 178–183. [CrossRef]
10. Arduino, P.; Carbone, M.; Della Ferrera, F.; Elia, A.; Conrotto, D.; Gambino, A.; Comba, A.; Calogiuri, P.; Broccoletti, R. Pimecrolimus vs. tacrolimus for the topical treatment of unresponsive oral erosive lichen planus: A 8 week randomized double-blind controlled study. *J. Eur. Acad. Dermatol. Venereol.* **2013**, *28*, 475–482. [CrossRef]
11. Gorouhi, F.; Solhpour, A.; Beitollahi, J.M.; Afshar, S.; Davari, P.; Hashemi, P.; Kashani, M.N.; Firooz, A. Randomized trial of pimecrolimus cream versus triamcinolone acetonide paste in the treatment of oral lichen planus. *J. Am. Acad. Dermatol.* **2007**, *57*, 806–813. [CrossRef] [PubMed]
12. Lodi, G.; Manfredi, M.; Mercadante, V.; Murphy, R.; Carrozzo, M. Interventions for treating oral lichen planus: Corticosteroid therapies. *Cochrane Database Syst. Rev.* **2020**, *2020*, CD001168. [CrossRef] [PubMed]
13. Thongprasom, K.; Carrozzo, M.; Furness, S.; Lodi, G. Interventions for treating oral lichen planus. *Cochrane Database Syst. Rev.* **2011**, *7*, CD001168. [CrossRef] [PubMed]
14. Yuan, P.; Qiu, X.; Ye, L.; Hou, F.; Liang, Y.; Jiang, H.; Zhang, Y.; Xu, Y.; Sun, Y.; Deng, X.; et al. Efficacy of topical administration for oral lichen planus: A network meta-analysis. *Oral Dis.* **2021**, *28*, 670–681. [CrossRef]
15. Hutton, B.; Salanti, G.; Caldwell, D.M.; Chaimani, A.; Schmid, C.H.; Cameron, C.; Ioannidis, J.P.A.; Straus, S.; Thorlund, K.; Jansen, J.P.; et al. The PRISMA Extension Statement for Reporting of Systematic Reviews Incorporating Network Meta-analyses of Health Care Interventions: Checklist and Explanations. *Ann. Intern. Med.* **2015**, *162*, 777–784. [CrossRef]
16. Higgins, J.P.T.; Green, S. Cochrane Handbook for Systematic Reviews of Interventions [Internet]. Available online: https://training.cochrane.org/handbook (accessed on 7 November 2022).
17. RoB 2: A Revised Cochrane Risk-of-Bias Tool for Randomized Trials [Internet]. Available online: https://methods.cochrane.org/bias/resources/rob-2-revised-cochrane-risk-bias-tool-randomized-trials (accessed on 6 February 2023).
18. Graphical Tools for Network Meta-Analysis in STATA | PLOS ONE [Internet]. Available online: https://journals.plos.org/plosone/article?id=10.1371/journal.pone.0076654 (accessed on 7 November 2022).
19. Veroniki, A.A.; Vasiliadis, H.S.; Higgins, J.P.T.; Salanti, G. Evaluation of inconsistency in networks of interventions. *Int. J. Epidemiol.* **2013**, *42*, 332–345. [CrossRef]
20. Higgins, J.P.T.; Jackson, D.; Barrett, J.K.; Lu, G.; Ades, A.E.; White, I.R. Consistency and inconsistency in network meta-analysis: Concepts and models for multi-arm studies. *Res. Synth. Methods* **2012**, *3*, 98–110. [CrossRef]

21. General Principles for Dealing with Missing Data [Internet]. Available online: https://handbook-5-1.cochrane.org/chapter_16/16_1_2_general_principles_for_dealing_with_missing_data.htm (accessed on 6 February 2023).
22. Higgins, J.P.T.; Thompson, S.G. Quantifying heterogeneity in a meta-analysis. *Stat. Med.* **2002**, *21*, 1539–1558. [CrossRef]
23. Higgins, J.P.T.; Thompson, S.G.; Deeks, J.J.; Altman, D.G. Measuring inconsistency in meta-analyses. *BMJ* **2003**, *327*, 557–560. [CrossRef]
24. Salanti, G.; Ades, A.E.; Ioannidis, J.P. Graphical methods and numerical summaries for presenting results from multiple-treatment meta-analysis: An overview and tutorial. *J. Clin. Epidemiol.* **2011**, *64*, 163–171. [CrossRef]
25. Voute ABSELangendijk, P.N.; Kostense, P.J.; van der Waal, I. Fluocinonide in an adhesive base for treatment of oral lichen planus. A double-blind, placebo-controlled clinical study. *Oral Surg. Oral Med. Oral Pathol.* **1993**, *75*, 181. [CrossRef] [PubMed]
26. Siponen, M.; Huuskonen, L.; Kallio-Pulkkinen, S.; Nieminen, P.; Salo, T. Topical tacrolimus, triamcinolone acetonide, and placebo in oral lichen planus: A pilot randomized controlled trial. *Oral Dis.* **2017**, *23*, 660–668. [CrossRef] [PubMed]
27. Arduino PGCMSciannameo, V.; Conrotto, D.; Gambino, A.; Cabras, M.; Ricceri, F.; Carossa, S.; Broccoletti, R.; Carbone, M. Randomized, placebo-controlled, double-blind trial of clobetasol propionate 0.05% in the treatment of oral lichen planus. *Oral Dis.* **2018**, *24*, 772. [CrossRef] [PubMed]
28. Samimi, M.; Le Gouge, A.; Boralevi, F.; Passeron, T.; Pascal, F.; Bernard, P.; Agbo-Godeau, S.; Leducq, S.; Fricain, J.C.; Vaillant, L.; et al. Topical rapamycin versus betamethasone dipropionate ointment for treating oral erosive lichen planus: A randomized, double-blind, controlled study. *J. Eur. Acad. Dermatol. Venereol.* **2020**, *34*, 2384–2391. [CrossRef]
29. Santonocito, S.; Polizzi, A.; De Pasquale, R.; Ronsivalle, V.; Giudice, A.L.; Isola, G. Analysis of the Efficacy of Two Treatment Protocols for Patients with Symptomatic Oral Lichen Planus: A Randomized Clinical Trial. *Int. J. Environ. Res. Public Heal.* **2020**, *18*, 56. [CrossRef]
30. Corrocher, G.; Di Lorenzo, G.; Martinelli, N.; Mansueto, P.; Biasi, D.; Nocini, P.F.; Lombardo, G.; Fior, A.; Corrocher, R.; Bambara, L.M.; et al. Comparative effect of tacrolimus 0.1% ointment and clobetasol 0.05% ointment in patients with oral lichen planus. *J. Clin. Periodontol.* **2008**, *35*, 244–249. [CrossRef]
31. Laeijendecker, R.; Tank, B.; Dekker, S.; Neumann, H. A Comparison of Treatment of Oral Lichen Planus with Topical Tacrolimus and Triamcinolone Acetonide Ointment. *Acta Derm.-Venereol.* **2006**, *86*, 227–229. [CrossRef]
32. Yoke, P.C.; Tin, G.B.; Kim, M.-J.; Rajaseharan, A.; Ahmed, S.; Thongprasom, K.; Chaimusik, M.; Suresh, S.; Machin, D.; Bee, W.H.; et al. A randomized controlled trial to compare steroid with cyclosporine for the topical treatment of oral lichen planus. *Oral Surg. Oral Med. Oral Pathol. Oral Radiol. Endod.* **2006**, *102*, 47–55. [CrossRef]
33. Sonthalia, S.S.A. Comparative efficacy of tacrolimus 0.1% ointment and clobetasol propionate 0.05% ointment in oral lichen planus: A randomized double-blind trial. *Int. J. Dermatol.* **2012**, *51*, 1371. [CrossRef]
34. Arunkumar, S.; Kalappa, S.; Kalappanavar, A.; Annigeri, R. Relative efficacy of pimecrolimus cream and triamcinolone acetonide paste in the treatment of symptomatic oral lichen planus. *Indian J. Dent.* **2015**, *6*, 14–19. [CrossRef]
35. Ezzatt, O.M.; Helmy, I.M. Topical pimecrolimus versus betamethasone for oral lichen planus: A randomized clinical trial. *Clin. Oral Investig.* **2018**, *23*, 947–956. [CrossRef] [PubMed]
36. Hettiarachchi, P.V.K.S.; Hettiarachchi, R.M.; Jayasinghe, R.D.; Sitheeque, M. Comparison of topical tacrolimus and clobetasol in the management of symptomatic oral lichen planus: A double-blinded, randomized clinical trial in Sri Lanka. *J. Investig. Clin. Dent.* **2016**, *8*, e12237. [CrossRef] [PubMed]
37. Pakfetrat, A.; Delavarian, Z.; Falaki, F.; Khorashadizadeh, M.; Saba, M. The effect of pimecrolimus cream 1% compared with triamcinolone acetonide paste in treatment of atrophic-erosive oral lichen planus. *Iran. J. Otorhinolaryngol.* **2015**, *27*, 119–126. [PubMed]
38. Thongprasom, K.; Chaimusig, M.; Korkij, W.; Sererat, T.; Luangjarmekorn, L.; Rojwattanasirivej, S. A randomized-controlled trial to compare topical cyclosporin with triamcinolone acetonide for the treatment of oral lichen planus. *J. Oral Pathol. Med.* **2007**, *36*, 142–146. [CrossRef]
39. Sivaraman, S.; Santham, K.; Nelson, A.; Laliytha, B.; Azhalvel, P.; Deepak, J.H. A randomized triple-blind clinical trial to compare the effectiveness of topical triamcinolone acetonate [0.1%], clobetasol propionate [0.05%], and tacrolimus orabase [0.03%] in the management of oral lichen planus. *J. Pharm. Bioallied. Sci.* **2016**, *8* (Suppl. 1), S86–S89. [CrossRef]
40. Revanappa, M.M.; Naikmasur, V.G.; Sattur, A.P. Evaluation of Efficacy of Tacrolimus 0.1% in Orabase and Triamcinolone Acetonide 0.1% in Orabase in the Management of Symptomatic Oral Lichen Planus Randomized Single Blind Control Study. *J. Indian Acad. Oral Med. Radiol.* **2012**, *24*, 269–273. [CrossRef]
41. Georgaki, M.; Piperi, E.; Theofilou, V.I.; Pettas, E.; Stoufi, E.; Nikitakis, N.G. A randomized clinical trial of topical dexamethasone vs. cyclosporine treatment for oral lichen planus. *Med. Oral Patol. Oral Cirugia Bucal.* **2022**, *27*, e113–e124. [CrossRef]
42. Malhotra, A.K.; Khaitan, B.K.; Sethuraman, G.; Sharma, V.K. Betamethasone oral mini-pulse therapy compared with topical triamcinolone acetonide [0.1%] paste in oral lichen planus: A randomized comparative study. *J. Am. Acad. Dermatol.* **2008**, *58*, 596–602. [CrossRef]
43. Dillenburg, C.S.; Martins, M.A.; Munerato, M.C.; Marques, M.M.; Carrard, V.C.; Sant'Ana Filho, M.; Castilho, R.M.; Martins, M.D. Efficacy of laser phototherapy in comparison to topical clobetasol for the treatment of oral lichen planus: A randomized controlled trial. *J. Biomed. Opt.* **2014**, *19*, 068002. [CrossRef]

44. Fu, J.; Zhu, X.; Dan, H.; Zhou, Y.; Liu, C.; Wang, F.; Li, Y.; Liu, N.; Chen, Q.; Xu, Y.; et al. Amlexanox is as effective as dexamethasone in topical treatment of erosive oral lichen planus: A short-term pilot study. *Oral Surg. Oral Med. Oral Pathol. Oral Radiol.* **2012**, *113*, 638–643. [CrossRef]
45. Bakhtiari, S.; Azari-Marhabi, S.; Mojahedi, S.M.; Namdari, M.; Rankohi, Z.E.; Jafari, S. Comparing clinical effects of photodynamic therapy as a novel method with topical corticosteroid for treatment of Oral Lichen Planus. *Photodiagnosis Photodyn. Ther.* **2017**, *20*, 159–164. [CrossRef] [PubMed]
46. Hashem, A.S.; Issrani, R.; Elsayed, T.E.; Prabhu, N. Topical hyaluronic acid in the management of oral lichen planus: A comparative study. *J. Investig. Clin. Dent.* **2019**, *10*, e12385. [CrossRef] [PubMed]
47. Kia, S.J.; Basirat, M.; Mortezaie, T.; Moosavi, M.-S. Comparison of oral Nano-Curcumin with oral prednisolone on oral lichen planus: A randomized double-blinded clinical trial. *BMC Complement. Med. Ther.* **2020**, *20*, 328. [CrossRef]
48. Ferri, E.P.; Cunha, K.R.; Abboud, C.S.; de Barros Gallo, C.; de Sousa Sobral, S.; de Fatima Teixeira da Silva, D.; Horliana, A.C.R.; Franco, A.L.D.S.; Rodrigues, M.F.S.D. Photobiomodulation is effective in oral lichen planus: A randomized, controlled, double-blind study. *Oral Dis.* **2021**, *27*, 1205–1216. [CrossRef] [PubMed]
49. Agha-Hosseini, F.; Borhan-Mojabi, K.; Monsef-Esfahani, H.-R.; Mirzaii-Dizgah, I.; Etemad-Moghadam, S.; Karagah, A. Efficacy of purslane in the treatment of oral lichen planus. *Phytother. Res.* **2009**, *24*, 240–244. [CrossRef] [PubMed]
50. Choonhakarn, C.; Busaracome, P.; Sripanidkulchai, B.; Sarakarn, P. The efficacy of aloe vera gel in the treatment of oral lichen planus: A randomized controlled trial. *Br. J. Dermatol.* **2008**, *158*, 573–577. [CrossRef] [PubMed]
51. Salazar-Sanchez, N.; Lopez-Jornet, P.; Camacho-Alonso, F.; Sanchez-Siles, M. Efficacy of topical Aloe vera in patients with oral lichen planus: A randomized double-blind study. *J. Oral Pathol. Med.* **2010**, *39*, 735–740. [CrossRef]
52. Nolan, A.; Badminton, J.; Maguire, J.; Seymour, R.A. The efficacy of topical hyaluronic acid in the management of oral lichen planus. *J. Oral Pathol. Med.* **2009**, *38*, 299–303. [CrossRef]
53. Eisen DECDuell, E.A.; Griffiths, C.E.; Voorhees, J.J. Effect of topical cyclosporine rinse on oral lichen planus. A double-blind analysis. *N. Engl. J. Med.* **1990**, *323*, 290. [CrossRef]
54. Swift, J.C.; Rees, T.D.; Plemons, J.M.; Hallmon, W.W.; Wright, J.C. The Effectiveness of 1% Pimecrolimus Cream in the Treatment of Oral Erosive Lichen Planus. *J. Periodontol.* **2005**, *76*, 627–635. [CrossRef]
55. Passeron, T.; Lacour, J.P.; Fontas, E.; Ortonne, J.P. Treatment of oral erosive lichen planus with 1% pimecrolimus cream: A double-blind, randomized, prospective trial with measurement of pimecrolimus levels in the blood. *Arch. Dermatol.* **2007**, *143*, 472–476. [CrossRef] [PubMed]
56. Volz, T.; Caroli, U.; Lüdtke, H.; Bräutigam, M.; Kohler-Späth, H.; Röcken, M.; Biedermann, T. Pimecrolimus cream 1% in erosive oral lichen planus—A prospective randomized double-blind vehicle-controlled study. *Br. J. Dermatol.* **2008**, *159*, 936–941. [CrossRef] [PubMed]
57. Bhatt, G.; Gupta, S.; Ghosh, S. Comparative efficacy of topical aloe vera and low-level laser therapy in the management of oral lichen planus: A randomized clinical trial. *Lasers Med. Sci.* **2021**, *37*, 2063–2070. [CrossRef] [PubMed]
58. Campisi, G.; Giandalia, G.; De Caro, V.; Di Liberto, C.; Arico, P.; Giannola, L.I. A new delivery system of clobetasol-17-propionate [lipid-loaded microspheres 0.025%] compared with a conventional formulation [lipophilic ointment in a hydrophilic phase 0.025%] in topical treatment of atrophic/erosive oral lichen planus. A Phase IV, randomized, observer-blinded, parallel group clinical trial. *Br. J. Dermatol.* **2004**, *150*, 984–990.
59. Carbone, M.; Arduino, P.G.; Carrozzo, M.; Caiazzo, G.; Broccoletti, R.; Conrotto, D.; Bezzo, C.; Gandolfo, S. Topical clobetasol in the treatment of atrophic-erosive oral lichen planus: A randomized controlled trial to compare two preparations with different concentrations. *J. Oral Pathol. Med.* **2009**, *38*, 227. [CrossRef]
60. Chainani-Wu, N.; Silverman, S.; Reingold, A.; Bostrom, A.; Mc Culloch, C.; Lozada-Nur, F.; Weintraub, J. A randomized, placebo-controlled, double-blind clinical trial of curcuminoids in oral lichen planus. *Phytomedicine Int. J. Phytother. Phytopharm.* **2007**, *14*, 437–446. [CrossRef]
61. Gaeta, G.M.; Serpico, R.; Femiano, F.; La Rotonda, M.I.; Cappello, B.; Gombos, F. Cyclosporin bioadhesive gel in the topical treatment of erosive oral lichen planus. *Int. J. Immunopath. Pharm.* **1994**, *7*, 125–132.
62. Ghabanchi, J.; Bahri Najafi, R.; Haghnegahdar, S. Treatment of oral inflammatory diseases with a new mucoadhesive prednisolone table versus triamcinolone acetonide paste. *Iran. Red Crescent Med. J.* **2009**, *11*, 155–159.
63. Hegarty, A.M.; Hodgson, T.A.; Lewsey, J.D.; Porter, S.R. Fluticasone propionate spray and betamethasone sodium phosphate mouthrinse: A randomized crossover study for the treatment of symptomatic oral lichen planus. *J. Am. Acad. Dermatol.* **2002**, *47*, 271–279. [CrossRef]
64. Wei, X.; Li, B.Q.; Zhou, X.D.; Chen, Q.M. Clinical effect of mycostatin paste plus dexamethasone paste in treatment of patients with OLP. *J. Clin. Stomatol.* **2003**, *19*, 568–569.
65. Lodi, G.; Tarozzi, M.; Sardella, A.; Demarosi, F.; Canegallo, L.; Di Benedetto, D.; Carrassi, A. Miconazole as adjuvant therapy for oral lichen planus: A double-blind randomized controlled trial. *Br. J. Dermatol.* **2007**, *156*, 1336. [CrossRef] [PubMed]
66. Lundquist, G.; Forsgren, H.; Gajecki, M.; Emtestam, L. Photochemotherapy of oral lichen planus. A controlled study. *Oral Surg. Oral Med. Oral Pathol. Oral Radiol. Endod.* **1995**, *79*, 554–558. [CrossRef] [PubMed]
67. Xiong, C.; Li, Q.; Lin, M.; Li, X.; Meng, W.; Wu, Y.; Zeng, X.; Zhou, H.; Zhou, G. The efficacy of topical intralesional BCG-PSN injection in the treatment of erosive oral lichen planus: A randomized controlled trial. *J. Oral Pathol. Med.* **2009**, *38*, 551. [CrossRef]

68. MMousavi, F.; Sherafati, S.; Mojaver, Y.N. Ignatia in the treatment of oral lichen planus. *Homeopath. J. Fac. Homeopath.* **2009**, *98*, 40–44. [CrossRef] [PubMed]
69. Rodstrom, P.-O.; Hakeberg, M.; Jontell, M.; Nordin, P. Erosive oral lichen planus treated with clobetasol propionate and triamcinolone acetonide in Orabase: A double-blind clinical trial. *J. Dermatol. Treat.* **1994**, *5*, 7–10. [CrossRef]
70. Xu, Y.Z.; Geng, Y.; Liu, Y.X.; Fuan, Y.Q.; Li, J. Clinical study on three-step treatment of oral lichen planus by integrated traditional and western medicine. *J. Mod. Stomatol.* **2002**, *16*, 344–346.
71. Sander, C.; Cooper, S.; Ali, I.; Dean, D.; Thiele, J.; Wojnarowska, F. Decreased antioxidant enzyme expression and increased oxidative damage in erosive lichen planus of the vulva. *BJOG Int. J. Obstet. Gynaecol.* **2005**, *112*, 1572–1575. [CrossRef]
72. Sezer, E.; Ozugurlu, F.; Ozyurt, H.; Sahin, S.; Etikan, I. Lipid peroxidation and antioxidant status in lichen planus. *Clin. Exp. Dermatol.* **2007**, *32*, 430–434. [CrossRef]
73. Khan, A.; Farah, C.S.; Savage, N.W.; Walsh, L.J.; Harbrow, D.J.; Sugerman, P.B. Th1 cytokines in oral lichen planus. *J. Oral Pathol. Med. Off. Publ. Int. Assoc. Oral Pathol. Am. Acad. Oral Pathol.* **2003**, *32*, 77–83. [CrossRef]
74. Eisen, D.; Carrozzo, M.; Sebastian, J.-V.B.; Thongprasom, K. Number V Oral lichen planus: Clinical features and management. *Oral Dis.* **2005**, *11*, 338–349. [CrossRef]
75. Shelton, R.M. Aloe vera. Its chemical and therapeutic properties. *Int. J. Dermatol.* **1991**, *30*, 679–683. [CrossRef]
76. Klein, A.D.; Penneys, N.S. Aloe vera. *J. Am. Acad. Dermatol.* **1988**, *18 Pt 1*, 714–720. [CrossRef] [PubMed]
77. Duansak, D.; Somboonwong, J.; Patumraj, S. Effects of Aloe vera on leukocyte adhesion and TNF-alpha and IL-6 levels in burn wounded rats. *Clin. Hemorheol. Microcirc.* **2003**, *29*, 239–246. [PubMed]
78. Eamlamnam, K.; Patumraj, S.; Visedopas, N.; Thong-Ngam, D. Effects of Aloe vera and sucralfate on gastric microcirculatory changes, cytokine levels and gastric ulcer healing in rats. *World J. Gastroenterol.* **2006**, *12*, 2034–2039. [CrossRef] [PubMed]
79. Hardinger, K.; Magee, C.C.; Brennan, D.C. Pharmacology of Cyclosporine and Tacrolimus [Internet]. Available online: https://www.medilib.ir/uptodate/show/7995 (accessed on 31 October 2022).
80. Al Johani, K.A.; Hegarty, A.M.; Porter, S.R.; Fedele, S. Calcineurin inhibitors in oral medicine. *J. Am. Acad. Dermatol.* **2009**, *61*, 829–840. [CrossRef] [PubMed]
81. Rebora, A. Treatment with Calcineurin Inhibitors of Oral Lichen Planus. An Attempt to Clarify the Issue. [Internet]. Available online: https://www.omicsonline.org/open-access/treatment-with-calcineurin-inhibitors-of-oral-lichen-planus-an-attempt-to-clarify-the-issue-100341.html (accessed on 8 November 2022).
82. Vohra, S.; Singal, A.; Sharma, S.B. Clinical and serological efficacy of topical calcineurin inhibitors in oral lichen planus: A prospective randomized controlled trial. *Int. J. Dermatol.* **2015**, *55*, 101–105. [CrossRef]
83. McCaughey, C.; MacHan, M.; Bennett, R.; Zone, J.J.; Hull, C.M. Pimecrolimus 1% cream for oral erosive lichen planus: A 6-week randomized, double-blind, vehicle-controlled study with a 6-week open-label extension to assess efficacy and safety. *J. Eur. Acad. Dermatol. Venereol.* **2011**, *25*, 1061–1067. [CrossRef]
84. Usatine, R.P.; Tinitigan, M. Diagnosis and treatment of lichen planus. *Am. Fam. Physician* **2011**, *84*, 53–60.
85. Pinas, L.; Garcia-Garcia, A.; Sayáns, M.P.; Suarez-Fernandez, R.; Alkhraisat, M.; Anitua, E. The use of topical corticosteroids in the treatment of oral lichen planus in Spain: A national survey. *Med. Oral Patol. Oral Cir. Buccal* **2017**, *22*, e264–e269. [CrossRef]
86. Carbone, M.; Goss, E.; Carrozzo, M.; Castellano, S.; Conrotto, D.; Broccoletti, R.; Gandolfo, S. Systemic and topical corticosteroid treatment of oral lichen planus: A comparative study with long-term follow-up. *J. Oral Pathol. Med.* **2003**, *32*, 323–329. [CrossRef]
87. Price, S.M.; Murrah, V.A. Why the general dentist needs to know how to manage oral lichen planus. *Gen. Dent.* **2015**, *63*, 16–22. [PubMed]
88. Carrozzo, M.; Thorpe, R. Oral lichen planus: A review. *Minerva Stomatol.* **2009**, *58*, 519–537. [PubMed]
89. Thongprasom, K.; Dhanuthai, K. Steriods in the treatment of lichen planus: A review. *J. Oral Sci.* **2008**, *50*, 377–385. [CrossRef]
90. Radwan-Oczko, M. Topical application of drugs used in treatment of oral lichen planus lesions. *Adv. Clin. Exp. Med. Off. Organ Wroclaw. Med. Univ.* **2013**, *22*, 893–898.

Disclaimer/Publisher's Note: The statements, opinions and data contained in all publications are solely those of the individual author(s) and contributor(s) and not of MDPI and/or the editor(s). MDPI and/or the editor(s) disclaim responsibility for any injury to people or property resulting from any ideas, methods, instructions or products referred to in the content.

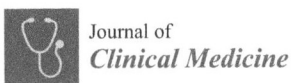

Review

It Is Time for a Multidisciplinary Rehabilitation Approach: A Scoping Review on Stomatognathic Diseases in Neurological Disorders

Angela Militi [1,†], Mirjam Bonanno [2,*,†] and Rocco Salvatore Calabrò [2]

1. Department of Biomedical and Dental Sciences and Morphological and Functional Imaging, University of Messina, 98125 Messina, Italy; amiliti@unime.it
2. IRCCS Centro Neurolesi "Bonino-Pulejo", Via Palermo, SS 113, C. Da Casazza, 98123 Messina, Italy; roccos.calabro@irccsme.it
* Correspondence: mirjam.bonanno@irccsme.it
† These authors contributed equally to this work.

Abstract: Patients affected by neurological disorders can develop stomatognathic diseases (SD) related to decreased bite force and quality of mastication, bruxism, severe clicking and other temporomandibular disorders (TMD), which deeply affect patients' swallowing, masticatory and phonation functions and, therefore, their quality of life. The diagnosis is commonly based on medical history and physical examination, paying attention to the temporomandibular joint (TMJ) range of movements, jaw sounds and mandibular lateral deviation. Diagnostic tools such as computed tomography and magnetic resonance imaging are used instead in case of equivocal findings in the anamnesis and physical evaluation. However, stomatognathic and temporomandibular functional training has not been commonly adopted in hospital settings as part of formal neurorehabilitation. This review is aimed at describing the most frequent pathophysiological patterns of SD and TMD in patients affected by neurological disorders and their rehabilitative approach, giving some clinical suggestions about their conservative treatment. We have searched and reviewed evidence published in PubMed, Google Scholar, Scopus and Cochrane Library between 2010 and 2023. After a thorough screening, we have selected ten studies referring to pathophysiological patterns of SD/TMD and the conservative rehabilitative approach in neurological disorders. Given this, the current literature is still poor and unclear about the administration of these kinds of complementary and rehabilitative approaches in neurological patients suffering from SD and/or TMD.

Keywords: stomatognathic disease; temporomandibular disorders; neurological patients; neurorehabilitation; multidisciplinary approach

1. Introduction

The stomatognathic system (SS) is defined as a functional complex including craniofacial structures with musculoskeletal and ligamentous components, the temporomandibular joint (TMJ), oral cavity, neck and masticatory muscles [1]. Patients affected by neurological disorders can develop stomatognathic diseases (SD) related to decreased bite force and quality of mastication, bruxism, severe clicking and other TMJ disorders (TMD), which deeply affect the patients' quality of life [2]. In fact, the integrity of SS is fundamental in activating the neuromuscular chain that initiates the swallow reflex. On the other hand, SD can also cause myofascial pain that may irradiate in different regions, such as dental arches, ears, temples, forehead, occiput, cervical spine and shoulders [3] (Figure 1), resembling atypical headaches and facial pain.

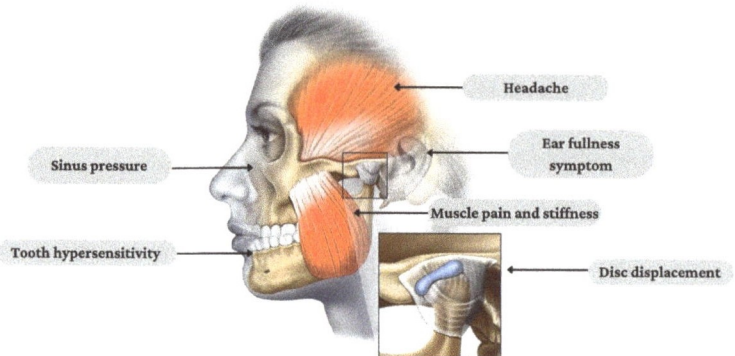

Figure 1. Clinical presentation of SD and TMD in people affected by neurological disorders.

Despite the presence of SD in neurological patients, functional training for SS and TMJ has not been commonly adopted in hospital settings as part of formal neurorehabilitation. Generally, the non-pharmacological treatment for SD and TMD aims to decrease pain, induce muscle release and stabilize muscle function and joint mobility through physical therapy (PT) and/or manual techniques (MT) [4]. Among the different PT modalities, electrophysical tools (ultrasound, LASER, TENS, interferential current) have analgesic and anti-inflammatory effects, as well as therapeutic exercise alone or in combination with MT. The latter consists of the administration of hands-on techniques to improve mobility and reduce pain in the cervical spine and its upper levels [5]. In this context, osteopathic manipulative treatment (OMT), which uses both direct and indirect MT, can be easily adapted to any type of patient [6]. The OMT can be useful in people complaining of orofacial pain as it induces muscle and fascial relaxation, promoting the release of endogenous opioids due to therapeutic touch [7,8]. Moreover, reticular formation and the brainstem are strictly involved in the coordination of the masticatory cycle, which is also controlled by a central pattern generator (CPG) which, in turn, influences gait rhythmicity too. In this way, the presence of SD and TMD is not only associated with pain or functional alterations, but it also involves the central nervous system, with a documented reduction of the grey matter volume in the somatosensory cortex and the premotor cortex [9,10]. Indeed, SS and TMJ dysfunction can be related to brain and muscle/joint alterations, so a multidisciplinary approach is required to deal with these complex problems. In current clinical practice, physiotherapists usually focus more on gait recovery and arm mobility, neglecting the role of TMJ in affecting posture and gait [11]. Patients affected by TMD could manifest a depressed head posture due to forces created by masticatory muscles. In this way, dysfunctional changes in the mandibular position, influenced by proprioceptive afferents, can have an impact on gait and balance stability through muscle connections provided by cervical muscles (i.e., sternocleidomastoid muscle, elevator scapulae), dorsal muscles (i.e., trapezius), lumbar spine (i.e., intrinsic spine muscles) and pelvic girdle [12–14]. Since this issue is often overlooked by professional figures of a neurorehabilitation team, our review is aimed to provide more awareness about this topic, describing the most frequent pathophysiological patterns of SD and TMD in patients affected by neurological disorders and their rehabilitative approach, and to give some clinical advice about their conservative interventions.

2. Methods

2.1. Search Strategy

The review was carried out by searching on PubMed, Google Scholar, Scopus and Cochrane Library using a combination of keywords that we have reported in Table 1.

Table 1. Search strategy used for the attrition of studies.

Neurological Disorders	Temporomandibular/ Stomatognathic Diseases	Conservative and Rehabilitative Approaches
"Parkinson's disease" OR "Multiple sclerosis" OR "Spino-cerebellar ataxia" OR "stroke" OR "oro-mandibular dystonia" OR "movement disorders"	"Temporomandibular joint disorders" OR "temporomandibular joint dysfunctions" OR "stomatognathic disease" OR "bruxism" OR "disc displacement" OR "temporomandibular myofascial pain" OR "orofacial pain"	"Physical exercise therapy" OR "manual therapy" OR "osteopathic manipulative treatment" OR "cranial-sacral therapy" OR "physical therapy" OR "occlusal splint therapy"

2.2. PICO Evaluation

Search terms were defined according to the PICO model (population, intervention, comparison and outcome) [15]. The population includes patients affected by neurological disorders such as Parkinson's disease, multiple sclerosis, spinocerebellar ataxia, oromandibular dystonia and stroke, and complaining about SD and/or TMD. Intervention included conservative and complementary therapies, such as physiotherapy, manual treatments, OMT and splint therapy. The comparison was referred to the absence of treatment and/or the administration of just one type of conservative treatment (as shown in Table 1). Lastly, the outcome included any improvements in pain perception and TMJ/SS function shown by the patients.

2.3. Inclusion and Exclusion Criteria

Then, the inclusion criteria were (i) neurological patients affected by SD/TMD; (ii) pain topic; (iii) English language; and (iv) publication in a peer-reviewed journal. We excluded articles that described theoretical models, methodological approaches, basic technical descriptions as well as animal studies and conference proceedings.

2.4. Literature Selection

We assessed the most relevant pilot studies, randomized controlled trials and case-control studies published between 2010 and 2023. Four hundred and twenty-nine articles were evaluated independently by two reviewers (MB and AM) according to title, abstract, text and scientific validity. The agreement assessment was performed using Cohen's kappa coefficient [16]. In case of disagreement, an independent reviewer (RSC) mediated to achieve consensus. After removing duplicates ($n = 264$), 149 papers were initially screened, and only 32 were found eligible for a full assessment. Finally, only 10 articles fulfilled the inclusion criteria, as reported in the new PRISMA flowchart (Figure 2) [17].

2.5. Study Risk of Bias Assessment

The risk of bias in controlled studies was assessed through a revised Cochrane risk of bias (RoB 2) [18], while cross-sectional and case-control studies were evaluated through Newcastle–Ottawa scale (NOS). Specifically, the risk of bias assessment was performed by two authors (A.M. and M.B.) without the use of automation tools.

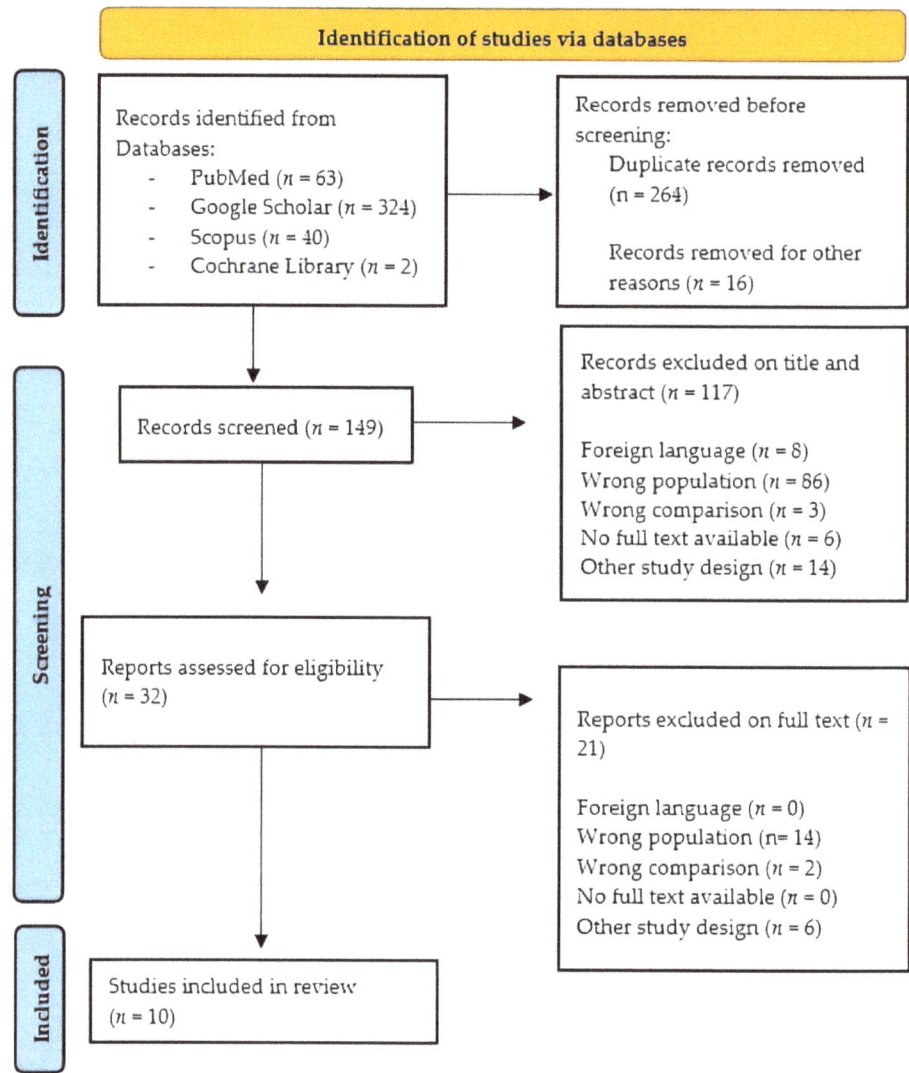

Figure 2. PRISMA flowchart for study selection.

3. Results

We analyzed the 10 selected pieces of evidence dealing with the presence and treatment of SD/TMD in patients affected by neurological disorders. The agreement of the judge's decision for the inclusion of the studies was Cohen's k = 0.82, which means a perfect agreement. In particular, we classified the studies according to the association between neurological disorders and TMD and its rehabilitation treatment, reporting a summary of results in a tabular form (see Table 2).

Table 2. Description of studies that dealt with SD/TMD in patients with neurological disorders.

Reference Number	Association between SD/TMD and Neurological Disorder (Yes or No)	Stomatognathic Disease	Diagnostic Tools	Musculoskeletal Structures Involved	Conservative and Complementary Treatments	Major Findings
Multiple sclerosis (MS)						
Costa et al. [19]	Yes	TMD, bruxism, tooth hypersensitivity and hyposalivation	Clinical intra- and extra-oral examination	Suboccipital and cervical muscles	Endodontic intervention, occlusal adjustment and behavioral education	The endodontic treatment met the aesthetic pleasing of the patient
Williams et al. [20]	Yes	Jaw clenching/bruxism	Ultrasonic pulsed phase-locked loop (PPLL) and change in acoustic pathlength (ΔL) as the measure of intracranial distance	Masticatory muscles, temporal bones and TMJ	NA	Jaw clenching/bruxism was associated with the displacement of the temporal bones and expansion of the cranial cavity in MS patients compared to healthy control
Spinocerebellar ataxia (SCA)						
Ferreira et al. [21]	Yes	Increased masticatory muscle activity and reduction of maximal molar bite force	RDCTMD, electromyographic activity, muscle thickness and maximum bite force	TMJ structures, masseter and temporalis	NA	SCA is characterized by functional and electromyographic alterations in SS, especially in chewing and bite force
Parkinson's disease (PD)						
Choi et al. [22]	Yes	Jaw tremor, bruxism amd TMJ rigidity	Diagnosis of TMD was considered using ICD-10 code K07.6	Masticatory muscles, TMJ structures and cervical spine	NA	The authors stated that PD patients have a high risk to develop TMD; conversely, individuals affected by TMD have more risk to develop PD in the future
Verhoeff et al. [23]	Yes	Bruxism (both sleep and awake bruxism), TMD and orofacial pain	The authors created an 18-item questionnaire, reporting: (i) chronic pain; (ii) the DC/TMD; (iii) oral behavior; (iv) DC/TMD symptom questionnaire; (v) TMD pain screener	Masticatory muscles, TMJ structures and cervical spine	NA	There are correlations between PD and bruxism, and PD with TMJ pain
Oromandibular dystonia (OMD)						
Handa et al. [24]	Yes	Myofascial pain in masticatory muscles and dental problems	Differential diagnosis between OMD and TMD by clinical examination and ICD-10	Masticatory muscles, TMJ structures and dental arches	NA	Since OMD shares clinical features with TMD, they are often misdiagnosed with the risk to receive unnecessary treatments
Stroke						
Alvater Ramos et al. [25]	Yes	Disc displacement and myogenous TMD	TMD diagnosis was performed using RDCTMD; physical mechanical pressure on trigger points was tested using the algometer Wagner PAIN TES and Pressure Pain Threshold Test, while cervical ROM was assessed using a Sanny Fleximeter	Cervical lateral-flexors muscles, TMJ and masticatory muscles	NA	The authors found that post-stroke patients manifested augmented muscle tone and reduced cervical ROM on the affected side, suggesting that the musculoskeletal alterations caused by a stroke can predispose to TMD
Choi et al. [26]	Yes	Dysphagia	Dysphagia was confirmed by a video-fluoroscopic swallowing study	Suprahyoid muscles (digastric and mylohyoid muscles) and hyoid bone movements	Jaw opening exercise (isometric and isotonic) and head lift exercise	JOE and HLE were useful to improve supra-hyoid muscle strength and thickness. However, JOE required less effort than HLF

Table 2. Cont.

Reference Number	Association between SD/TMD and Neurological Disorder (Yes or No)	Stomatognathic Disease	Diagnostic Tools	Musculoskeletal Structures Involved	Conservative and Complementary Treatments	Major Findings
Oh et al. [27]	Yes	Decreased TMJ function	Clinical examination with craniomandibular index and limited range in opening mouth; swallowing function was assessed using MASA	TMJ structures, masticatory muscles, neck and shoulder muscles	Stomatognathic alignment exercise program (exercises to increase the mobility of the neck and TMJ), head and neck posture exercises and anterior chest stretching exercise)	Stomatognathic alignment exercises were useful to improve TMJ and swallowing functions
Umay et al. [28]	Yes	Swallowing dysfunction, masticatory and swallowing muscles weakness	Swallowing intervals and motor action potentials (MAPs) of trigeminal, facial and hypoglossal nerves were measured	Swallowing muscles, masticatory muscles, hyoid bone and neck structures	Thermal stimulation (to radix of tongue, palate, tonsillar plica, and oral mucosa); oral motor strength exercises for labial, intrinsic tongue and masticatory muscles; intermittent galvanic stimulation	After four weeks of treatment, significant recovery in swallowing, motor and general functional levels of the patients was provided

Legend: SD (stomatognathic disease), TMD (temporomandibular disorder), TMJ (temporomandibular joint), RDCTMD (Research Diagnostic Criteria for Temporomandibular Disorders), JOE (jaw opening exercise), HLF (head lift exercise), MASA (Mann assessment of swallowing ability).

The risk of bias assessment of randomized controlled trials, cross-sectional studies and case-control studies was evaluated, respectively, with RoB 2 (Table 3) and NOS (Table 4).

Table 3. Risk of bias assessment of randomized trials with RoB 2.

Reference	Randomization Process	Effect of Assignment on Intervention	Effect of Adhering to Intervention	Missing Outcome Data	Measurement of the Outcome	Selection of the Reported Results
Choi et al. [26]	SC	SC	L	SC	SC	SC
Oh et al. [27]	L	L	L	L	SC	SC
Umay et al. [28]	L	L	L	L	L	L

Legend: L (low); H (high); SC (some concerns).

Table 4. Risk of bias assessment of cross-section and case-control studies through Newcastle–Ottawa Scale (NOS).

Reference	NOS
Williams et al. [20]	4
Ferreira et al. [21]	4
Choi et al. [22]	6
Verhoeff et al. [23]	7
Handa et al. [24]	5
Alvater Ramos [25]	3

The general quality of the included studies ranged from low [19–22,24,25,27,28] to moderate [27,29]. It should be considered that the low quality of the selected evidence is likely related to the great heterogeneity among studies for the methodologies, diagnostic tools and rehabilitation treatment administered. Additionally, we excluded one study from the risk of bias assessment [19], since it is a case report.

4. Pathophysiology of Stomatognathic and Temporomandibular Joint Disorders in Neurological Disorders

The etiology of SD and TMD is linked to a wide range of functional, psychological and environmental factors, especially in neurological disorders in which the underlying pathology is complex. People affected by multiple sclerosis (MS) are more susceptible to developing TMD disorders [30,31]. Indeed, the concomitant presence of psychological disturbances (i.e., anxiety, depression, behavioral alteration) can exacerbate TMD disorders, as confirmed by a systematic review [30]. In this vein, it has been recently reported that patients who suffer from psychological distress are less responsive to conventional treatments for TMD, requiring a longer duration of therapy [32]. MS patients can manifest three common orofacial alterations: facial palsy, trigeminal neuralgia and/or paresthesia. However, Costa, C. et al. [19] described an unusual pattern of SD in a MS patient, which included tooth hypersensitivity, hyposalivation associated with caries, halitosis and bruxism. The latter tends to increase when occlusion is impaired, also contributing to head and neck pain. In this context, some studies hypothesized that the augmented mobility of cranial bones due to reduced bone mass density, especially in the temporal ones, expands and contracts during bruxism, increasing intracranial pressure, which can favor brain damage [20]. Another mechanism that can be involved in the pathogenesis of TMD or SD in MS patients is cerebellar dysfunction. In fact, cerebellar plaques and proprioceptive changes may lead to an increased propensity to fatigue of TMJ structures in addition to a lack of coordination of mandibular movements [30,33]. In a similar way, SD is present in patients with spinocerebellar ataxia (SCA), who often present dysarthric speech and swallowing difficulties. According to Ferreira et al. [21], SCA subjects showed a decreased bite force and hypotrophy of the masseter and temporalis muscles, with an augmented electromyographic activity. The underlying hypothesis for these electromyographic changes can be related to an increase in the amplitude and duration of motor unit action potentials, in addition to reduced muscle recruitment [34]. Moreover, the lack of coordination, especially during lateral mandibular movements in SCA patients, can be explained by the pathological alteration in cerebellum pathways, affecting the synchrony and precision of movements [35]. Furthermore, patients affected by Parkinson's disease (PD) can manifest SD and TMD due to the presence of rigidity. Body muscle rigidity could also affect masticatory muscles in association with augmented muscle tone during sleep [22]. This condition could favor the repetitive jaw muscle activity and grinding of the teeth, named bruxism, which is considered a factor for developing TMD. Bruxism can occur both during sleep (sleep bruxism) and wakefulness (awake bruxism) [36], and its pathogenesis seems to be related to central nervous structure alterations. In fact, some antidepressant drugs, such as Selective Serotonin Reuptake Inhibitors (SSRI), can cause bruxism as a side-effect of inhibiting dopaminergic neurons [23]. This could explain why bruxism is frequent in PD patients due to the reduction of dopamine presence in basal ganglia [29]. TMD and SD were also found in other movement disorders, including dystonia. The term "dystonia" refers to prolonged or intermittent muscle contractions, causing repetitive and abnormal movements and/or postures [37]. In this context, oromandibular dystonia (OMD) is often misdiagnosed due to shared clinical features with TMD [24]. In fact, OMD is associated with masticatory disturbances such as limited mouth opening, orofacial pain and TMJ dislocations that can simulate an isolated TMD, overlooking the real etiology of the disturbance or pain. Today, six subtypes of OMD are recognized: jaw closing (i), opening (ii), deviation (iii), protrusion (iv), lingual (v) and lip (vi) dystonia. In particular, the jaw-closing subtype is related to a loss of reciprocal muscle inhibition that greatly limits mouth opening, especially during speaking or eating, worsening the patient's quality of life. In addition, dystonia tends to expand to other muscles, including orbicularis oculi, neck and shoulder muscles [38]. The pathophysiology of SD in OMD patients is still unclear, although some studies found that functional movement disorders, as well as dystonia, present a hypoactivation of the supplementary motor area and abnormal connectivity of those brain areas designed to select or inhibit movements [39]. The onset of SD and TMD in stroke patients depends on the extent and site of the vascular lesion, which can affect cortical areas, or motor-neuron pools of cranial nerves in the brain stem, causing sensorimotor deficits in SS. The presence of facial and masticatory muscle dysfunctions has been demonstrated in post-stroke patients, including weakness and hypotonus of the masseter, orbicularis oris, mylohyoid and digastric with an increase of thickness in these muscles [40]. In detail, the most common TMD in post-stroke patients seems to be related to disc displacement, which alters the structural relationship with condyle, thus producing a click sound when the mouth opens due to translation movements. This alteration could be chronic as it interferes with the simple opening of the mouth during speech or eating, and the disc becomes progressively more dislocated. Another hypothesis is that forward head posture, due to inefficacy to maintain postural alignment, causes an overload in posterior cervical muscles that can influence the TMJ by changing the position of the mandibular condyle and, consequentially, its functioning [25,41,42].

5. Diagnostic Methods and Tools for TMD

When orofacial pain occurs, patients commonly consult dentists or gnathologists, although osteopaths or physiotherapists can primarily identify a TMD during a physical examination and manual treatment [43]. In fact, the diagnosis of TMD is based on medical history and physical evaluation findings (Figure 3).

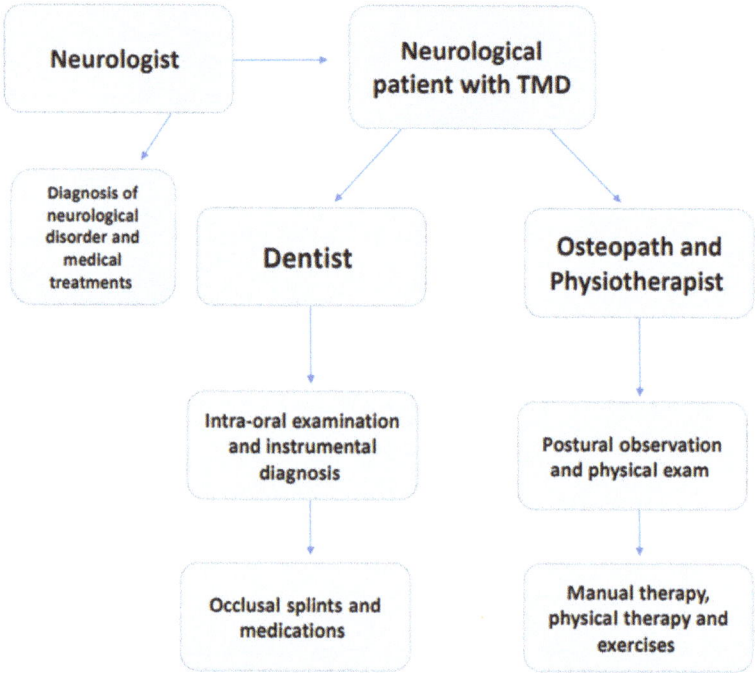

Figure 3. Theoretical diagnostic and therapeutic paradigm for neurological patients affected by TMD.

An in-depth anamnesis is the first fundamental step to guide the clinician to carry out the most relevant physical examination and diagnosis. A comprehensive history for a patient with orofacial pain includes the main complaint, medical history, dental history and psychosocial history. The patient should provide the dentist with a full description of the symptoms and the reason why the patient is seeking care. In this context, clinicians should investigate the quality of pain (i.e., burning, stabbing and blocking pain), which movements or activity exacerbates the pain and how long it has been present. In addition, clinicians should ask patients to indicate their pain point(s) with their fingers, figuring out the pain localization [44]. To more objectively rate the pain, different scales can be used in current clinical practice, such as the McGill Pain Questionnaire (MPQ), for the multidimensional detailed evaluation of orofacial pain. However, it takes a lot of time and requires good patient compliance. As an alternative, the short form of the MPQ (SF-MPQ) can be easily administered since it measures the pain intensity through the scores from the Present Pain Intensity (PPI) and the Visual Analogical Scale (VAS), also including sensory and affective scores that form the MPQ descriptors [44,45]. Otherwise, unidimensional pain scales are widely used in clinical evaluation routines and include VAS, the Verbal Rating Scale (VRS), which contains a list of adjectives marked up with a number describing five different levels of pain intensity; the Numerical Rating Scale (NRS), which ranges from 0 (no pain) to 10 (worst possible pain); and the Face Pain Scale (FPS), which uses seven emoticons to describe the pain sensation and is particularly useful in those patients with reduced compliance and/or aphasia [45]. As an adjunct, the Helkimo Clinical Dysfunction Index (HCDI) is a quick and simple test for the specific evaluation of TMD, assessing limitations in mandibular movements, joint function and also pain [46]. For research purposes, the neurophysiological methods, including laser-evoked potentials (LEPs), could be reliable assessment tools for painful syndromes, including TMD. According to de Tommaso [47], LEPs in trigeminal neuralgia and TMD present a smaller amplitude than healthy controls, suggesting trigeminal nociceptive system dysfunctions and neuropathic pain.

Furthermore, clinicians should observe the patient's head and neck alignment with the whole body, hemifacial asymmetry, paying attention to abnormal mandibular movements, decreased joint range of motion and jaw sounds (i.e., clicking, popping, crepitus and grating), which can be related to anterior disc displacement (i.e., the click is produced during mouth opening) or to recapture the displaced disc (i.e., a second click is heard during mouth closing) [48]. In particular, the maximum mouth opening (MMO) is determined by measuring the interincisal distance, which is considered restricted when it is inferior to 35 mm. Restriction in MMO from 25 to 30 mm can be caused by intracapsular problems, such as disc displacement blocking the translation of the condyle. In this condition, the clinician describes the end-feel, which identifies the characteristics of TMJ restriction, as "hard". Otherwise, a restricted mouth opening of 8 to 10 mm associated with a "soft" end-feel is most certainly of muscle origin. During MMO, two types of alteration can occur: deviations and deflections [47]. A deviation refers to any shift of the jaw midline that disappears during continued opening movement. Generally, it is caused by disc displacement with a reduction in one or both TMJs. A deflection consists of any shift of the midline to one side that becomes great during opening and does not return to the midline, and it reflects a restriction in one joint [49,50]. Indeed, lateral jaw movements should be about 12 mm. Moreover, dentists and gnathologists should consider both static and dynamic components of the patient's occlusal scheme (see Table 5).

Table 5. Description of the main occlusal physiological parameters that dentists can measure during physical examination.

Main Occlusal Physiological Parameters	Description
Centric occlusion	Consists of a full occlusal contact between upper and lower teeth in habitual occlusion.
Incisal guidance	Consists of the influence of the contacting surfaces of the mandibular and maxillary anterior teeth on mandibular movements.
Canine guidance	Vertical displacement of the mandible due to gliding contact of the canine teeth, preventing potential damages.
Overjet	Defined as the horizontal overlap of the incisors, which can be augmented in the second occlusion class or reduced in the third class.
Overbite	Defined as the vertical distance between the incisal margins of the upper incisors and the incisal margins of the lower incisors. It can be increased in case of a deep bite or reduced in an open bite.
Occlusal vertical dimension (OVD)	Also known as the vertical dimension of occlusion and indicates the occlusion position of teeth in maximum intercuspation. A common trick is to ask the patient to say the word "Emma", and after completing the word, the clinician has an estimate of OVD.
Resting vertical dimension (RVD)	Refers to a resting position of the mandibula. It happens when the maxillary and mandibular arches are not in contact with each other.
Freeway space	Defined as the neutral position attained by the mandibula as it is involuntarily suspended by the reciprocal coordination of masticatory muscles, with the maxillary and mandibular teeth separated.

A static occlusal examination includes detecting teeth rotation, spacing, overjet and overbite (see Table 4) (including open-bites and cross-bites) that can reveal occlusal instability due to the presence of recurrently fracturing teeth and changes in tooth shape or position associated with indentations on lateral borders of the tongue and buccal mucosa related to bruxism tendency. In addition, dentists usually measure resting vertical dimension (RVD) and occlusal vertical dimension (OVD) through the Willis gauge, which is a tool that registers, in millimeters, the distance between the maxilla and mandibula. On the other hand, a dynamic occlusion examination refers to the study of teeth contact during mandibular movements, assessing the centric occlusion and intercuspal contacts marked up using articulating paper or a photographic record [51]. It should not be underestimated that physiological occlusion in adults can deviate in one or more occlusal parameters (Table 2) from the theoretically ideal one. Since this "well-adapted" occlusion is also aesthetically pleasing to the patient and has no pathological manifestations, it does not require any medical or orthodontic intervention. In fact, dentists should respect the biological variation in form and appearance of occlusion coherently with its function [52].

Actually, physical examination also includes palpation, following the direction of muscle fibers causing pain that can radiate into neighbor areas (periauricular, occiput, neck, shoulders) [53]. The palpation should address masticatory muscles (i.e., temporalis, superficial and deep masseter) and the surrounding neck and shoulder muscles that can highlight the location of pain and myogenous TMD. Notably, the temporalis muscle is divided into three portions (anterior, medial and posterior) that should be evaluated individually, as well as the digastric muscle during the opening movement, sub-occipital and sternocleidomastoid. Since lateral and medial pterygoids are not directly touchable, clinicians should therefore examine them using the resistance of hands during contractions. Interestingly, it has been hypothesized that medial pterygoid muscles could influence the opening pressure of the auditory tube, causing the "ear fullness" symptom in those patients with ear-related TMD. In detail, the dentist or therapist (both physiotherapist and osteopath) should bilaterally palpate masticatory muscles, placing one finger extra-orally and another one intra-orally, to detect hypertrophy, tenderness or pain, especially in muscle insertions. Moreover, postural evaluation should consider the upper cervical vertebral spine (C1, C2 and C3) and the cranial morphology of TMD patients since cervical dysfunctions could play a pivotal role in the development and maintenance of SD and TMD symptoms [54]. In fact, the TMJ degenerative process induces a backward-positioned jaw, which reduces pharyngeal airway capacity, altering the cervical posture in a compensatory forward head position for the decreased airway volume in the upright position [55]. Finally, clinicians should not overlook the psychological and stress status of the patients, since it can be involved in the etiology of some TMD, including bruxism [56]. When medical history and physical examination are equivocal, imaging instruments such as radiographic examinations (i.e., panoramic, planography and transcranial radiography), Computed Tomography (CT) and Magnetic Resonance Imaging (MRI) can be valid tools in the diagnostic path. TMJ radiographs are useful to collect information about morphological and anatomical characteristics between the condyle, articular tubercle and fossa. In detail, panoramic radiography is used to reveal osteophytes, fractures or other bone alterations, whereas planography is more accurate than panoramic radiography in spotting details in the styloid and mastoid process and the zygomatic arch. In the sagittal and coronal planes, the planography can also document the position of the condyle in relationship to the fossa during the MMO. Transcranial radiography provides a detailed evaluation imaging of the condyle, fossa and articular tubercle, with a large overlap in skull bones [57]. Notably, the most performed variation of CT in dentistry is the cone-beam (CBCT), which is useful to view skeletal and dental tissues involved in degenerative joint processes (osteoarthritis) using a low dose of radiation. MRI can instead confirm any disc-related TMD due to its ability to detect early abnormalities in the location and morphology of TMJ. Additionally, ultrasonography is less expensive than MRI and allows the diagnosis of an internal TMJ derangement [58,59]. However, these instruments are typically reserved for patients with persistent symptoms and for those in which conservative therapy has been ineffective.

6. Cranial–Temporomandibular and Stomatognathic Rehabilitation Approach

Multidisciplinary management with a focus on conservative and complementary therapies is currently recommended for patients who present TMD or orofacial pain. However, evidence about cranial–temporomandibular and stomatognathic rehabilitation (CTS-R) in patients affected by neurological disorders is still lacking (see Table 2).

Conservative and rehabilitative management should aim to decrease orofacial pain and muscle contractures/spasms, improving TMJ function, despite the variety of TMD and SD types that clinicians could find in the population of neurological patients. Notably, Zapata-Soria et al. [60] identified some CTS-R interventions in post-stroke patients, including therapeutic jaw exercises. It seems that both jaw opening and head lift exercises can improve digastric and mylohyoid muscle thickness as well as hyoid bone movements. In fact, the digastric muscle assists the depression and retrusion of the mandible during the following breathing, swallowing and chewing activity [26]. According to Oh et al. [27], the administration of postural alignment exercises can be a promising approach to restore neck mobility and TMJ opening function, especially in post-stroke patients. It is not surprising that a postural re-education approach can be effective in TMJ pain relief because of the strictly biomechanical relationship among stomatognathic skeletal elements, the cervical spine and the shoulder girdle [26]. In this context, postural exercises, such as head posture adjustments and the correction of the mandibular position and tongue [61], can be easily adapted and administered to a variety of neurological diseases.

Indeed, specific coordination exercises, including open-close or lateral mandibular movements [62], can be more useful in SCA and MS patients with cerebellum impairments since these exercises are effective to promote balanced and synchronized muscle activity, reducing muscle pain. Moreover, muscle strengthening exercises contribute to increasing the range of motion of the mandibula by the administration of isotonic jaw opening exercises with resistance, which inhibits jaw-closing muscles (i.e., masseter and temporalis), improving TMJ opening range and pain relief [63]. In this vein, it has been [64] suggested that exercise therapy, in addition to manual treatments, postural exercises and jaw mobilization, can be the most effective conservative and complementary management for orofacial pain and TMJ mobility. In particular, TMJ can be manipulated through myofascial release (MFR), in which the operator palpates muscles and soft tissues, producing a compression in tenderness points. Balanced ligamentous tension (BLT) comprises a series of techniques that provides both compression and passive approaches to place a joint in "balance" when moved in different planes. Among the manual treatments, cranial–sacral therapy (CST) consists of hands-on gentle manipulation of the skull and sacrum, which are bidirectionally linked through dural attachments [65]. Using this light pressure, the osteopath should release myofascial restrictions, identified through palpation, and restore mobility and reduce pain for patients [66]. Generally, the five-finger bilateral grip or "Sutherland's technique" is a common means for the evaluation and treatment of cranial dysfunctions. The patient is supine and relaxed, while the osteopath is sitting behind him/her, with his/her hands bilaterally placed on the head of the patient. In detail, the fingers are placed in the following manner: (i) the index finger on the pterion, (ii) the middle finger in front of the ear's tragus, (iii) the ring finger on the mastoid of the temporal bone, (iv) the little finger in the inferior-posterior part of the occiput, (v) while the thumb is placed gently on the cranial vault [67] (as shown in Figure 4).

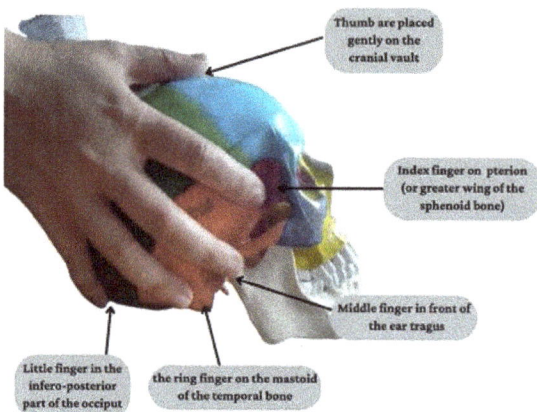

Figure 4. Illustration of how "Sutherland technique" is practically performed on a skeletal model.

Actually, the use of the occlusal splint to treat TMD is common in dentistry. In fact, these devices promote the correction of vertical dimension, TMJ realignment and repositioning, also providing cognitive awareness [68]. The mechanism of action consists of reducing electromyographic jaw muscle activity in the short term; however, long-term outcomes are still unclear due to the adaptive mechanisms of muscles [69].

Interestingly, Umay et al. [28] performed a combined protocol in post-stroke patients using intra-oral cold stimulation, strengthening oral exercises and intermittent galvanic stimulation to the masseter muscles for thirty minutes a day. The administration of functional electric stimulation prevented muscle atrophy, promoting compensatory mechanisms and coordination.

Another conservative and complementary approach that needs to be mentioned is the psychological management of pain, which should be included in the multimodal rehabilitation approach of TMD patients [70]. In fact, neurological disorders can cause psychological sequelae (i.e., anxiety and depression symptoms), which can exacerbate the TMD's or SD's symptoms. Breathing and relaxing exercises in which therapists guide the diaphragmatic inspiration, through hands on the rectus abdominis, are useful to promote muscle release and psychological wellness [71,72]. This is why counseling and behavioral approaches and relaxation techniques to manage pain could be adjunctive promising treatments, personalizing rehabilitation in a more centered-care way.

7. Discussion

As far as we know, this is one of the few reviews [11,60] that deal with SD and TMD and their rehabilitative approach in patients affected by neurological disorders. In fact, this issue is often overlooked by clinicians and therapists when it would need more attention, especially for the possible improvements in the most important functions of life: speech, eating and breathing, besides the postural alignment. It is noteworthy that evidence highlighted the correlation and the relationship between the neurological disorder and the onset of SD or TMD [14,22,36–38], while the literature about CTS-R intervention remains poor or limited to physical exercises for the post-stroke population [25–27,60] (see Table 2). Indeed, we have focused not only on the pathophysiological mechanism but also on the diagnostic work-up and treatment, pointing out the importance of a multidisciplinary and personalized approach.

Understanding the loading of SS and the existence of myofascial tension, articular dysfunctions and parafunctions such as bruxism are fundamental in delivering the most tailored functional evaluation and training in these patients. In fact, in neurological patients, it is not easy to address the right diagnosis due to patient compliance and the common overlapping between neurological disorders and SD or TMD. Physical examination should be meticulously performed, investigating patterns of occlusal contacts, mandibular opening movement and muscle tenderness. In this way, clinicians can collect indispensable information for planning primary and tempestive treatment.

Additionally, Botox injection and dry needling have been suggested to manage orofacial pain in myogenous TMD, especially when other strategies have already failed [73]. In particular, dry needling is less invasive than Botox injection, and it seems to be superior in reducing pain and improving the jaw range of motion, as confirmed by Kütük et al. [74]. Other kinds of medications, including corticosteroids, benzodiazepines and antidepressants, can also be used in TMD patients [75]. However, neurological patients have already taken many of these drugs for their pathology, and when ineffective, non-pharmacological approaches such as therapeutic exercises, manual techniques and physical therapy, as well as occlusal splints, should be considered as the primary intervention in these patients. Given that most medications induce muscle relaxation to reduce spasms and contractures, some authors [76] proposed the administration of relaxation exercises of masticatory muscles to improve TMD range of motion and reduce pain. In this context, static relaxation exercises can be more effective than standard active exercises.

Today, clinicians and therapists should consider the whole person as a unique and global system in which muscular and fascial components can influence body posture, SS and its functions (chewing, speaking and swallowing), which are almost impaired in neurological patients. Some authors stated [77,78] that the SS should be considered a part of the proprioceptive system, among balance, sight and postural control of the whole body. This could explain why manual treatments (such as OMT), physical exercise and postural re-education can be more effective than other pharmacological or non-conservative treatments. In fact, these treatments have been shown to act on the proprioceptive system and then sensorimotor integration, including the brainstem, subcortical and cortical centers, cervical region, proprioception and body posture. Given that, posture and gait training should be used with CTS-R since cervical, TMJ structures and lower muscles could influence each other through the fascial system; thus, it forms a single body system [79,80].

Consequentially, an altered pattern of movements in TMJ may cause an overload in masticatory muscles (i.e., posterior temporalis, ipsilateral external pterygoid and contralateral temporal anterior pterygoid, contralateral internal pterygoid). These alterations have repercussions on the upper trapezius and contralateral sternocleidomastoid, which determine flexion and side deviation of the head, also involving the ipsilateral shoulder (levator scapulae, omohyoid) and spine muscles (such as gran dorsi and iliopsoas) that have insertions on the lumbar tract and ileum. In this way, the cranial–mandibular structures could influence lower body extremity, not only in static posture but also during gait [11,81]. However, the relationship between human posture and TMD remains one of the unsolved research questions. Future studies should consider the chance for conservative and complementary approaches to induce appropriate neuroplastic changes, integrating them with neurologic exams, monitoring of body balance and coordination control systems.

Furthermore, a multidisciplinary approach is strongly recommended, as patients can benefit from complementary therapies, including OMT, posture re-education, physical exercises and occlusal splint therapy, for SD and TMD. Finally, a co-work among gnathologists (or even dentists), physiotherapists, osteopaths and neurologists is extremely important in achieving better outcomes and avoiding unnecessary treatments.

Since a standardized protocol for the evaluation and treatment of SD/TMD in neurological disorders is still lacking, herein, we have reported some evidence-based clinical advice about the administration of multidisciplinary conservative approaches for neurological patients who have SD/TMD:

- Parafunctional activities, such as bruxism and day clenching, have been found in PD and MS patients [11,19,22,23], causing muscle pain and harmful effects on tooth enamel. Currently, there are no treatment methods to make these alterations stop. Occlusal splint therapy can reduce bruxism and clenching symptoms, acting on a

negative feedback mechanism that greatly decreases muscle activity, maintaining a normal activation threshold for the muscle protective reflex. In addition, MT and MFR could be useful to induce masseter, temporalis and neck muscle relaxation that are associated with these symptoms [65];
- Reduction in TMJ movements due to painful muscle contractions is a common TMD feature in neurological conditions, especially in OMD, PD and SCA [21,24,29,35,37,38]. However, evidence-based treatments have been documented only for OMD subjects, suggesting the use of Botox injections in specific head and neck muscles, such as platysma, lateral pterygoid and temporalis, to reduce muscle spasms [38]. Coordination exercises of TMJ through opening and closing the mouth, using a mirror or fingers bilaterally, to promote symmetrical movements may also be of help [62,82,83]. Additionally, MT and/or OMT could induce muscle release and restore pain thanks to the discharge of endogenous opioids due to therapeutic touch [9,65];
- Muscle weakness and reduced TMJ functions were found in post-stroke survivors as a result of the acute onset of the brain damage [25–28]. In this clinical condition, authors [26,27,60] suggested the administration of specific isometric and isotonic exercises to improve jaw muscle strength and postural programs [61,84], including exercises to increase TMJ and neck mobility. To restore oral muscle strength, some evidence supported the administration of specific exercises for labial, intrinsic tongue and masticatory muscles, which can be helpful in managing dysphagic symptoms [28].

8. Conclusions

To summarize, although SD and TMD in neurological patients do not seem to be uncommon, a standard diagnostic or rehabilitation approach is still lacking. Clinicians and therapists should consider the role of SS and TMJ structures during functional training, given their fundamental role in swallowing, chewing, breathing and speaking. To better manage SD/TMD, neurological patients should be seen as a single unit, in which the stomatognathic complex works together with the cervical spine and lower extremity in maintaining body posture and spinal alignment. Future studies are needed to fill this existing gap in the individuation and treatment of SD and/or TMD in the neurorehabilitation field.

Author Contributions: Conceptualization, A.M. and M.B.; methodology, A.M. and M.B.; software, M.B.; validation, all authors; formal analysis, M.B.; investigation, A.M. and M.B.; resources, R.S.C.; data curation, M.B.; writing—original draft preparation, A.M. and M.B.; writing—review and editing, R.S.C.; visualization, all authors; supervision, R.S.C.; project administration, A.M. and R.S.C.; funding acquisition, R.S.C. All authors have read and agreed to the published version of the manuscript.

Funding: This study was supported by Current Research Funds 2023, Ministry of Health, Italy.

Institutional Review Board Statement: Not applicable.

Informed Consent Statement: Not applicable.

Data Availability Statement: Not applicable.

Acknowledgments: The authors wish to thank Elena Barbera for her contribution to this work and Agata Grosso for English editing.

Conflicts of Interest: The authors declare no conflict of interest.

Abbreviations

SS	Stomatognathic system
TMJ	Temporomandibular joint
TMD	Temporomandibular dysfunction
SD	Stomatognathic disease
PT	Physiotherapy
MT	Manual therapy
OMT	Osteopathic manipulative treatment
CPG	Central pattern generator
MS	Multiple sclerosis
SCA	Spinocerebellar ataxia
PD	Parkinson's disease
OMD	Oromandibular dystonia
RoB	Revised Cochrane risk of bias
NOS	Newcastle–Ottawa Scale
MPQ	McGill Pain Questionnaire
SF-MPQ	Short form McGill Pain Questionnaire
PPI	Present pain intensity
VAS	Visual analogical scale
VRS	Verbal rating scale
NRS	Numerical rating scale
FPS	Faces pain scale
HCDI	Helkimo Clinical Dysfunction Index
OVD	Occlusal vertical dimension
RVD	Resting vertical dimension
MMO	Maximum mouth opening
LEP	Laser-evoked potential
CT	Computed tomography
MRI	Magnetic Resonance Imaging
CBCT	Cone-beam computed tomography
CTS-R	Cranial–temporomandibular and stomatognathic rehabilitation
MFR	Myofascial release
CST	Cranial–sacral therapy
BLT	Balanced ligamentous tension

References

1. Zieliński, G.; Filipiak, Z.; Ginszt, M.; Matysik-Woźniak, A.; Rejdak, R.; Gawda, P. The Organ of Vision and the Stomatognathic System—Review of Association Studies and Evidence-Based Discussion. *Brain Sci.* **2022**, *12*, 14. [CrossRef] [PubMed]
2. Dai, R.; Lam, O.L.; Lo, E.C.; Li, L.S.; Wen, Y.; McGrath, C. Orofacial functional impairments among patients following stroke: A systematic review. *Oral. Dis.* **2015**, *21*, 836–849. [CrossRef] [PubMed]
3. Wieckiewicz, M.; Boening, K.; Wiland, P.; Shiau, Y.-Y.; Paradowska-Stolarz, A. Reported concepts for the treatment modalities and pain management of temporomandibular disorders. *J. Headache Pain* **2015**, *16*, 106. [CrossRef] [PubMed]
4. McNeely, M.; Armijo Olivo, S.; Magee, D. A systematic review of physical therapy intervention for temporomandibular dis-orders. *Phys. Ther.* **2006**, *86*, 710–720. [CrossRef] [PubMed]
5. Bialosky, J.E.; Bishop, M.D.; Price, D.D.; Robinson, M.E.; George, S.Z. The mechanisms of manual therapy in the treatment of musculoskeletal pain: A comprehensive model. *Man Ther.* **2009**, *14*, 531–538. [CrossRef]
6. Armijo-Olivo, S.; Pitance, L.; Singh, V.; Neto, F.; Thie, N.; Michelotti, A. Effectiveness of Manual Therapy and Therapeutic Exercise for Temporomandibular Disorders: Systematic Review and Meta-Analysis. *Phys. Ther.* **2016**, *96*, 9–25. [CrossRef]
7. Easterbrook, S.; Keys, J.; Talsma, J.; Pierce-Talsma, S. Osteopathic Manipulative Treatment for Temporomandibular Disorders. *J. Am. Osteopat. Assoc.* **2019**, *119*, e29–e30. [CrossRef]
8. Gesslbauer, C.; Vavti, N.; Keilani, M.; Mickel, M.; Crevenna, R. Effectiveness of osteopathic manipulative treatment versus osteopathy in the cranial field in temporomandibular disorders—A pilot study. *Disabil. Rehabil.* **2018**, *40*, 631–636. [CrossRef]
9. McParlin, Z.; Cerritelli, F.; Friston, K.J.; Esteves, J.E. Therapeutic Alliance as Active Inference: The Role of Therapeutic Touch and Synchrony. *Front. Psychol.* **2022**, *13*, 783694. [CrossRef]
10. Yin, Y.; He, S.; He, N.; Zhang, W.; Luo, L.; Chen, L.; Liu, T.; Tian, M.; Xu, J.; Chen, S.; et al. Brain alterations in sensorimotor and emotional regions associated with temporomandibular disorders. *Oral. Dis.* **2022**. [CrossRef]

11. Minervini, G.; Franco, R.; Marrapodi, M.M.; Crimi, S.; Badnjević, A.; Cervino, G.; Bianchi, A.; Cicciù, M. Correlation between Temporomandibular Disorders (TMD) and Posture Evaluated trough the Diagnostic Criteria for Temporomandibular Disorders (DC/TMD): A Systematic Review with Meta-Analysis. *J. Clin. Med.* **2023**, *12*, 2652. [CrossRef] [PubMed]
12. An, J.-S.; Jeon, D.-M.; Jung, W.-S.; Yang, I.-H.; Lim, W.H.; Ahn, S.-J. Influence of temporomandibular joint disc displacement on craniocervical posture and hyoid bone position. *Am. J. Orthod. Dentofac. Orthop.* **2015**, *147*, 72–79. [CrossRef] [PubMed]
13. Paço, M.; Duarte, J.; Pinho, T. Orthodontic Treatment and Craniocervical Posture in Patients with Temporomandibular Disor-ders: An Observational Study. *Int. J. Environ. Res. Public. Health* **2021**, *18*, 3295. [CrossRef] [PubMed]
14. Garstka, A.A.; Brzózka, M.; Bitenc-Jasiejko, A.; Ardan, R.; Gronwald, H.; Skomro, P.; Lietz-Kijak, D. Cause-Effect Relationships between Painful TMD and Postural and Functional Changes in the Musculoskeletal System: A Preliminary Report. *Pain Res. Manag.* **2022**, *2022*, 1429932. [CrossRef] [PubMed]
15. Brown, D. A Review of the PubMed PICO Tool: Using Evidence-Based Practice in Health Education. *Health Promot. Pract.* **2019**, *21*, 496–498. [CrossRef] [PubMed]
16. Więckowska, B.; Kubiak, K.B.; Jóźwiak, P.; Moryson, W.; Stawińska-Witoszyńska, B. Cohen's Kappa Coefficient as a Measure to Assess Classification Improvement following the Addition of a New Marker to a Regression Model. *Int. J. Environ. Res. Public. Health* **2022**, *19*, 10213. [CrossRef]
17. Page, M.J.; McKenzie, J.E.; Bossuyt, P.M.; Boutron, I.; Hoffmann, T.C.; Mulrow, C.D.; Shamseer, L.; Tetzlaff, J.M.; Akl, E.A.; Brennan, S.E. The PRISMA 2020 statement: An updated guideline for reporting systematic reviews. *BMJ* **2021**, *372*, n71. [CrossRef] [PubMed]
18. Sterne, J.A.C.; Savović, J.; Page, M.J.; Elbers, R.G.; Blencowe, N.S.; Boutron, I.; Cates, C.J.; Cheng, H.Y.; Corbett, M.S.; Eldridge, S.M.; et al. RoB 2: A revised tool for assessing risk of bias in randomised trials. *BMJ* **2019**, *366*, l4898. [CrossRef]
19. Costa, C.; Santiago, H.; Pereira, S.; Castro, A.R.; Soares, S.C. Oral Health Status and Multiple Sclerosis: Classic and Non-Classic Manifestations—Case Report. *Diseases* **2022**, *10*, 62. [CrossRef]
20. Williams, D.E.; Lynch, J.E.; Doshi, V.; Singh, G.D.; Hargens, A.R. Bruxism and Temporal Bone Hypermobility in Patients with Multiple Sclerosis. *Cranio®* **2011**, *29*, 178–186. [CrossRef]
21. Ferreira, B.; Palinkas, M.; Gonçalves, L.; Da Silva, G.; Arnoni, V.; Regalo, I.H.; Vasconcelos, P.; Júnior, W.; Hallak, J.; Regalo, S.C.H.; et al. Spinocerebellar ataxia: Functional analysis of the stomatognathic system. *Med. Oral Patol. Oral Cir. Bucal* **2019**, *24*, e165–e171. [CrossRef]
22. Choi, H.-G.; Yoon, J.-H.; Chung, T.-H.; Min, C.; Yoo, D.-M.; Wee, J.-H.; Kang, S.-Y.; Choi, Y.; Hong, S.-J.; Byun, S.-H. Association between Temporomandibular Joint Disorder and Parkinson's Disease. *Brain Sci.* **2021**, *11*, 747. [CrossRef] [PubMed]
23. Beers, E.; Van Grootheest, A.C. Bruxisme als bijwerking van serotonineheropnameremmers. *Ned. Tijdschr. Tandheelkd.* **2007**, *114*, 388–390. [PubMed]
24. Handa, S.; Shaefer, J.R.; Keith, D.A. Oromandibular dystonia and temporomandibular disorders. *J. Am. Dent. Assoc.* **2022**, *153*, 899–906. [CrossRef] [PubMed]
25. Ramos, M.A.; Moura, B.G.; Araujo, C.C.; Del Antonio, T.T.; Da Silva, J.K.M. Temporomandibular dysfunction in patients with a history of stroke. *Man. Ther. Posturol. Rehabil. J.* **2020**, *17*, 1–5. [CrossRef]
26. Choi, J.B.; Jung, Y.J.; Park, J. Comparison of 2 types of therapeutic exercise: Jaw opening exercise and head lift exercise for dysphagic stroke: A pilot study. *Medicine* **2020**, *99*, e22136. [CrossRef]
27. Oh, D.-W.; Kang, T.-W.; Kim, S.-J. Effect of Stomatognathic Alignment Exercise on Temporomandibular Joint Function and Swallowing Function of Stroke Patients with Limited Mouth Opening. *J. Phys. Ther. Sci.* **2013**, *25*, 1325–1329. [CrossRef]
28. Umay, E.K.; Yilmaz, V.; Gundogdu, I.; Ozturk, E.; Gurcay, E.; Karaahmet, O.; Saylam, G.; Ceylan, T.; Cakci, A. What happens to swallowing muscles after stroke? A prospective randomized controlled electrophysiological study. *Neurol. India* **2019**, *67*, 1459–1466. [CrossRef]
29. Verhoeff, M.C.; Lobbezoo, F.; Wetselaar, P.; Aarab, G.; Koutris, M. Parkinson's disease, temporomandibular disorders and bruxism: A pilot study. *J. Oral. Rehabil.* **2018**, *45*, 854–863. [CrossRef]
30. Minervini, G.; Mariani, P.; Fiorillo, L.; Cervino, G.; Cicciù, M.; Laino, L. Prevalence of temporomandibular disorders in people with multiple sclerosis: A systematic review and meta-analysis. *Cranio®* **2022**, 1–9. [CrossRef]
31. Manchery, N.; Henry, J.D.; Nangle, M.R. A systematic review of oral health in people with multiple sclerosis. *Community Dent. Oral. Epidemiol.* **2020**, *48*, 89–100. [CrossRef] [PubMed]
32. Jung, W.; Lee, K.-E.; Suh, B.-J. Influence of psychological factors on the prognosis of temporomandibular disorders pain. *J. Dent. Sci.* **2021**, *16*, 349–355. [CrossRef] [PubMed]
33. Carvalho, L.; Matta, A.; Nascimento, O. Temporomandibular disorders (TMD) and multiple sclerosis (MS)(P1. 120). *Cranio* **2015**, *84*, 120.
34. Liang, L.; Chen, T.; Wu, Y. The electrophysiology of spinocerebellar ataxias. *Neurophysiol. Clin.* **2016**, *46*, 27–34. [CrossRef]
35. Velázquez-Pérez, L.C.; Rodríguez-Labrada, R.; Fernandez-Ruiz, J. Spinocerebellar Ataxia Type 2: Clinicogenetic Aspects, Mechanistic Insights, and Management Approaches. *Front. Neurol.* **2017**, *8*, 472. [CrossRef] [PubMed]
36. Verhoeff, M.C.; Koutris, M.; Berendse, H.W.; van Dijk, K.D.; Lobbezoo, F. Parkinson's disease, temporomandibular disorder pain and bruxism and its clinical consequences: A protocol of a single-centre observational outpatient study. *BMJ Open.* **2022**, *12*, e052329. [CrossRef]

37. Albanese, A.; Bhatia, K.; Bressman, S.B.; DeLong, M.R.; Fahn, S.; Fung, V.S.; Hallett, M.; Jankovic, J.; Jinnah, H.A.; Klein, C.; et al. Phenomenology and classification of dystonia: A consensus update. *Mov. Disord.* **2013**, *28*, 863–873. [CrossRef]
38. Yoshida, K. Botulinum Toxin Therapy for Oromandibular Dystonia and Other Movement Disorders in the Stomatognathic System. *Toxins* **2022**, *14*, 282. [CrossRef]
39. Yoshida, K. Clinical Characteristics of Functional Movement Disorders in the Stomatognathic System. *Front. Neurol.* **2020**, *11*, 123. [CrossRef]
40. Schimmel, M.; Leemann, B.; Christou, P.; Kiliaridis, S.; Herrmann, F.R.; Müller, F. Quantitative assessment of facial muscle impairment in patients with hemispheric stroke. *J. Oral. Rehabil.* **2011**, *38*, 800–809. [CrossRef]
41. Lau, K.T.; Cheung, K.Y.; Chan, K.B.; Chan, M.H.; Lo, K.Y.; Chiu, T.T.W. Relationships between sagittal postures of thoracic and cervical spine, presence of neck pain, neck pain severity and disability. *Man. Ther.* **2010**, *15*, 457–462. [CrossRef] [PubMed]
42. Corrêa, E.C.; Bérzin, F. Temporomandibular disorder and dysfunctional breathing. *Braz. J. Oral. Sci.* **2004**, *3*, 498–502.
43. Saran, S.; Saccomanno, S.; Petricca, M.T.; Carganico, A.; Bocchieri, S.; Mastrapasqua, R.F.; Caramaschi, E.; Levrini, L. Physiotherapists and Osteopaths' Attitudes: Training in Management of Temporomandibular Disorders. *Dent. J.* **2022**, *10*, 210. [CrossRef] [PubMed]
44. Bender, S.D. Assessment of the Orofacial Pain Patient. *Dent. Clin.* **2018**, *62*, 525–532. [CrossRef] [PubMed]
45. Sirintawat, N.; Sawang, K.; Chaiyasamut, T.; Wongsirichat, N. Pain measurement in oral and maxillofacial surgery. *J. Dent. Anesth. Pain Med.* **2017**, *17*, 253–263. [CrossRef]
46. Alonso-Royo, R.; Sánchez-Torrelo, C.M.; Ibáñez-Vera, A.J.; Zagalaz-Anula, N.; Castellote-Caballero, Y.; Obrero-Gaitán, E.; Rodríguez-Almagro, D.; Lomas-Vega, R. Validity and Reliability of the Helkimo Clinical Dysfunction Index for the Diagnosis of Temporomandibular Disorders. *Diagnostics* **2021**, *11*, 472. [CrossRef]
47. De Tommaso, M. Laser-evoked potentials in primary headaches and cranial neuralgias. *Expert. Rev. Neurother.* **2008**, *8*, 1339–1345. [CrossRef]
48. Małgorzata, P.; Małgorzata, K.-M.; Karolina, C.; Gala, A. Diagnostic of Temporomandibular Disorders and Other Facial Pain Conditions—Narrative Review and Personal Experience. *Medicina* **2020**, *56*, 472. [CrossRef]
49. Krasińska-Mazur, M.; Homel, P.; Gala, A.; Stradomska, J.; Pihut, M. Differential diagnosis of temporomandibular disorders—A review of the literature. *Folia Med. Cracov.* **2022**, *62*, 121–137. [CrossRef]
50. Okeson, J.P.; de Leeuw, R. Differential Diagnosis of Temporomandibular Disorders and Other Orofacial Pain Disorders. *Dent. Clin.* **2011**, *55*, 105–120. [CrossRef]
51. Mehta, S.B.; Rizzo, D.; Paulose, B.; Botbol, A.; Vijay, S.; Arjuna, A.; Banerji, S. An evaluation of dental practitioner habits with occlusal assessment and the clinical application of practical techniques in occlusion, amongst a cohort of participants based in the UK, South Africa, Malta, and Malaysia. *J. Oral. Rehabil.* **2022**, *49*, 944–953. [CrossRef] [PubMed]
52. de Kanter, R.J.A.M.; Battistuzzi, P.G.F.C.M.; Truin, G.-J. Temporomandibular Disorders: "Occlusion" Matters! *Pain Res. Manag.* **2018**, *2018*, 8746858. [CrossRef] [PubMed]
53. De Rossi, S.S.; Stern, I.; Sollecito, T.P. Disorders of the Masticatory Muscles. *Dent. Clin.* **2013**, *57*, 449–464. [CrossRef] [PubMed]
54. Kang, J.-H. Associations Among Temporomandibular Joint Osteoarthritis, Airway Dimensions, and Head and Neck Posture. *J. Oral. Maxillofac. Surg.* **2020**, *78*, 2183.e1–2183.e12. [CrossRef]
55. Opris, H.; Baciut, M.; Bran, S.; Onisor, F.; Almasan, O.; Manea, A.; Tamas, T.; Stoia, S.; Gabriel, A.; Baciut, G.; et al. Lateral Cephalometric Analytical Uses for Temporomandibular Joint Disorders: The Importance of Cervical Posture and Hyoid Position. *Int. J. Environ. Res. Public. Health* **2022**, *19*, 11077. [CrossRef]
56. Manfredini, D.; Lobbezoo, F. Role of psychosocial factors in the etiology of bruxism. *J. Orofac. Pain* **2009**, *23*, 153–166.
57. Ferreira, L.A.; Grossmann, E.; Januzzi, E.; de Paula, M.V.Q.; Carvalho, A.C.P. Diagnosis of temporomandibular joint disorders: Indication of imaging exams. *Braz. J. Otorhinolaryngol.* **2016**, *82*, 341–352. [CrossRef]
58. Gauer, R.L.; Semidey, M.J. Diagnosis and treatment of temporomandibular disorders. *Am. Fam. Physician* **2015**, *91*, 378–386.
59. Chan, N.H.Y.; Ip, C.K.; Li, D.T.S.; Leung, Y.Y. Diagnosis and Treatment of Myogenous Temporomandibular Disorders: A Clinical Update. *Diagnostics* **2022**, *12*, 2914. [CrossRef]
60. Zapata-Soria, M.; Cabrera-Martos, I.; López-López, L.; Ortiz-Rubio, A.; Granados-Santiago, M.; Ríos-Asín, I.; Valenza, M.C. Clinical Characteristics and Rehabilitation Strategies for the Stomatognathic System Disturbances in Patients with Stroke: A Systematic Review. *Int. J. Environ. Res. Public. Health* **2023**, *20*, 657. [CrossRef]
61. Carini, F.; Mazzola, M.; Fici, C.; Palmeri, S.; Messina, M.; Damiani, P.; Tomasello, G. Posture and posturology, anatomical and physiological profiles: Overview and current state of art. *Acta Bio Med. Atenei Parm.* **2017**, *88*, 11–16. [CrossRef]
62. Haketa, T.; Kino, K.; Sugisaki, M.; Takaoka, M.; Ohta, T. Randomized Clinical Trial of Treatment for TMJ Disc Displacement. *J. Dent. Res.* **2010**, *89*, 1259–1263. [CrossRef] [PubMed]
63. Tuncer, A.B.; Ergun, N.; Tuncer, A.H.; Karahan, S. Effectiveness of manual therapy and home physical therapy in patients with temporomandibular disorders: A randomized controlled trial. *J. Bodyw. Move Ther.* **2013**, *17*, 302–308. [CrossRef] [PubMed]
64. Shimada, A.; Ishigaki, S.; Matsuka, Y.; Komiyama, O.; Torisu, T.; Oono, Y.; Sato, H.; Naganawa, T.; Mine, A.; Yamazaki, Y.; et al. Effects of exercise therapy on painful temporomandibular disorders. *J. Oral. Rehabil.* **2019**, *46*, 475–481. [CrossRef]
65. Roberts, A.; Harris, K.; Outen, B.; Bukvic, A.; Smith, B.; Schultz, A.; Bergman, S.; Mondal, D. Osteopathic Manipulative Medicine: A Brief Review of the Hands-On Treatment Approaches and Their Therapeutic Uses. *Medicines* **2022**, *9*, 33. [CrossRef]

66. Brantingham, J.W.; Cassa, T.K.; Bonnefin, D.; Pribicevic, M.; Robb, A.; Pollard, H.; Tong, V.; Korporaal, C. Manipulative and Multimodal Therapy for Upper Extremity and Temporomandibular Disorders: A Systematic Review. *J. Manip. Physiol. Ther.* **2013**, *36*, 143–201. [CrossRef]
67. Bordoni, B.; Zanier, E. Sutherland's legacy in the new millennium: The osteopathic cranial model and modern osteopathy. *Adv. Mind Body Med.* **2015**, *29*, 15–21.
68. Zhang, L.; Xu, L.; Wu, D.; Yu, C.; Fan, S.; Cai, B. Effectiveness of exercise therapy versus occlusal splint therapy for the treatment of painful temporomandibular disorders: A systematic review and meta-analysis. *Ann. Palliat. Med.* **2021**, *10*, 6122–6132. [CrossRef]
69. de Paula Gomes CA, F.; El Hage, Y.; Amaral, A.P.; Politti, F.; Biasotto-Gonzalez, D.A. Effects of massage therapy and occlusal splint therapy on electromyographic activity and the intensity of signs and symptoms in individuals with temporomandibular disorder and sleep bruxism: A randomized clinical trial. *Chiropr. Man. Ther.* **2014**, *22*, 43. [CrossRef]
70. Penlington, C.; Bowes, C.; Taylor, G.; Otemade, A.A.; Waterhouse, P.; Durham, J.; Ohrbach, R. Psychological therapies for temporomandibular disorders (TMDs). *Cochrane Database Syst. Rev.* **2022**, *8*, CD013515. [CrossRef]
71. Urbański, P.; Trybulec, B.; Pihut, M. The Application of Manual Techniques in Masticatory Muscles Relaxation as Adjunctive Therapy in the Treatment of Temporomandibular Joint Disorders. *Int. J. Environ. Res. Public. Health* **2021**, *18*, 12970. [CrossRef] [PubMed]
72. De Melo, L.A.; Medeiros, A.; Campos, M.D.F.T.P.; De Resende, C.M.B.M.; Barbosa, G.A.S.; De Almeida, E.O. Manual Therapy in the Treatment of Myofascial Pain Related to Temporomandibular Disorders: A Systematic Review. *J. Oral. Facial Pain. Headache* **2020**, *34*, 141–148. [CrossRef] [PubMed]
73. Gil-Martinez, A.; Paris-Alemany, A.; López-De-Uralde-Villanueva, I.; La Touche, R. Management of pain in patients with temporomandibular disorder (TMD): Challenges and solutions. *J. Pain Res.* **2018**, *11*, 571–587. [CrossRef] [PubMed]
74. Kütük, S.G.; Özkan, Y.; Kütük, M.; Özdaş, T. Comparison of the Efficacies of Dry Needling and Botox Methods in the Treatment of Myofascial Pain Syndrome Affecting the Temporomandibular Joint. *J. Craniofacial Surg.* **2019**, *30*, 1556–1559. [CrossRef]
75. Ouanounou, A.; Goldberg, M.; Haas, D.A. Pharmacotherapy in Temporomandibular Disorders: A Review. *J. Canadian Dent. Assoc.* **2017**, *83*, h7.
76. Bae, Y.; Park, Y. The Effect of Relaxation Exercises for the Masticator Muscles on Temporomandibular Joint Dysfunction (TMD). *J. Phys. Ther. Sci.* **2013**, *25*, 583–586. [CrossRef]
77. Cuccia, A.M.; Caradonna, C.; Caradonna, D. Manual therapy of the mandibular accessory ligaments for the man-agement of temporomandibular joint disorders. *J. Osteopath. Med.* **2011**, *111*, 102–112.
78. Yin, C.S.; Lee, Y.J. Neurological influences of the temporomandibular joint. *J. Bodyw. Mov. Ther.* **2007**, *11*, 285–294. [CrossRef]
79. Schleip, R.; Klingler, W.; Lehmann-Horn, F. Active fascial contractility: Fascia may be able to contract in a smooth muscle-like manner and thereby influence musculoskeletal dynamics. *Med. Hypotheses* **2005**, *65*, 273–277. [CrossRef]
80. Schleip, R.; Gabbiani, G.; Wilke, J.; Naylor, I.; Hinz, B.; Zorn, A.; Jäger, H.; Breul, R.; Schreiner, S.; Klingler, W. Fascia Is Able to Actively Contract and May Thereby Influence Musculoskeletal Dynamics: A Histochemical and Mechanographic Investigation. *Front. Physiol.* **2019**, *10*, 336. [CrossRef]
81. Stecco, A.; Giordani, F.; Fede, C.; Pirri, C.; De Caro, R.; Stecco, C. From Muscle to the Myofascial Unit: Current Evidence and Future Perspectives. *Int. J. Mol. Sci.* **2023**, *24*, 4527. [CrossRef] [PubMed]
82. Saito, E.T.; Akashi, P.M.H.; Sacco, I.D.C.N. Global Body Posture Evaluation in Patients with Temporomandibular Joint Disorder. *Clinics* **2009**, *64*, 35–39. [CrossRef] [PubMed]
83. Moraes, A.D.R.; Sanches, M.L.; Ribeiro, E.C.; Guimarães, A.S. Therapeutic exercises for the control of temporomandibular disorders. *Dent. Press J. Orthod.* **2013**, *18*, 134–139. [CrossRef] [PubMed]
84. Craane, B.; Dijkstra, P.U.; Stappaerts, K.; De Laat, A. Randomized Controlled Trial on Physical Therapy for TMJ Closed Lock. *J. Dent. Res.* **2012**, *91*, 364–369. [CrossRef] [PubMed]

Disclaimer/Publisher's Note: The statements, opinions and data contained in all publications are solely those of the individual author(s) and contributor(s) and not of MDPI and/or the editor(s). MDPI and/or the editor(s) disclaim responsibility for any injury to people or property resulting from any ideas, methods, instructions or products referred to in the content.

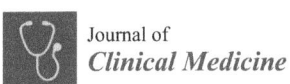

Article

Expression of Interleukin 17A and 17B in Gingival Tissue in Patients with Periodontitis

Małgorzata Mazurek-Mochol [1], Karol Serwin [2], Tobias Bonsmann [1], Małgorzata Kozak [3], Katarzyna Piotrowska [2], Michał Czerewaty [2], Krzysztof Safranow [4] and Andrzej Pawlik [2,*]

1. Department of Periodontology, Pomeranian Medical University, 70-111 Szczecin, Poland; malgorzata.mazurek@poczta.onet.pl (M.M.-M.); tobias.bonsmann1@gmail.com (T.B.)
2. Department of Physiology, Pomeranian Medical University, 70-111 Szczecin, Poland; karol.serwin@pum.edu.pl (K.S.); piot.kata@gmail.com (K.P.); michal.czerewaty@wp.pl (M.C.)
3. Department of Dental Prosthetics, Pomeranian Medical University, 70-111 Szczecin, Poland; gosia-ko@o2.pl
4. Department of Biochemistry and Medical Chemistry, Pomeranian Medical University, 70-111 Szczecin, Poland; chrissaf@mp.pl
* Correspondence: pawand@poczta.onet.pl

Abstract: Periodontitis (PD) is a chronic inflammatory disease that is initiated by oral microorganisms. The pathogens induce the production of cytokines, such as interleukin (IL)-17, which enhances the inflammatory response and progression of the disease. The aim of this study was to examine the expression and localization in gingival tissue of IL-17A and IL-17B in patients with periodontitis. This study included 14 patients with periodontal disease and 14 healthy subjects without periodontal disease as a control group. There were no statistically significant differences in the expression of *IL-17A* mRNA between patients with periodontitis and control subjects. The expression of *IL-17B* mRNA was statistically significantly lower in patients with periodontitis in comparison with healthy subjects ($p < 0.048$). The expression of *IL-17A* correlated significantly with the approximal plaque index. The *IL-17B* expression in gingival tissue correlated with the clinical attachment level. This correlation reached borderline statistical significance ($p = 0.06$). In immunohistochemical analysis, we have shown the highest expression of IL-17 protein in inflamed connective tissue, epithelium, and granulation tissue from gingival biopsy specimens from patients with periodontitis. In biopsy specimens from healthy individuals, no IL-17 was found in the epithelium, while an expression of IL-17 was found in the connective tissue. The results of our study confirm the involvement of IL-17 in the pathogenesis of periodontitis. Our results suggest that an increase in IL-17 protein expression in the gingival tissue of patients with periodontitis occurs at the post-translational stage.

Keywords: IL-17; periodontal disease; inflammation

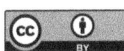

1. Introduction

Periodontitis (PD) is a chronic inflammatory state caused by bacterial infection in the periodontal tissues. Susceptibility to periodontitis may be caused by genetic factors as well as environmental factors, such as smoking and oral hygiene [1]. In periodontal tissue, bacterial infections induce the immune response leading to the production of inflammatory mediators, such as proinflammatory cytokines, and subsequently to tissue destruction [2,3]. The body's immune response to eliminate the bacterial infection can lead to an abnormal immune response causing the destruction of periodontal tissues, including the alveolar process. The cellular immune response plays an important role in the inflammatory process in PD, and Th17 cells and the IL-17 they produce are an important component of this response. IL-17 is a multidirectional cytokine and exists as six isoforms IL-17A-IL-17F. IL-17 is primarily produced by T helper 17 (Th17) cells, which also secrete other cytokines involved in the immune response. Previous studies have shown that interleukin (IL)-17 is a cytokine involved in the pathogenesis of PD and other inflammatory diseases [4–6].

IL-17 plays an important role in immune processes on the surfaces of mucous membranes, providing an important element of protection against bacterial infections. In the inflammatory state, IL-17 can affect various types of cells including endothelial cells, fibroblasts, osteoblasts, and keratinocytes [7–9]. It can stimulate these cells to synthesize numerous pro-inflammatory cytokines that aggravate the inflammatory process [10–12]. IL-17 can also inhibit osteoblasts, leading to the reduction in alveolar bone [13].

Many studies to date have shown an important role for IL-17 in periodontitis [14]. Previous studies have indicated elevated levels of IL-17, particularly in saliva and gingival fluid, in patients with periodontitis. However, these findings vary depending on patient selection criteria, disease severity, or diagnostic criteria. Increased levels of IL-17 were found, especially in patients with an aggressive form of periodontitis. To date, there have been few studies evaluating IL-17 in the gingival tissue of patients with periodontitis. In addition, most of the studies did not evaluate individual IL-17 isoforms, but only total IL-17. The results of previous studies suggest that IL-17A and IL-17B isoforms may play the most important role in the development of periodontitis [7–9].

The aim of this study was to examine the expression and localization in gingival tissue of IL-17A and IL-17B in patients with periodontitis.

2. Materials and Methods
2.1. Patients

This study included 14 patients with periodontitis (5 male, 9 female; mean age 54.2 ± 12.5 years) diagnosed according to the 2017 classification system of periodontal diseases [15], and 14 healthy subjects (5 male, 9 female; mean age 52.8 ± 11.3 years) without periodontal disease who had small oral surgery as a control group.

In patients with periodontitis, the gingival tissue for examination was obtained during flap procedures, gingivaosteoplasty, as well as through a distal wedge or trapezoidal excision at the last molar.

In patients with healthy periodontium, the gingival tissue was obtained during aesthetic lengthening of clinical tooth crowns before prosthetic, conservative, or orthodontic treatment. The procedure was performed under local anesthesia, during which the removed gingival tissue, normally disposed of, was used in our study.

The patients with diagnosed periodontitis were defined if interdental CAL $\geq$ 2 mm was detectable at two or more than two non-adjacent teeth or buccal or oral CAL $\geq$ 3 mm and periodontal pockets > 3 mm were detectable at two or more than two teeth and the observed CAL could not be attributed to non-periodontal causes [16]. We also observed bleed on probing with deep probing pocket depth (PPD $\geq$ 5 mm). A minimum of 15% radiographic bone loss was required. When more than 30% of the teeth were affected, periodontitis was considered as generalized in relation to extent and distribution.

Exclusion criteria were as follows: (1) smoking within the past 5 years; (2) antibiotic therapies during the previous 6 months; (3) pregnancy; (4) chronic apical periodontitis; and (5) any systemic condition that could affect the progression of periodontitis (e.g., immunologic disorders, diabetes, and osteoporosis).

Gingival tissues were collected using a scalpel. The tissue samples were taken from a single tooth in each participant. The excised tissues were washed with PBS and immediately placed in a commercial reagent for RNA isolation for gene expression assays. The study was approved by the local ethics committee (BN-001/93/08) and is in accordance with the Declaration of Helsinki. Patients were informed about the study and their written consent was obtained.

2.2. Periodontal Examination

Periodontal evaluation included probing pocket depth (PPD), clinical attachment level (CAL), the approximal plaque index (API), and bleeding on probing (BoP).

Clinical measurements were taken in homogeneous conditions in a dental clinic. Probing pocket depth (PPD) and clinical attachment level (CAL) were assessed at six sites per tooth, using an UNC 15 periodontal probe calibrated with 1 mm (Hu-Friedy Mfg Co., Inc., Chicago, IL, USA). A UNC-15 Color-Coded Probe was used for all explorations. Pressure of approximately 20 g was applied for probing.

2.3. Quantitative Real-Time Reverse Transcription PCR (qRT-PCR) Analysis

Total RNA was extracted from 50–100 mg tissue samples using an RNeasy Lipid Tissue Mini Kit (Qiagen, Hilden, Germany) in accordance with the manufacturer's protocol. The obtained RNA was used for the reverse transcription reaction. A quantity of 1 µg of RNA from each sample was reverse transcribed into cDNA with the RevertAid First Strand cDNA Synthesis Kit (Thermo Scientific, Waltham, MA, USA) according to the manufacturer's instructions.

Quantitative assessment of mRNA levels was performed by real-time RT-PCR using an ABI 7500 Fast instrument with Power SYBR Green PCR Master Mix reagent. Real-time conditions were as follows: 95 °C (15 s), 40 cycles at 95 °C (15 s) and 60 °C (1 min).

In the next step, the $2^{-\Delta Ct}$ method was used to calculate the values. The values were normalized to the B2M (β2-microglobulin) gene. The primer sequences used in the study were prepared according to the sequence information obtained from the NCBI database, and were synthesized by Oligo.pl (IBB PAN, Warsaw, Poland). Primers used for gene expression analysis by qRT PCR were as follow: B2M-F 5′-AATGCGGCATCTTCAAACCT-3′, B2M-R 5′-TGACTTTGTCACAGCCCAAGA-3′, IL17A-F 5′-AGATTACTACAACCGATCCAC-3′, IL17A-R 5′-GGGGACAGAGTTCATGTGGT-3′, IL17B-F 5′-GAGCCCCAAAAGCAAGAGGA-3′, IL17B-R 5′-TGCGGGCATACGGTTTCATC-3′.

2.4. Immunohistochemical Analysis of IL17

After deparaffinization in Xylene (ChemPour, Tarnowskie Góry, Poland), sections of gingival or granulation tissue from the inflammatory site (3 µm thick) were hydrated in gradually decreasing ethanol (100–70%) and rinsed in tap water for 5 min. Next, heat epitope retrieval was performed in retrieval solution buffer pH = 6 (DAKO, Glostrup, Denmark), in a microwave oven for 10 min. After cooling to room temperature (RT), all the slides were incubated with 0.3% solution of H_2O_2 for inhibition of endogenous peroxidase, washed twice with PBS, and then incubated with 2.5% horse serum to prevent unspecific antibody bounding (Vector Laboratories, Newark, CA, USA). After incubation with serum, slides were incubated in a humid chamber with primary antibody of rabbit anti-human IL-17 (ab2) (Sigma-Aldrich, Burlington, MA, USA) for 1 h at RT. After washing in PBS, immunoreactions were visualized with ImmPRESS UNIVERSAL REAGENT and Vector NovaRED Substrate KIT FOR PEROXIDASE (Vector Laboratories, Newark, CA, USA) according to protocols provided by the manufacturer. Nuclei were counterstained with Mayer hematoxylin (Sigma-Aldrich, Burlington, MA, USA). As a negative control, the primary antibody was replaced with PBS on the specimen. Positive staining was defined by visual identification of a yellow/brown pigmentation in a bright field microscope. Images were collected with an Olympus IX81 inverted microscope (Olympus, Hamburg, Germany) with a color camera and with CellSens image processing software (Olympus, Germany).

2.5. Statistical Analysis

Non-parametric tests were used for statistical analysis of quantitative variables ($p < 0.05$; Shapiro–Wilk test). The Mann–Whitney U test was used for comparisons between two groups, and Spearman's rank correlation coefficient for assessment of associations between variables. Normalized expression values are presented as medians with lower and upper quartiles (Q1–Q3). Values of $p < 0.05$ were considered to indicate statistical significance. The study had a statistical power of 80% to detect the true effect size corresponding to (1) the difference between group means equal to 1.3 standard deviations, and (2) the correlation coefficient between parameters measured in patients equal to ±0.67.

3. Results

In the first step of our study, we compared the expression of *IL-17A* and *IL-17B* at the mRNA level in gingival tissue in patients with periodontitis and control subjects. As shown in Figure 1, there were no statistically significant differences in expression of *IL-17A* between patients with periodontitis and control subjects (median: 0.00039, Q1–Q3: 0.000068–0.00088 vs. median: 0.00088, Q1–Q3: 0–0.0023, respectively, $p = 0.81$). The expression of *IL-17B* was statistically significantly lower in patients with periodontitis in comparison with healthy subjects (median: 0.00017, Q1–Q3: 0.000087–0.0021 vs. median: 0.0042, Q1–Q3: 0.00076–0.012, respectively, $p = 0.048$), (Figure 2).

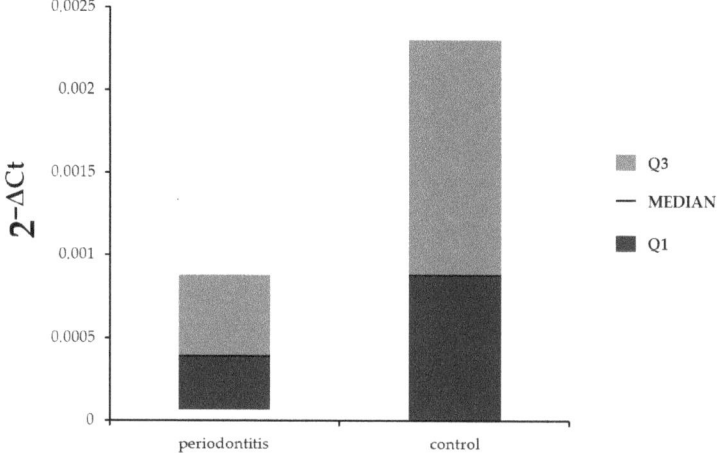

Figure 1. Expression of *IL-17A* mRNA in gingival tissue of patients with periodontitis and control subjects.

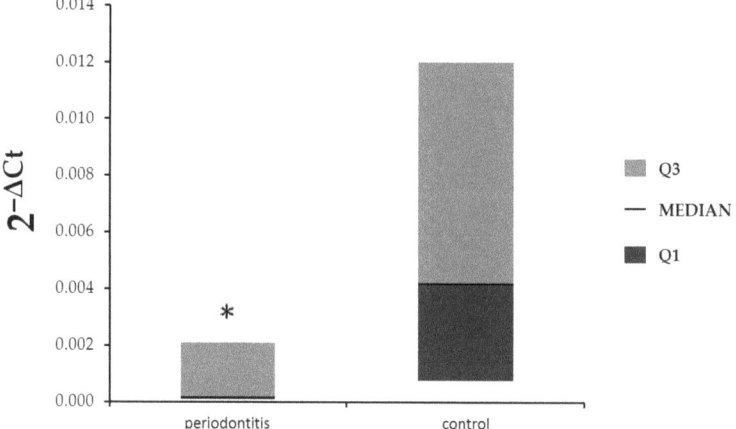

Figure 2. Expression of *IL-17B* mRNA in gingival tissue of patients with periodontitis and control subjects, * $p = 0.048$, Mann–Whitney U test.

Additionally, we examined the correlations between expression of *IL-17A* and *IL-17B* and clinical parameters such as PPD, API, CAL, and BoP. As shown in Table 1 the expression of *IL-17A* correlated significantly with API values. Moreover, the *IL-17B* expression in gingival tissue correlated with CAL values. This correlation reached borderline statistical significance ($p = 0.06$). There were no statistically significant correlations between the other clinical parameters noted above and expression of *IL-17A* and *IL-17B* in gingival tissues.

Table 1. Correlation between *IL-17A* and *IL-17B* expression and clinical parameters.

Clinical Parameters	IL-17A		IL-17B	
	Rs	p	Rs	p
Age [years]	−0.0221	0.94	0.1850	0.52
NRT	−0.0598	0.83	0.0066	0.98
API	0.6099	0.02	0.3300	0.24
BoP	0.0818	0.78	0.0770	0.79
PPD	−0.2539	0.38	−0.0681	0.81
CAL	0.1392	0.63	0.5061	0.06

Rs—Spearman rank correlation coefficient; NRT—Number of remaining teeth; API—approximal plaque index; BoP—bleeding on probing; PPD—probing pocket depth; CAL—clinical attachment level.

We also performed immunohistochemical analysis of IL-17 protein expression in gingival tissue from PD patients and controls. Figure 3 shows the expression of IL-17 protein in gingival tissue from PD patients and controls.

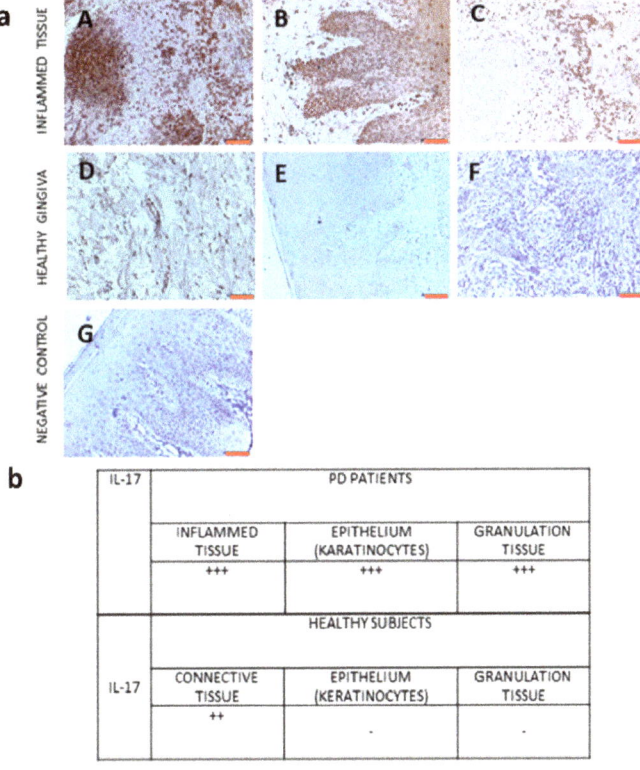

Figure 3. The expression of IL-17 protein in gingival tissue from: panel (**a**) (**A**–**C**): PD patients (inflamed tissue: (**A**)—connective tissue, (**B**)—epithelial tissue, (**C**)—granular tissue;); panels (**D**–**E**): controls (healthy gingiva): (**D**)—connective tissue, (**E**)—epithelial tissue, (**F**)—granular tissue; negative primary antibody control, where primary antibody was replaced with PBS (negative control—panel (**G**)). Original objective magnification ×20, scale bar = 50 µm, only representative images are presented. Panel (**b**): cellular immunolocalization of IL-17; +++ very high expression, ++ high expression, - no expression.

The expression of proinflammatory markers was observed in all samples of inflammatory tissues. The pigmentation was observed in the cytoplasm of cells in connective tissue and in keratinocytes. In the case of granulation tissue, the immunoreaction was observed in the cytoplasm of inflammatory cells. According to the saturation and color of pigmentation, the result was described as +++ very high expression, ++ high expression, - no expression.

4. Discussion

Periodontitis is a chronic inflammation of periodontal tissues initiated by a bacterial infection. However, mechanisms to eliminate the bacterial infection can develop into chronic inflammation that causes damage to periodontal tissues, including the alveolar process. Numerous immune response cells that secrete a number of pro-inflammatory mediators are involved in the development of this inflammation. Among the cells that play an important role in this process are Th-17 lymphocytes, which produce IL-17 [10,11]. IL-17 is an important component of the inflammatory cascade in periodontitis. It exhibits a number of direct actions in periodontal tissues, such as stimulating immune response cells to synthesize other cytokines (interleukin-6, interleukin-8, TNF and G-CSF) that are involved in the development of periodontitis [13].

IL-17 is an important cytokine that plays a multidirectional function in periodontal tissues. Under physiological conditions, IL-17 plays an important role in the mucosal barrier that protects against bacterial infections. IL-17 is mainly produced by Th-17 cells; however, the expression of this cytokine was also found on other immune cells such as neutrophils and natural killer cells [9,10]. IL-17 increases the recruitment and stimulation of other immune response cells, mainly neutrophils, which play an important role in the development of periodontitis. This cytokine also increases the synthesis of metalloproteinases, which cause periodontal tissue destruction. IL-17 influences the expression of RANKL and osteoprotegerin, thereby affecting the destruction of alveolar bone [10].

The role of IL-17 in the pathogenesis of PD has been investigated in animal models and in clinical studies [4–6]. Previous studies have indicated increased expression of IL-17 in serum, gingival cervical fluid, and saliva of patients with various forms of PD [4–6]; however, the studies examining the expression of IL-17 in gingival tissue are limited. These studies analyzed various forms of periodontal disease and periodontitis (aggressive and chronic according to the previous classification). Most of the studies evaluated total IL-17 without identifying the different isoforms of this cytokine. Most studies have shown increased expression of IL-17, especially in saliva and gingival fluid in patients with acute forms of periodontitis [17–19]. In the study by Awang et al., serum, saliva, and gingival crevicular fluid IL-17 levels were higher in periodontitis patients and correlated positively with clinical parameters of attachment loss, pocket depth, and bleeding on probing [20]. Liukkonen et al. indicated that salivary concentrations of IL-17 were elevated significantly in patients with local periodontal disease compared with controls and patients with generalized periodontal disease [21]. Furthermore, in the study by Mitani et al., IL-17 levels were significantly higher in gingival crevicular fluid from patients with periodontitis [6].

The studies also examined IL-17 serum concentrations in patients with PD [22,23]. Duarte et al. [14] reported significantly higher levels of IL-17 in the serum of patients with chronic PD. Similar results were presented by Cifcibasi et al., who also observed increased levels of IL-17 in patients with aggressive PD [24]. However, the mechanisms causing the increase in IL-17 in systemic circulation remain unclear. Duarte et al. demonstrated elevated serum IL-17 levels in patients with generalized aggressive periodontitis, which were reduced by therapy [25]. These studies suggest that local inflammatory changes in gingival tissue caused an increase in the IL-17 level in systemic circulation.

Increased numbers of IL-17-producing cells were detected in gingival tissue in patients with periodontitis [26]. These results suggest that the degree of infiltration with IL-17-producing cells is correlated with the severity of inflammation in PD.

In our study, we examined the expression of *IL-17A* and *IL-17B* at the mRNA level, as well as IL-17 protein expression in gingival tissue from patients with periodontitis as well as in healthy subjects. Our results did not detect statistically significant differences in *IL-17A* expression at the mRNA level in the gingival tissue of periodontitis patients and healthy subjects, but *IL-17A* expression correlated with the proximate plaque index. We have shown lower expression of *IL-17B* at the mRNA level in patients with periodontitis in comparison with healthy subjects. The gingival expression of *IL-17B* at the mRNA level correlated with clinical attachment loss. Clinical attachment loss is a parameter indicating the severity of periodontal disease. Clinical attachment loss is caused by inflammation and the secretion of cytokines, chemokines, metalloproteinases, and other mediators by cells of the immune system, causing the destruction of periodontal tissues. IL-17B has been shown to enhance neutrophil migration, thereby increasing inflammation [8]. It is possible that *IL-17B* expression at the mRNA level in gingival tissue may be inhibited by other mediators involved in the development of periodontitis.

In immunohistochemical analysis, we analyzed the IL-17 protein expression in gingival tissue from PD patients and healthy subjects. The highest expression of IL-17 was shown in inflamed connective tissue, epithelium (karatinocytes), and granulation tissue from gingival biopsy specimens from patients with periodontitis. In biopsy specimens from healthy individuals, no IL-17 was found in the epithelium (keratinocytes), while an expression of IL-17 was found in the connective tissue.

One limitation of our study is the lack of a positive control in immunohistochemical analysis.

The results of this study indicated that *IL-17A* expression in gingival tissue at the mRNA level did not differ between PD patients and controls, while *IL-17B* expression at the mRNA level is lower in PD patients than in controls. In contrast, we showed increased IL-17 expression at the protein level in the gingival tissue of PD patients compared to the healthy group. The results of our study suggest that the increase in IL-17 expression in the gingival tissue of PD patients occurs at the post-translational stage. Likewise, inflammatory mediators involved in the development of periodontitis cause stimulation of IL-17 protein expression, which increases the amount of IL-17 protein in gingival tissue. Periodontitis is a chronic inflammatory condition in which the immune response is disrupted. Multiple immune response pathways are activated, leading to the synthesis of pro-inflammatory mediators and the formation of numerous feedback loops. These results suggest that IL-17 is part of the inflammatory cascade present in periodontitis. Previous studies have indicated that IL-17 increases the production of other cytokines, so it also appears that other pro-inflammatory mediators may affect IL-17 expression [4,5].

Previous studies have shown increased IL-17 expression in the serum, gingival fluid, and saliva of patients with various forms of periodontal disease [17–22]. These studies often used previous criteria for classifying periodontal disease, which may be a factor in the results. In our study, patients were classified according to new criteria in accordance with the 2017 periodontal disease classification system [15]. It has been shown that IL-17 expression can vary in different tissues. IL-17 is demonstrated to be part of a complex inflammatory cascade occurring in periodontitis. There is a mutual influence of individual pro-inflammatory mediators, which interact with each other. Elevated expression of IL-17 protein in gingival tissue may indicate the involvement of IL-17 in the inflammatory process in the periodontal tissues.

Although a number of previous studies have confirmed an important role in the development of periodontal diseases, it seems that a full understanding of the involvement of this cytokine and its individual isoforms in the inflammatory cascade present in periodontitis, especially in light of the new classification of periodontal diseases, requires further research.

5. Conclusions

The results of our study confirm the involvement of IL-17 in the pathogenesis of periodontitis.

Our results suggest that an increase in IL-17 protein expression in the gingival tissue of patients with periodontitis occurs at the post-translational stage.

Author Contributions: Investigation, M.M.-M., K.S. (Karol Serwin), M.K., K.P. and M.C.; software, K.S. (Krzysztof Safranow); formal analysis, T.B. and A.P.; manuscript preparation, A.P.; conceptualization, A.P. All authors have read and agreed to the published version of the manuscript.

Funding: This work was supported by the Polish National Science Centre Miniatura-2 Grant DEC-2018/02/X/NZ3/00871 to K.S. (Karol Serwin).

Institutional Review Board Statement: The study was approved by the local ethics committee (BN-001/93/08) and is in accordance with the Declaration of Helsinki.

Informed Consent Statement: Informed consent was obtained from all subjects involved in the study.

Data Availability Statement: Not applicable.

Conflicts of Interest: The authors declare no conflict of interest.

References

1. Kinane, D.F.; Peterson, M.; Stathopoulou, P.G. Environmental and other modifying factors of the periodontal diseases. *Periodontology 2000* **2006**, *40*, 107–119. [CrossRef] [PubMed]
2. Di Benedetto, A.; Gigante, I.; Colucci, S.; Grano, M. Periodontal disease: Linking the primary inflammation to bone loss. *Clin. Dev. Immunol.* **2013**, *2013*, 503754. [CrossRef] [PubMed]
3. Sandros, J.; Karlsson, C.; Lappin, D.F.; Madianos, P.N.; Kinane, D.F.; Papapanou, P.N. Cytokine responses of oral epithelial cells to Porphyromonas gingivalis infection. *J. Dent. Res.* **2000**, *79*, 1808–1814. [CrossRef] [PubMed]
4. Cheng, W.C.; Hughes, F.J.; Taams, L.S. The presence, function and regulation of IL-17 and Th17 cells in periodontitis. *J. Clin. Periodontol.* **2014**, *41*, 541–549. [CrossRef] [PubMed]
5. Cheng, W.C.; van Asten, S.D.; Burns, L.A.; Evans, H.G.; Walter, G.J.; Hashim, A.; Hughes, F.J.; Taams, L.S. Periodontitis-associated pathogens P. gingivalis and A. actinomycetemcomitans activate human CD14(+) monocytes leading to enhanced Th17/IL-17 responses. *Eur. J. Immunol.* **2016**, *46*, 2211–2221. [CrossRef]
6. Mitani, A.; Niedbala, W.; Fujimura, T.; Mogi, M.; Miyamae, S.; Higuchi, N.; Abe, A.; Hishikawa, T.; Mizutani, M.; Ishihara, Y.; et al. Increased expression of interleukin (IL)-35 and IL-17, but not IL-27, in gingival tissues with chronic periodontitis. *J. Periodontol.* **2015**, *86*, 301–309. [CrossRef]
7. Gaffen, S.L. Structure and signalling in the IL-17 receptor family. *Nat. Rev. Immunol.* **2009**, *9*, 556–567. [CrossRef]
8. Gu, C.; Wu, L.; Li, X. IL-17 family: Cytokines, receptors and signaling. *Cytokine* **2013**, *64*, 477–485. [CrossRef]
9. Miossec, P.; Kolls, J.K. Targeting IL-17 and TH17 cells in chronic inflammation. *Nat. Rev. Drug. Discov.* **2012**, *11*, 763–776. [CrossRef]
10. Zenobia, C.; Hajishengallis, G. Basic biology and role of interleukin-17 in immunity and inflammation. *Periodontology 2000* **2015**, *69*, 142–159. [CrossRef]
11. Iyoda, M.; Shibata, T.; Kawaguchi, M.; Hizawa, N.; Yamaoka, T.; Kokubu, F.; Akizawa, T. IL-17A and IL-17F stimulate chemokines via MAPK pathways (ERK1/2 and p38 but not JNK) in mouse cultured mesangial cells: Synergy with TNF-alpha and IL-1beta. *Am. J. Physiol. Renal. Physiol.* **2010**, *298*, 779–787. [CrossRef] [PubMed]
12. Koenders, M.I.; Marijnissen, R.J.; Devesa, I.; Lubberts, E.; Joosten, L.A.; Roth, J.; van Lent, P.L.; van de Loo, F.A.; van den Berg, W.B. Tumor necrosis factor-interleukin-17 interplay induces S100A8, interleukin-1β, and matrix metalloproteinases, and drives irreversible cartilage destruction in murine arthritis: Rationale for combination treatment during arthritis. *Arthritis Rheum.* **2011**, *63*, 2329–2339. [CrossRef] [PubMed]
13. Behfarnia, P.; Birang, R.; Andalib, A.R.; Asadi, S. Comparative Evaluation of IFNγ, IL4 and IL17 Cytokines in Healthy Gingiva and Moderate to Advanced Chronic Periodontitis. *J. Dent. Res.* **2010**, *7*, 45–50.
14. Duarte, P.M.; Miranda, T.S.; Lima, J.A.; Dias Gonçalves, T.E.; Santos, V.R.; Bastos, M.F.; Ribeiro, F.V. Expression of immune-inflammatory markers in sites of chronic periodontitis in patients with type 2 diabetes. *J. Periodontol.* **2012**, *83*, 426–434. [CrossRef]
15. Dietrich, T.; Ower, P.; Tank, M.; West, N.X.; Walter, C.; Needleman, I.; Hughes, F.J.; Wadia, R.; Milward, M.R.; Hodge, P.J.; et al. Periodontal diagnosis in the context of the 2017 classification system of periodontal diseases and conditions—Implementation in clinical practice. *Br. Dent. J.* **2019**, *226*, 16–22. [CrossRef]
16. Papapanou, P.N.; Sanz, M.; Buduneli, N.; Dietrich, T.; Feres, M.; Fine, D.H.; Flemmig, T.F.; Garcia, R.; Giannobile, W.V.; Graziani, F.; et al. Periodontitis: Consensus report of workgroup 2 of the 2017 World Workshop on the Classification of Periodontal and Peri-Implant Diseases and Conditions. *J. Periodontol.* **2018**, *89*, S173–S182. [CrossRef]
17. Özçaka, Ö.; Nalbantsoy, A.; Buduneli, N. Interleukin-17 and interleukin-18 levels in saliva and plasma of patients with chronic periodontitis. *J. Periodont. Res.* **2011**, *46*, 592–598.
18. Shaker, O.G.; Ghallab, N.A. IL-17 and IL-11 GCF levels in aggressive and chronic periodontitis patients: Relation to PCR bacterial detection. *Mediat. Inflamm.* **2012**, *2012*, 174764. [CrossRef]
19. Vernal, R.; Dutzan, N.; Chaparro, A.; Puente, J.; Antonieta Valenzuela, M.; Gamonal, J. Levels of interleukin-17 in gingival crevicular fluid and in supernatants of cellular cultures of gingival tissue from patients with chronic periodontitis. *J. Clin. Periodontol.* **2005**, *32*, 383–389. [CrossRef]

20. Awang, R.A.; Lappin, D.F.; MacPherson, A.; Riggio, M.; Robertson, D.; Hodge, P.; Ramage, G.; Culshaw, S.; Preshaw, P.M.; Taylor, J.; et al. Clinical associations between IL-17 family cytokines and periodontitis and potential differential roles for IL-17A and IL-17E in periodontal immunity. *Inflamm. Res.* **2014**, *63*, 1001–1012. [CrossRef]
21. Liukkonen, J.; Gürsoy, U.K.; Pussinen, P.J.; Suominen, A.L.; Könönen, E. Salivary Concentrations of Interleukin (IL)-1β, IL-17A, and IL-23 Vary in Relation to Periodontal Status. *J. Periodontol.* **2016**, *87*, 1484–1491. [CrossRef] [PubMed]
22. Schenkein, H.A.; Koertge, T.E.; Brooks, C.N.; Sabatini, R.; Purkall, D.E.; Tew, J.G. IL-17 in sera from patients with aggressive periodontitis. *J. Dent. Res.* **2010**, *89*, 943–947. [CrossRef]
23. Qi, Y.; Feng, W.; Song, A.; Song, H.; Yan, S.; Sun, Q.; Yang, P. Role of serum IL-23/IL-17 axis in the relationship between periodontitis and coronary heart disease. *Int. J. Periodontics Restor. Dent.* **2013**, *33*, 185–191. [CrossRef] [PubMed]
24. Cifcibasi, E.; Koyuncuoglu, C.; Ciblak, M.; Badur, S.; Kasali, K.; Firatli, E.; Cintan, S. Evaluation of Local and Systemic Levels of Interleukin-17, Interleukin-23, and Myeloperoxidase in Response to Periodontal Therapy in Patients with Generalized Aggressive Periodontitis. *Inflammation* **2015**, *38*, 1959–1968. [CrossRef]
25. Duarte, P.M.; da Rocha, M.; Sampaio, E.; Mestnik, M.J.; Feres, M.; Figueiredo, L.C.; Bastos, M.F.; Faveri, M. Serum levels of cytokines in subjects with generalized chronic and aggressive periodontitis before and after non-surgical periodontal therapy: A pilot study. *J. Periodontol.* **2010**, *81*, 1056–1063. [CrossRef] [PubMed]
26. Adibrad, M.; Deyhimi, P.; Ganjalikhani Hakemi, M.; Behfarnia, P.; Shahabuei, M.; Rafiee, L. Signs of the presence of Th17 cells in chronic periodontal disease. *J. Periodontal. Res.* **2012**, *47*, 525–531. [CrossRef]

Disclaimer/Publisher's Note: The statements, opinions and data contained in all publications are solely those of the individual author(s) and contributor(s) and not of MDPI and/or the editor(s). MDPI and/or the editor(s) disclaim responsibility for any injury to people or property resulting from any ideas, methods, instructions or products referred to in the content.

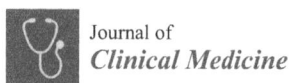 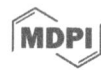

Opinion

COVID-19 and Oral Lichen Planus: Between an "Intriguing Plot" and the "Fata Morgana Effect"

Gaetano Scotto [1,†], Vincenzina Fazio [2,†], Salvatore Massa [3], Lorenzo Lo Muzio [4] and Francesca Spirito [4,*]

1. Infectious Diseases Unit, University Hospital "OORR" Foggia, 71122 Foggia, Italy; gaetano.scotto@unifg.it
2. Clinical Chemistry Laboratory, Virology Unit, University Hospital "OORR" Foggia, 71122 Foggia, Italy; vincenzina.fazio@unifg.it
3. Department of Agriculture, Food, Natural Resource and Engineering, University of Foggia, 71122 Foggia, Italy; salvatore.massa@unifg.it
4. Department of Clinical and Experimental Medicine, University of Foggia, 71122 Foggia, Italy; lorenzo.lomuzio@unifg.it
* Correspondence: francesca.spirito@unifg.it
† Retired.

Abstract: The COVID-19 pandemic, caused by the SARS-CoV-2 virus, has led to significant morbidity and mortality worldwide since its declaration as a global pandemic in March 2020. Alongside the typical respiratory symptoms, unusual clinical manifestations such as oral lichen planus (OLP) have been observed. OLP is a chronic inflammatory mucocutaneous dermatosis that results from a cell-mediated reaction, and its pathogenesis involves the loss of immunological tolerance. OLP has been associated with several triggering factors, such as certain drugs, stress, smoking, and even some viruses. Exposure to the spike protein antigen of SARS-CoV-2 during an infection can trigger autoimmune reactions and lead to the onset or flare of OLP. The E3 protein ligase TRIM21, which is identified in the lamina propria of OLP lesions, is overexpressed in COVID-19 patients and plays a critical role in autoimmune pathologies. Furthermore, the psychological stress of the lockdown and quarantine can be a trigger for the onset or exacerbation of OLP. However, the diagnosis of OLP is complex and requires a biopsy in order to confirm a clinical diagnosis, rule out other pathologies, and establish the most appropriate therapeutic procedure. Further research is needed to understand the potential link between Co-19 and OLP.

Keywords: COVID-19; SARS-CoV-2; oral lichen planus

It has been about three years since the World Health Organization (WHO) declared coronavirus disease-19, COVID-19 (Co-19), as a global pandemic on 11 March 2020. Co-19 is an acute respiratory disease that is caused by the SARS-CoV-2 virus. COVID-19 exhibits a wide range of clinical manifestations that vary from asymptomatic or mildly symptomatic cases, which feature upper respiratory tract involvement, to severe forms that feature lung impairment and life-threatening conditions that are caused by critical respiratory distress. In mild cases, Co-19 symptoms are similar to the flu, and the most commonly observed symptoms of COVID-19 include fever, fatigue, dry cough, headache, hemoptysis, anorexia, and sore throat [1]; in the most critical cases, it is a systemic disease with severe acute respiratory syndrome. However, in addition to the "classic" clinical features, there have been reports linking Co-19 infection or Co-19 therapy to less common pathologies, including atypical manifestations that affect various systems such as the neurological, psychiatric, neuropsychiatric, cardiovascular, gastrointestinal, and dermatological systems [2]. The virus enters host cells through the binding of the homotrimeric spike glycoprotein on the viral surface to the angiotensin-converting enzyme 2 (ACE2) receptor, which is found in different organs and systems of the human body [3]. This mechanism of viral entry contributes to the characteristic multiorgan tropism of the virus. SARS-CoV-2 demonstrates a particular tropism for head and neck tissues, and it leads to distinct extrapulmonary manifestations that have become notable features of the disease [4]. These manifestations include dysfunctions in the sense of smell (anosmia) and taste (ageusia, dysgeusia) [5]. Indeed, the receptors and enzymes that are required for SARS-CoV-2 cell entry, such as the ACE2 receptor [6], transmembrane protease serine 2 (TMPRSS2), and furin [7,8], are highly expressed in oral and nasal cavity tissues, including the epithelial cells of the tongue, taste buds (particularly fungiform papillae), major and minor salivary glands, and nasal mucosa. The virus enters target cells through the interaction between the spike protein (S protein) and the ACE2 receptor [6,9], and TMPRSS2 plays a priming role in this process [5]. Therefore, this specific tropism manifests through the development of oral cavity pathologies [10–12] and other maxillofacial conditions, such as the well-known association with mucormycosis [13,14]. Indeed, during SARS-CoV-2 infection, the oral mucosa can serve as a potential route for the virus, and regional pathologies in the oral cavity may arise [15–17]. These pathologies can manifest as ulcerative lesions, vesicles, blisters, petechiae, erythema multiforme-like lesions, aphthous-like lesions, and herpetiform lesions, which typically concurrently appear with general symptoms or within one week [10,17–20]. Oral manifestations can also be a result of COVID-19 therapies, such as the long-term use of antibiotics or mechanical ventilation devices in severely affected patients, which can lead to Candida infections in the form of red or white plaque lesions [21]. Delayed onset oral lesions, including ulcerations, bullous angina, petechiae, and late-onset erythema multiforme-like lesions, have also been reported following the initiation of therapy [20]. The prolonged hospitalization of patients can contribute to poor oral hygiene and be combined with compromised overall health, states of immunosuppression, and physical and psychological stress, which can lead to the development of plaque-related diseases, such as ulcer-necrotic gingivitis [22]. Regarding certain oral cavity diseases, some reports have recently appeared in the literature that must be examined with a touch of curiosity and pinch of skepticism as they discuss the onset or exacerbation of oral lichen planus (OLP) during Co-19 infection [23].

OLP—a clinical variant of lichen planus (LP), which is a chronic inflammatory muco-cutaneous dermatosis of immune etiology—results in an inflammatory state that affects the stratified squamous epithelium of the oral cavity and the underlying lamina propria [24]. OLP is a cell-mediated reaction in which CD8 cytotoxic lymphocytes play the primary role against an unknown keratinocyte antigen that is no longer recognized as self. Consequently, the lesions can be seen as the manifestation of various oral diseases and conditions that are caused by the loss of immunological tolerance. Both LP and OLP can arise or be exacerbated in the presence of triggering factors such as certain drugs (non-steroidal anti-inflammatory drugs (NSAIDs), antihypertensives, antimalarials, etc.), psycho-organic stress, smoking, and even some viruses [25–27]. In fact, an association between the presence of OLP and infection by citomegalovirus (CMV), herpes simplex (HSV) type 1, 4, and 6, hepatitis B virus (HBV), papilloma virus and, above all, hepatitis C virus (HCV) has been identified [26,27]. This is probably due to the extra-hepatic manifestations of HCV, such as cryoglobulinemia [27]. Data on the inductive mechanisms of the potential triggers and on the identities of the target antigens are still not conclusive; however, the immune dysregulation alludes to the hypothesis of an autoimmune-based chronic inflammatory reaction.

As far as Co-19/OLP is concerned, this hypothesis seems plausible, as immune dysregulation with hints of autoimmunity would seem to be a common finding by it playing a fundamental role in the pathogenesis of OLP and underlying the cytokine storm that is a hallmark of Co-19. There are several theories linking the pathogenesis of oral lichen planus with Co-19, starting from the fact that SARS-CoV-2 infection has been linked to an imbalance in the signaling pathway of the mammalian target of rapamycin (mTOR), which is known to contribute to the abnormal proliferation of T-cells and the development of OLP. It has been hypothesized that exposure to the spike protein antigen during a Co-19 infection can trigger an autoimmune reaction. Increased levels of inflammatory mediators such as cytokines, matrix metalloproteinases, and chemokines, as well as the recruitment and alteration of the activity of cytotoxic CD8+ T cells (CTLs), would mediate the onset or flare of OLP [28]. Furthermore, Co-19 seems to trigger the overexpression of the tripartite motif-containing protein 21 (E3 protein ligase TRIM21), which belongs to a tripartite motif protein family that is encoded by gene 21 and is an important autoantigen in autoimmune pathologies (Sjogren syndrome, systemic lupus erythematosus (SLE)). This stimulates CTL and increases cytokine production with enhanced IL-6 secretion; the trait d'union would be the identification of E3TRIM21 as also being in the lamina propria of OLP lesions [29,30]. Furthermore, the cytokine storms that are characterized by increased levels of interleukin-1 (IL-1), interleukin-6 (IL-6), interleukin-12 (IL-12), interferon y (IFN-γ), and tumor necrosis factor α (TNF-α) are a prominent feature of SARS-CoV-2 infection, and they contribute to tissue damage and inflammation; it should also be added that, in COVID-19 patients, there is a high level of interleukin-2 (IL-2), interleukin-4 (IL-4), interleukin-7 (IL-7), interleukin-10 (IL-10), interleukin-13 (IL-13), and interleukin-17 (IL-17) [31]. Several interleukins (ILs), including IL-1, IL-2, IL-4, IL-5, IL-6, IL-8, IL-10, IL-12, IL-17, and IL-18, have been implicated in the development and progression of OLP [32]. Genetic variations in IL-18, TNFα, IFN-γ, IL-10, IL-17, IL-1ß, IL-12, IL-8, and IL-4 have also been associated with OLP [28]. These cytokines damage the basement membrane and cause extensive tissue destruction, which results in the formation of observable lesions. The increased levels of cytokines, malfunctioning T-cells, and activation of TRIM21 in individuals that are affected by or recovering from COVID-19 may make them more vulnerable to developing oral lichen planus.

A further hypothesis, although very suggestive, is that Co-19 may not directly contribute to OLP, but when combined with psychological stress with depressive elements that are linked to the lockdown and/or quarantine, it can be a trigger for the onset or exacerbation of OLP. It is known that stress can be a cause for the alteration of various parameters of the endocrine system and immune dysregulation in subjects that are affected by OLP [25,33]. In fact, a high increase in stress can activate the sympathetic nervous system and the hypothalamic–pituitary–adrenocortical axis, causing a significant influx of inflammatory cytokines such as interleukin-6 (IL-6), interleukin-1 (IL-1) and tumor necrosis factor (TNF), as well as an alteration of CTL activity. As a result of this influx, changes in kynurenine metabolites lead to neurotoxic changes in the brain. This is likely to result in an autoimmune reaction, which can trigger the onset or exacerbation of OLP [34,35]. This seems to happen preferentially in women, as demonstrated in an Indian study that was carried out on socially frail women during the pandemic. The reason for this is that female hormonal changes, in addition to the increase in cytokines, make them more susceptible to systemic disorders that are induced by a state of stress or depression [36,37]. Considering the above, there is a high probability of an "intriguing mix" between the two pathologies of Co-19 and OLP; however, in medicine, there is usually a catch.

The diagnosis of OLP is typically based on a combination of clinical objectivity and histopathological features. Exclusively defining the diagnosis on clinical criteria presents critical issues, as studies have shown possible interpretative variability. The lesions that present themselves in OLP in an erosive, atrophic, bullous, reticular, and plaque form can, in fact, also be found in other clinical conditions, such as lupus erythematosus, syphilis, candidiasis, aphthous ulcers, pemphigoid mucosa, and carcinoma of the oral cavity [24]. Therefore, a biopsy is necessary to confirm a clinical diagnosis to exclude other pathologies and establish the most appropriate therapeutic procedure. In 2003, van der Meij and van der Waal [38] proposed a modification of the diagnostic criteria that were previously recommended by the WHO in order to reduce this variability. The complete correspondence of the clinical criteria (presence of bilateral lesions, presence of reticular striae) and histopathological criteria (presence of a well-defined area of cellular infiltration with a "band" arrangement that is limited to the superficial part of the connective tissue; signs of degeneration in the layer of basal cells; absence of epithelial dysplasia) constituted and still constitutes the necessary check for a diagnosis of OLP [38,39]. After analyzing the scientific literature published between 2020 and 2022, it was possible to highlight the prevalence of the Co-19/OLP association and the criteria that led to the diagnoses.

We screened Medline via the PubMed, Web of Science, Scopus and Google scholar databases for articles investigating the association between COVID and oral lichen that were published between 1, January 2020 and 31 May 2023. Several combinations of keywords were used in the following orders to conduct the search strategy: (1) "Lichen Planus" OR "Oral Lichen Planus"; and (2) "COVID-19" OR "Co-19" OR "SARS-CoV-2" OR "Coronavirus".

All clinical studies, case series, and case reports that reported cases of OLP in association with COVID-19 were considered as potentially admissible. To date, 17 cases of post-infection OLP have been described, including individual case reports, which constitute the vast majority, as well as case series and observational studies. Only five cases provide more detailed clinical characteristics, which are reported in Table 1 [40–43]. From a strictly clinical-morphological point of view, four out of five subjects presented a papulo-reticular form with evident Wicham's striae and one out of five subjects presented painful erosive areas surrounded by white radiating striae. Three out of five patients were symptomatic, and three patients had cutaneous involvement. In one case, there was information about the histopathology included: a hyperparakeratinized, stratified epithelium; partial ulceration; mild degree of acanthosis; liquefactive degeneration of basal cells; and prominent band-like sub-epithelial lymphocytic infiltration. The remaining 12 cases were part of an observational study [23] that considered all oral lesions that were found in a cohort of patients with COVID-19. In this study by Fidan et al. [23], oral lichen planus represented 20.6% of the lesions found in the 74 included patients. Considering all the cases, the manifestations of significance were observed in various locations of the oral cavity, where it was observed in the tongue for four cases, buccal mucosa for nine cases, gums for five cases, and palate for one case [23,40–44].

The diagnosis seems to have been made by clinical observation in 16 cases and only in 1 case was it confirmed by a histopathology from oral biopsy; the vast majority of authors did not mention a biopsy of the lesions, so it is assumed that the diagnoses were only based on clinical observations. Describing it as OLP is questionable in such cases, as various oral pathologies can present similar clinical observations. Furthermore, in 12 out of 17 cases, the descriptions of the lesions were directed towards single localizations, an aspect that should not be typical of OLP. In fact, one of its most relevant clinical characteristics is its frequent bilateral expression and ability to spread to several areas in the oral cavity; this aspect often helps the clinician to arrive at a correct diagnosis of OLP and exclude, in differential diagnosis, other lesions with unique and monolateral topographical characteristics. From this literature analysis, it is evident that there is a lack of data along with reporting bias, as confirmed by a recent literature review that indicates that, when considering all the data regarding lichen planus occurring after infection or vaccination, there are more cases that have been reported post-vaccination than post-infection in the literature [45].

To conclude, while our intention is not to criticize the scientific rigor of our colleagues' research, the critical issue with these reports lies in the small number of cases and the limited use of histological tests for confirmation. These biases, when combined with other clinical descriptors, could cause confusion and make the diagnosis extremely uncertain, a drawback of which that is also highlighted by some authors of these reports. Therefore, additional reports of cases with confirmatory histological tests are required. This will lead to a discussion of an "intriguing Co-19/OLP plot" and not of a "Fata Morgana mirage effect", which causes us to see what we want to see and not what it actually is.

Table 1. Case report and cases series reporting OLP after COVID-19 infection.

Article	Case	Sex	Age (Years)	After Infection, Days to Onset of Symptoms	Location of Lesions	Lesions Morphology and Symptomatology	Cutaneous Manifestation	Histopathology (Oral Biopsy)	Treatment for Oral Lesions	Outcomes of Oral Lesions
[40]	Case 1	F	56	42 days	Bilateral buccal mucosae	Papules with lace-like pattern	Widespread papulosquamous eruption on the trunk	NR	NR	NR
[41]	Case 2	F	52	NR	Bilateral buccal mucosae	Papules with lace-like pattern	Black annular plaque with a whitish rim on the right shin that measured 2 cm in diameter	NR	None	NR
[42]	Case 3	M	63	30 days	Dorsum linguae + buccal mucosae	Painful erosive areas surrounded by white radiating striae	Brown pruritic macules on the flexure surface of the arm	Hyper-parakeratinized stratified epithelium, partial ulceration, mild degree of acanthosis, liquefactive degeneration of basal cells, and prominent band-like sub-epithelial lymphocytic infiltration	Topical corticosteroids	Symptom remission and reduction of the extent of lesion (4 weeks)
[43]	Case 5	M	41	14 days	Buccal and gingival mucosae	Lichenoid striations with erythema + oral sensitivity	NR	NR	Topical corticosteroids	Symptom remission (4 weeks)
										Reduction of the extent of lesions
	Case 6	F	56	NR	Bilateral buccal mucosa	Lichenoid striations with erythema + oral sensitivity	NR	NR	Topical corticosteroids	NR

Funding: This research received no external funding.

Institutional Review Board Statement: Not applicable.

Informed Consent Statement: Not applicable.

Data Availability Statement: No new data were created.

Conflicts of Interest: The authors declare no conflict of interest.

References

1. Hu, B.; Guo, H.; Zhou, P.; Shi, Z.L. Characteristics of SARS-CoV-2 and COVID-19. *Nat. Rev. Microbiol.* **2021**, *19*, 141–154. [CrossRef] [PubMed]
2. Nelwan, E.J.; Tunjungputri, R.N.; Tetrasiwi, E.N.; Lauditta, R.K.; Nainggolan, L. Extrapulmonary Manifestations COVID-19. *Acta Med. Indones.* **2022**, *54*, 314–315. [PubMed]
3. Lan, J.; Ge, J.; Yu, J.; Shan, S.; Zhou, H.; Fan, S.; Zhang, Q.; Shi, X.; Wang, Q.; Zhang, L.; et al. Structure of the SARS-CoV-2 spike receptor-binding domain bound to the ACE2 receptor. *Nature* **2020**, *581*, 215–220. [CrossRef] [PubMed]
4. Spirito, F.; Leuci, S.; Di Cosola, M.; Lo Muzio, L. New emerging pandemic: Head and neck manifestations. *Minerva Med.* **2022**, *113*, 905–909. [CrossRef]
5. Scotto, G.; Fazio, V.; Lo Muzio, E.; Lo Muzio, L.; Spirito, F. SARS-CoV-2 Infection and Taste Alteration: An Overview. *Life* **2022**, *12*, 690. [CrossRef]
6. Xu, H.; Zhong, L.; Deng, J.; Peng, J.; Dan, H.; Zeng, X.; Li, T.; Chen, Q. High expression of ACE2 receptor of 2019-nCoV on the epithelial cells of oral mucosa. *Int. J. Oral Sci.* **2020**, *12*, 8. [CrossRef] [PubMed]
7. Song, J.; Li, Y.; Huang, X.; Chen, Z.; Li, Y.; Liu, C.; Chen, Z.; Duan, X. Systematic analysis of ACE2 and TMPRSS2 expression in salivary glands reveals underlying transmission mechanism caused by SARS-CoV-2. *J. Med. Virol.* **2020**, *92*, 2556–2566. [CrossRef]
8. Zhong, M.; Lin, B.; Pathak, J.L.; Gao, H.; Young, A.J.; Wang, X.; Liu, C.; Wu, K.; Liu, M.; Chen, J.M.; et al. ACE2 and Furin Expressions in Oral Epithelial Cells Possibly Facilitate COVID-19 Infection via Respiratory and Fecal-Oral Routes. *Front. Med.* **2020**, *7*, 580796. [CrossRef] [PubMed]
9. Walls, A.C.; Park, Y.J.; Tortorici, M.A.; Wall, A.; McGuire, A.T.; Veesler, D. Structure, Function, and Antigenicity of the SARS-CoV-2 Spike Glycoprotein. *Cell* **2020**, *181*, 281–292.e86. [CrossRef]
10. Iranmanesh, B.; Khalili, M.; Amiri, R.; Zartab, H.; Aflatoonian, M. Oral manifestations of COVID-19 disease: A review article. *Dermatol. Ther.* **2021**, *34*, e14578. [CrossRef]
11. Santacroce, L.; Pia Cazzolla, A.; Lovero, R.; Brescia, V.; Ciavarella, D.; Spirito, F.; Colella, M.; Bilancia, M.; Lo Muzio, L.; Di Serio, F. Neurosensory alterations and Interleukins Cascade in SARS-CoV-2 Infection—Results from a Retrospective Cohort of COVID-19 Inpatients. *Endocr. Metab. Immune Disord. Drug Targets* **2023**, *23*, 1162–1172. [CrossRef]
12. Favia, G.; Barile, G.; Tempesta, A.; Copelli, C.; Novielli, G.; Dell'Olio, F.; Capodiferro, S.; Spirito, F.; Brienza, N.; Ribezzi, M.; et al. Relationship between oral lesions and severe SARS-CoV-2 infection in intensive care unit patients. *Oral Dis.* **2023**, 1–8. [CrossRef] [PubMed]
13. Al-Tawfiq, J.A.; Alhumaid, S.; Alshukairi, A.N.; Temsah, M.H.; Barry, M.; Al Mutair, A.; Rabaan, A.A.; Al-Omari, A.; Tirupathi, R.; AlQahtani, M.; et al. COVID-19 and mucormycosis superinfection: The perfect storm. *Infection* **2021**, *49*, 833–853. [CrossRef]
14. Kumar, M.; Alagarsamy, R.; Madi, M.; Pentapati, K.C.; Vineetha, R.; Shetty, S.R.; Sharma, A. Rhinocerebral mucormycosis: A systematic review of case reports and case series from a global perspective. *Oral Surg. Oral Med. Oral Pathol. Oral Radiol.* **2022**, *134*, 708–716. [CrossRef]
15. Abdelgawad, N.; Elsayed, S.A.; Babkair, H.; Dar-Odeh, N. Verrucous leukoplakia affecting the tongue of a patient recovered from COVID-19. *Minerva Dent. Oral Sci.* **2021**, *70*, 128–130. [CrossRef] [PubMed]
16. Cicciu, M.; Fiorillo, L.; Laino, L. Oral signs and symptoms of COVID-19 affected patients: Dental practice as prevention method. *Minerva Dent. Oral Sci.* **2021**, *70*, 3–6. [CrossRef]
17. Surboyo, M.D.; Ernawati, D.S.; Budi, H.S. Oral mucosal lesions and oral symptoms of the SARS-CoV-2 infection. *Minerva Dent. Oral Sci.* **2021**, *70*, 161–168. [CrossRef]
18. Amorim Dos Santos, J.; Normando, A.G.C.; Carvalho da Silva, R.L.; Acevedo, A.C.; De Luca Canto, G.; Sugaya, N.; Santos-Silva, A.R.; Guerra, E.N.S. Oral Manifestations in Patients with COVID-19: A Living Systematic Review. *J. Dent. Res.* **2021**, *100*, 141–154. [CrossRef]
19. Farid, H.; Khan, M.; Jamal, S.; Ghafoor, R. Oral manifestations of COVID-19-A literature review. *Rev. Med. Virol.* **2022**, *32*, e2248. [CrossRef]
20. Favia, G.; Tempesta, A.; Barile, G.; Brienza, N.; Capodiferro, S.; Vestito, M.C.; Crudele, L.; Procacci, V.; Ingravallo, G.; Maiorano, E.; et al. COVID-19 Symptomatic Patients with Oral Lesions: Clinical and Histopathological Study on 123 Cases of the University Hospital Policlinic of Bari with a Purpose of a New Classification. *J. Clin. Med.* **2021**, *10*, 757. [CrossRef]
21. Nambiar, M.; Varma, S.R.; Jaber, M.; Sreelatha, S.V.; Thomas, B.; Nair, A.S. Mycotic infections—Mucormycosis and oral candidiasis associated with COVID-19: A significant and challenging association. *J. Oral Microbiol.* **2021**, *13*, 1967699. [CrossRef]
22. Patel, J.; Woolley, J. Necrotizing periodontal disease: Oral manifestation of COVID-19. *Oral Dis.* **2021**, *27* (Suppl. 3), 768–769. [CrossRef] [PubMed]

23. Fidan, V.; Koyuncu, H.; Akin, O. Oral lesions in COVID 19 positive patients. *Am. J. Otolaryngol.* **2021**, *42*, 102905. [CrossRef] [PubMed]
24. Alrashdan, M.S.; Cirillo, N.; McCullough, M. Oral lichen planus: A literature review and update. *Arch. Dermatol. Res.* **2016**, *308*, 539–551. [CrossRef]
25. Rojo-Moreno, J.L.; Bagan, J.V.; Rojo-Moreno, J.; Donat, J.S.; Milian, M.A.; Jimenez, Y. Psychologic factors and oral lichen planus. A psychometric evaluation of 100 cases. *Oral Surg. Oral. Med. Oral Pathol. Oral Radiol. Endod.* **1998**, *86*, 687–691. [CrossRef]
26. Lucchese, A.; Di Stasio, D.; Romano, A.; Fiori, F.; De Felice, G.P.; Lajolo, C.; Serpico, R.; Cecchetti, F.; Petruzzi, M. Correlation between Oral Lichen Planus and Viral Infections Other Than HCV: A Systematic Review. *J. Clin. Med.* **2022**, *11*, 5487. [CrossRef] [PubMed]
27. Calvaruso, V.; Craxi, A. Immunological alterations in hepatitis C virus infection. *World J. Gastroenterol.* **2013**, *19*, 8916–8923. [CrossRef] [PubMed]
28. Sood, A.; Raghavan, S.; Batra, P.; Sharma, K.; Talwar, A. Rise and exacerbation of oral lichen planus in the background of SARS-CoV-2 infection. *Med. Hypotheses* **2021**, *156*, 110681. [CrossRef]
29. Caddy, S.L.; Vaysburd, M.; Papa, G.; Wing, M.; O'Connell, K.; Stoycheva, D.; Foss, S.; Terje Andersen, J.; Oxenius, A.; James, L.C. Viral nucleoprotein antibodies activate TRIM21 and induce T cell immunity. *EMBO J.* **2021**, *40*, e106228. [CrossRef]
30. Wei, W.; Wang, Y.; Sun, Q.; Jiang, C.; Zhu, M.; Song, C.; Li, C.; Du, G.; Deng, Y.; Nie, H.; et al. Enhanced T-cell proliferation and IL-6 secretion mediated by overexpression of TRIM21 in oral lesions of patients with oral lichen planus. *J. Oral Pathol. Med.* **2020**, *49*, 350–356. [CrossRef]
31. Tang, Y.; Liu, J.; Zhang, D.; Xu, Z.; Ji, J.; Wen, C. Cytokine Storm in COVID-19: The Current Evidence and Treatment Strategies. *Front. Immunol.* **2020**, *11*, 1708. [CrossRef] [PubMed]
32. Lu, R.; Zhang, J.; Sun, W.; Du, G.; Zhou, G. Inflammation-related cytokines in oral lichen planus: An overview. *J. Oral Pathol. Med.* **2015**, *44*, 1–14. [CrossRef]
33. Cerqueira, J.D.M.; Moura, J.R.; Arsati, F.; Lima-Arsati, Y.B.O.; Bittencourt, R.A.; Freitas, V.S. Psychological disorders and oral lichen planus: A systematic review. *J. Investig. Clin. Dent.* **2018**, *9*, e12363. [CrossRef]
34. Ivanovski, K.; Nakova, M.; Warburton, G.; Pesevska, S.; Filipovska, A.; Nares, S.; Nunn, M.E.; Angelova, D.; Angelov, N. Psychological profile in oral lichen planus. *J. Clin. Periodontol.* **2005**, *32*, 1034–1040. [CrossRef] [PubMed]
35. Krasowska, D.; Pietrzak, A.; Surdacka, A.; Tuszynska-Bogucka, V.; Janowski, K.; Rolinski, J. Psychological stress, endocrine and immune response in patients with lichen planus. *Int. J. Dermatol.* **2008**, *47*, 1126–1134. [CrossRef] [PubMed]
36. Stein, D.J.; Szatmari, P.; Gaebel, W.; Berk, M.; Vieta, E.; Maj, M.; de Vries, Y.A.; Roest, A.M.; de Jonge, P.; Maercker, A.; et al. Mental, behavioral and neurodevelopmental disorders in the ICD-11: An international perspective on key changes and controversies. *BMC Med.* **2020**, *18*, 21. [CrossRef]
37. Routray, S.; Mishra, P. A probable surge in oral lichen planus cases under the aura of coronavirus in females in India. *Oral Oncol.* **2020**, *109*, 104714. [CrossRef]
38. van der Meij, E.H.; van der Waal, I. Lack of clinicopathologic correlation in the diagnosis of oral lichen planus based on the presently available diagnostic criteria and suggestions for modifications. *J. Oral Pathol. Med.* **2003**, *32*, 507–512. [CrossRef]
39. van der Meij, E.H.; Schepman, K.P.; Plonait, D.R.; Axell, T.; van der Waal, I. Interobserver and intraobserver variability in the clinical assessment of oral lichen planus. *J. Oral Pathol. Med.* **2002**, *31*, 95–98. [CrossRef]
40. Burgos-Blasco, P.; Fernandez-Nieto, D.; Selda-Enriquez, G.; Melian-Olivera, A.; De Perosanz-Lobo, D.; Dominguez-Santas, M.; Alonso-Castro, L. COVID-19: A possible trigger for oral lichen planus? *Int. J. Dermatol.* **2021**, *60*, 882–883. [CrossRef]
41. Diaz-Guimaraens, B.; Dominguez-Santas, M.; Suarez-Valle, A.; Fernandez-Nieto, D.; Jimenez-Cauhe, J.; Ballester, A. Annular lichen planus associated with coronavirus SARS-CoV-2 disease (COVID-19). *Int. J. Dermatol.* **2021**, *60*, 246–247. [CrossRef] [PubMed]
42. Saleh, W.; Shawky, E.; Halim, G.A.; Ata, F. Oral lichen planus after COVID-19, a case report. *Ann. Med. Surg.* **2021**, *72*, 103051. [CrossRef] [PubMed]
43. Alabdulaaly, L.; Sroussi, H.; Epstein, J.B. New onset and exacerbation of oral lichenoid mucositis following SARS-CoV-2 infection or vaccination. *Oral Dis.* **2022**, *28* (Suppl. 2), 2563–2567. [CrossRef] [PubMed]
44. Zou, H.; Daveluy, S. Lichen planus after COVID-19 infection and vaccination. *Arch. Dermatol. Res.* **2023**, *315*, 139–146. [CrossRef] [PubMed]
45. Nguyen, B.; Perez, A.G.; Elgart, G.W.; Elman, S.A. Lichen planus after COVID-19 infection and vaccination: A systematic review. *J. Eur. Acad. Dermatol. Venereol.* **2023**, *37*, e278–e281. [CrossRef] [PubMed]

Disclaimer/Publisher's Note: The statements, opinions and data contained in all publications are solely those of the individual author(s) and contributor(s) and not of MDPI and/or the editor(s). MDPI and/or the editor(s) disclaim responsibility for any injury to people or property resulting from any ideas, methods, instructions or products referred to in the content.

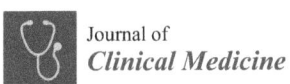

Systematic Review

Subgingival Use of Air-Polishing Powders: Status of Knowledge: A Systematic Review

Dorin Nicolae Gheorghe [1,*,†], Francesco Bennardo [2,*], Margarita Silaghi [3,†], Dora-Maria Popescu [1], George-Alexandru Maftei [4], Marilena Bătăiosu [5,†] and Petra Surlin [1]

[1] Department of Periodontology, Research Center of Periodontal-Systemic Interactions, Faculty of Dental Medicine, University of Medicine and Pharmacy of Craiova, 200349 Craiova, Romania; popescu131@yahoo.com (D.-M.P.); surlinpetra@gmail.com (P.S.)
[2] Department of Health Sciences, School of Dentistry, Magna Graecia University of Catanzaro, 88100 Catanzaro, Italy
[3] Faculty of Dental Medicine, University of Medicine and Pharmacy of Craiova, 200349 Craiova, Romania; margaritasil@outlook.com.gr
[4] Department of Dento-Alveolar Surgery and Oral Pathology, "Grigore T. Popa" University of Medicine and Pharmacy, 700115 Iași, Romania; george-alexandru.maftei@umfiasi.ro
[5] Department of Pedodontics, University of Medicine and Pharmacy of Craiova, 200349 Craiova, Romania; marilena.bataiosu@umfcv.ro
* Correspondence: dorin.gheorghe@umfcv.ro (D.N.G.); francesco.bennardo@unicz.it (F.B.)
† These authors contributed equally to this work.

Abstract: Effective subgingival biofilm removal is crucial for achieving positive and stable outcomes in periodontal therapy, forming an indispensable part of any periodontal treatment approach. The development of air-polishing tools has emerged as a promising alternative to hand and ultrasonic scalers for dental biofilm removal. The objective of this systematic review was to assess existing literature regarding the subgingival use of various types of air-polishing powders, as an effective method of subgingival biofilm control. For this, 55 articles on this subjected were sourced from searched databases and subjected to an evaluation process of their contained information, which was subsequently structured and compiled into this manuscript. The existing literature acknowledges that good subgingival biofilm control is essential for the success of periodontal therapy, including through subgingival air-polishing, as an adjunctive procedure. This approach has the potential to enhance patient comfort during and after subgingival mechanical plaque removal, thereby mitigating damage to periodontal structures. Consequently, it may lead to improved healing capabilities within the periodontal tissues and the formation of a more stable reparative gingival junctional epithelium.

Keywords: periodontal; air-polishing; subgingival; periodontal therapy; glycine; erythritol

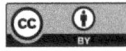

1. Introduction

Periodontitis is a chronic and multifactorial inflammatory condition characterized by the gradual loss of teeth-supporting structures, including alveolar bone and the periodontal ligament, resulting from the accumulation of dental plaque or biofilm [1]. Typical clinical signs of periodontitis include gingival inflammation, radiographic evidence of alveolar bone loss, clinical attachment loss, deep probing depths, bleeding on probing, mobility, and pathologic migration [2]. The staging system for periodontitis categorizes the disease into four stages (stage I, stage II, stage III, and IV) based on the severity, complexity, extent, and distribution of the disease, as determined based on clinical attachment loss, radiographic bone loss, and tooth loss [3]. The grading system (grade A, grade B, grade C) reflects the biological aspects of the infection, such as indicators or risks of rapid disease progression, anticipated treatment outcomes, and consequences for systemic health [4]. The development of this new classification system has been the first step towards the implementation of a pan-European clinical guideline for the treatment of stage 1–3 and stage

4 periodontitis [3]. Thus, the guideline issued by the European Federation of Periodontology offers clinicians valuable recommendations for the treatment of periodontitis, using both non-surgical and surgical means. Despite the different treatment options, the guideline emphasizes the paramount role of efficient biofilm control [4]. Consequently, this could be achieved through the subgingival use of air-polishing, as an adjunctive procedure to subgingival instrumentation.

The primary causative factor of periodontitis is the accumulation of dental biofilm. However, the disease pathogenesis is multifactorial and involves complex interactions among specific bacterial infections (red-complex bacteria, including *Porphyromonas gingivalis*, *Tannerella forsythia*, and *Treponema denticola*, which are predominantly found in deep periodontal pockets), dysregulated host immune responses, and environmental factors, such as smoking [5]. These interrelated factors contribute to the progression of the disease through intricate and dynamic interactions [6].

Smoking represents the most significant environmental risk factor for periodontitis. Individuals who smoke exhibit a higher prevalence and quantity of red-complex periodontal bacteria within their subgingival biofilm when compared to nonsmokers or former smokers [7,8]. Additionally, smoking has been implicated in the impairment of host immune cell function, particularly that of neutrophils, which increases susceptibility to periodontitis [9]. Both active periodontal therapy and long-term maintenance periodontal therapy are affected by the adverse effects of smoking. Therefore, it is crucial for patients to be continually reminded of the importance of smoking cessation in achieving effective periodontitis care [10].

The development of air-polishing tools has emerged as a viable alternative to hand and ultrasonic scalers for the removal of dental biofilm [11,12]. These tools function by projecting a stream of compressed air, mixed with water and abrasive particles such as sodium bicarbonate, glycine, trehalose, and erythritol, onto the tooth surface, effectively eliminating the biofilm [13,14]. Unlike hand and ultrasonic instruments, air-polishing equipment only removes biofilm, reducing clinical time and causing less discomfort to patients. Air-polishing can be used alone or in combination with hand instrumentation to eliminate residual pockets during initial or supportive periodontal therapy [15].

The food industry has embraced erythritol, an alcohol sugar, as an artificial sweetener [16]. This sugar substitute is not metabolized after consumption and is excreted intact in urine, making it a safe daily dietary option [17,18]. Erythritol has a sweet taste, which makes it safe for use in the oral cavity, and it is well-tolerated by individuals [18]. Additionally, erythritol is not cariogenic, which means that it does not contribute to tooth decay [19,20]. Although erythritol has limitations in removing large and firmly attached deposits of calculus and other hard substances, it is a suitable alternative to supportive periodontal therapy when used as an adjuvant to active periodontal therapy [21,22]. Moreover, erythritol exhibits antimicrobial properties that inhibit the growth of periodontal infections, as suggested by research [23].

The objective of this review was to address three main questions. Firstly, the review aimed to determine whether subgingival air-polishing is a viable alternative to ultrasonic scalers or whether it is more effective when used in combination with other tools. Secondly, the review sought to identify the most effective and least traumatic airflow powder for subgingival air-polishing. Finally, the review aimed to assess whether subgingival air-polishing can be safely used on both natural teeth and implant structures.

2. Materials and Methods

This systematic review adhered to the Preferred Reporting Items for Systematic Review and Meta-Analyses (PRISMA) guidelines and followed a PICO framework to answer the research questions (Figure 1).

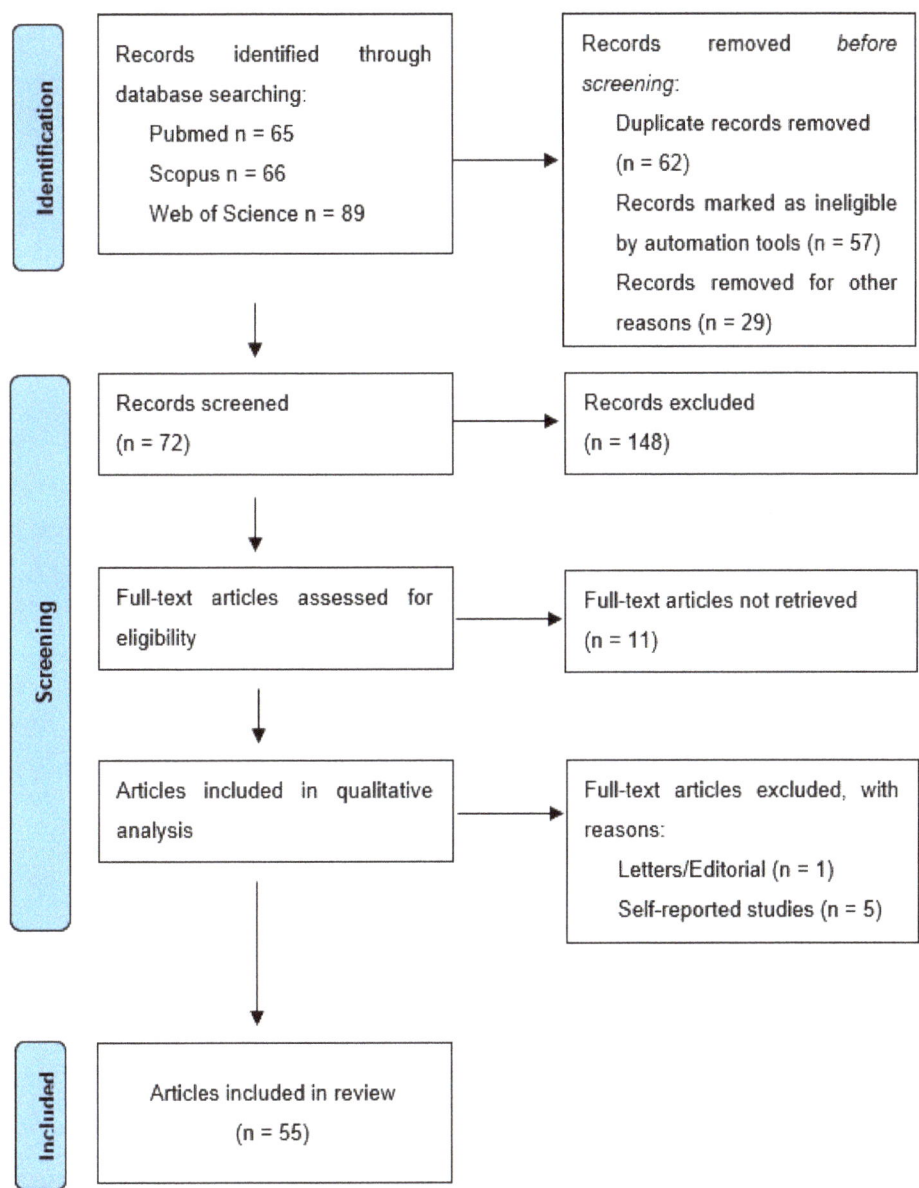

Figure 1. PRISMA flow diagram.

2.1. PICO Questions

The PICO question for this systematic review is as follows: "In patients with periodontal disease, can professional-mechanical plaque removal with sub-gingival air-polishing have the same efficiency as ultrasonic devices for effective control of subgingival biofilm deposits during periodontal therapy?" (Population: patients with periodontal disease; intervention: professional-mechanical plaque removal with subgingival air-polishing; comparison: ultrasonic subgingival professional mechanical-plaque removal; outcome: effective control of subgingival biofilm deposits.)

2.2. Search Strategy

To conduct this review, the authors (two independent researchers, M.S. and D.N.G.) performed an electronic search of relevant scientific databases using PubMed, Web of Science, and Scopus, limiting results to papers published between 1990 and 2022. The search, performed from January to February 2023, was conducted using keywords, such as "periodontitis", "periimplantitis", "subgingival air polishing", "glycine powder air-polishing", "GPAP", "trehalose powder air-polishing", "TPAP", "erythritol powder air-polishing", "EPAP", and "air polishing devices". (Table 1) The papers included for future analysis included randomized clinical trials (RCTs) or controlled clinical trials (CCTs), clinical trials, transversal and cohort studies, case reports, and meta-analyses.

Table 1. Terms used in the research.

Database	Key Word Search
PUBMED	("glycine powder, air-polishing"[Mesh]) AND "Periodontitis"[Mesh]; ("erythritol powder, air-polishing"[Mesh]) AND "Periodontal Diseases"[Mesh]; ("trehalose powder, air-polishing"[Mesh]) AND "Periodontal Status"[Mesh]; ("air-polishing, device"[Mesh]) AND "Periodontitis"[Mesh]; ("subgingival, air-polishing"[Mesh]) AND "Periimplantitis"[Mesh];
Web of Science	TS = ("subgingival air-polishing") AND TS = ("Periodontal Diseases"); TS = ("subgingival air-polishing") AND TS = ("Periodontitis"); TS = ("subgingival air-polishing") AND TS = ("Periimplantitis").
SCOPUS	ALL("Subgingival air-polishing") AND ALL("Periodontal Diseases"); ALL("Subgingival air-polishing") AND ALL("Periodontitis"); TITLE-ABS-KEY("Subgingival air-polishing") AND TITLE-ABS-KEY("Periodontal Diseases"); TITLE-ABS-KEY("Subgingival air-polishing") AND TITLE-ABS-KEY("Periimplantitis").

2.3. Exclusion Criteria for Studies

Some articles were excluded based on the following criteria: studies with outcomes and conclusions that were not relevant to the main goal of this review; studies with limited follow-up periods; studies that did not involve the type of interventions being investigated in this review; monographs; letters to the editor, due to the low grade of evidence or absence of a peer-reviewing process.

2.4. Information Extraction and Review Structuring

The risk of bias was appreciated using the JADAD modified scale, with only papers scoring a minimum of grade 4 being further processed. After carefully selecting relevant articles, the information was extracted (by two independent researchers, M.S. and D.N.G., and a mediator, F.B.) and then organized into three parts for this review. The first part included studies that compared the efficiency of air-polishing powders to ultrasonic root smoothing, in addition to evaluating the abrasiveness of air-polishing powders on tooth tissues. The second part focused on the efficiency of various types of air-polishing powders for controlling subgingival biofilm formation on both tooth surfaces and implants. Finally, the third part examined the limitations of using subgingival air-polishing alone or in combination with other therapies, such as SRP and ultrasonic devices. The registration of the review was not possible, as data extraction and review structuring had already been initiated at the time of the attempted registration.

3. Results

3.1. Basics of Periodontal Therapy

3.1.1. Patient Motivation and Education

The initial stage of cause-related therapy involves educating patients about the primary etiological factor of periodontal disease: the accumulation of plaque both above and below the gumline [24]. This education is essential for enhancing patients' comprehension of the disease and empowering them to effectively manage and prevent it [25,26]. Enhancing oral care practices at home holds significant importance in the prevention of periodontal disease, successful periodontal therapy, and the sustained maintenance of positive outcomes. Emphasizing the significance of meticulous home maintenance should remain a central focus throughout all stages of periodontal therapy [27].

3.1.2. Professional Mechanical Plaque Removal

Professional mechanical plaque removal, as part of the secondary prevention of periodontitis (PMPR+), entails the regular removal of the subgingival plaque and calculus, accompanied by subgingival debridement down to the depth of the sulcus/pocket [28]. This procedure constitutes a crucial element of supportive periodontal therapy (SPT), which should encompass various components: an evaluation of oral hygiene practices, motivational and instructional guidance, counseling for smoking cessation, management of co-existing health conditions, and promotion of healthy lifestyles [28,29]. Furthermore, a comprehensive periodontal examination should be performed to detect early indications of deepening pockets (pocket depth ≥ 5 mm) that necessitate active periodontal intervention [30].

3.1.3. Adjunctive Procedures

Scaling and root planing (SRP) are performed in areas where the periodontal probing depth measures 5 mm or more [28]. In conjunction with SRP, active carious lesions should be addressed, irreparable teeth should be extracted, and local contributing factors need to be managed [31,32].

As an adjunct to SRP for patients with moderate-to-severe periodontitis, systemic antibiotics can be employed [28,33]. The benefits of antibiotic use encompass decreased bleeding upon probing, a lower prevalence of lingering periodontal pockets, and the enhanced closure of such pockets [34]. The most notable advantage was evident with amoxicillin and metronidazole, administered at the highest effective dosage for the shortest feasible duration to mitigate the risk of antibiotic resistance. It is important to note that there are insufficient data to establish the superiority of any specific dosing regimen [35].

3.1.4. Periodontal Reevaluation

Following the initial scaling and root planing, a re-evaluation should be conducted within four to six weeks to assess the extent of improvement [28]. This process entails updating the periodontal charting and comparing it to the original charting. Additionally, it is crucial to assess the patient's adherence to the prescribed at-home oral care routine. In cases of relatively shallow probing depths (1–5 mm), non-surgical interventions, including periodic periodontal maintenance therapy, repeated root planing as required, and consistent encouragement of home care, may be considered [36].

However, for sites with deeper probing depths (≥ 6 mm), the effectiveness of subgingival calculus removal diminishes, and surgical periodontal therapy might be recommended. It is important to carefully evaluate each case to determine the most appropriate course of action for optimal periodontal health [36].

3.2. Subgingival Use of Air-Polishing Powders

3.2.1. Effectiveness of Subgingival Air-Polishing

In a study conducted by Wenzler et al., subgingival air-polishing powders based on glycine and trehalose were found to possess antimicrobial properties capable of reducing periopathogenic bacteria, such as *Porphyromonas gingivalis* and *Tannerella forsythia* [37]. Comparing air-polishing using the trehalose powder to sonic scalers, a study by Kruse et al. revealed that it was equally effective while causing less discomfort and presenting a lower risk of damaging the tooth structure [38].

For the removal of biofilm in patients with periodontal pockets up to 5 mm, low-abrasive glycine powder can prove effective when used in conjunction with hand instruments or scalers. This treatment is considered comfortable and safe not only for periodontitis and peri-implantitis, but also in the fields of operative dentistry and orthodontics [39,40]. While this article primarily focuses on the air-polishing powder, it gives comparatively less emphasis on the device type. However, Kruse et al. cast doubt on the efficacy of trehalose powder in effectively removing subgingival biofilm, as their study found it had no impact on the microbiome of the regrown biofilm [38]. In a study by Sekino et al., it was observed that inflammation could still persist even in cases of supportive periodontal therapy when air-polishing with glycine powder and a special subgingival application nozzle was employed at 30-day intervals [41].

Regarding peri-implantitis, treatment with glycine air-polishing (GPAP) can be effective, although Jiang and Tong suggest that the improvement might be short-term [42]. Jing et al. concluded that subgingival glycine air-polishing, ultrasonic scaling, and 0.12% chlorhexidine rinsing were equally effective in treating early peri-implant diseases, with early treatment potentially being more effective in controlling inflammation [43]. Using air-polishing as the primary treatment without combining it with scaling and root planing in cases with a probing depth ≥ 6 mm may yield a successful short-term gain in the clinical attachment level (CAL), according to Schlagenhauf et al. [44]. Petersilka et al. noted that using GPAP alone does not improve the clinical outcome of periodontal maintenance compared to mechanical plaque removal [45]. Furthermore, using GPAP to address furcation defects appears to be contraindicated [45].

Zhao et al. indicated that air-polishing with 65 μm glycine powder is comparable to ultrasonic scaling combined with polishing paste in terms of clinical effects, but it should be limited to patients with shallow pockets and no visible tooth calculus [46]. Petersilka et al. demonstrated that the low-abrasive air-polishing powder is superior to curettes for removing subgingival plaque at interdental locations with probing depths up to 5 mm during periodontal maintenance therapy [40]. According to Laleman et al., no specific treatment demonstrates a preferable therapeutic advantages or significant microbiological variations, but methods, like laser therapy, photodynamic therapy, or air-polishing, cause less discomfort compared to hand- and/or (ultra)sonic instrumentation [47].

Bühler et al. suggested that powders containing glycine lead to less discomfort when performing both supra- and subgingival air-polishing as part of non-surgical periodontal therapy [48]. Petersilka et al. found that the innovative low-abrasive air-polishing powder is more effective than curettes for removing subgingival plaque from pockets that are 3–5 mm deep during supportive periodontal therapy and provides higher patient comfort [39]. Finally, according to Wennström et al., air-polishing was perceived as less uncomfortable during treatment compared to ultrasonic debridement [49]. Both methods significantly reduced BOP, PPD, and attachment loss at two months after treatment [49].

According to Lu et al., supragingival glycine air-polishing consistently proves effective in removing dental plaque biofilm during the maintenance phase, suggesting that a three-month interval may be appropriate for pockets no deeper than 5 mm [50]. Seidel et al. found that while powered scalers used in conventional mechanical debridement were the most efficient, air-polishing was faster [51]. The findings from Zhu et al. suggest that GPAP may have the potential to replace conventional treatments for gingival inflammation due to its potential for quicker treatment and reduced discomfort [52]. However, higher-quality studies are still necessary to comprehensively assess its effects [52].

The study conducted by Kargas et al. did not establish the superiority of GPAP over SRP or subgingival ultrasonic scaling as sole treatments, based on clinical or microbiological data [53]. Furthermore, research by Petersilka et al. provides additional evidence of the safety of GPAP, demonstrating that it results in less gingival erosion than sodium bicarbonate air-polishing (SBAP) or hand instrumentation [54]. Zhang et al. found that local periodontal therapy has a short-term impact on blood microbiota stability. Full-mouth SRP followed by adjunctive GPAP appears to be a potential method to reduce bacterial entry into the bloodstream during the procedure [55]. While SRP is effective in treating halitosis and periodontitis, using GPAP with mechanical instruments does not improve periodontal or halitosis characteristics, as reported by Caygur et al. [56].

In an in vitro investigation, Poornima et al. determined that hand root surface smoothing with curettes is more effective than ultrasonic root smoothing [57]. The addition of GPAP for 5 s to hand scaling or ultrasonic scaling during periodontal maintenance therapy improves the smoothness of the root surface. Both ultrasonic scaling (US) and air-polishing (AP) treatments effectively reduce the pathogenicity of the subgingival microbiome by lowering microbial diversity, decreasing the proportion of microbiota associated with periodontitis, and inhibiting pathogenic metabolism [57]. Lu et al. reported that this contributes to maintaining a balanced subgingival community and a stable periodontal state over a three-month maintenance period [58]. According to Flemmig et al., GPAP is more effective than SRP at removing subgingival biofilm in moderate-to-deep periodontal pockets [59]. Full-mouth GPAP is well-tolerated and can lead to a positive change in the oral microbiota [59].

3.2.2. Differences in the Type of Powder

According to a study by Jentsch et al., the use of erythritol air-polishing powder as an adjunct to subgingival instrumentation does not supplementarily reduce bleeding on probing (BOP) [60]. However, it may exert positive effects, such as reducing the frequency of residual periodontal pockets with a probing depth of 5 mm [60]. Resnik et al. discovered that during the initial phase of non-surgical periodontal therapy, subgingival airflow therapy combined with an erythritol powder air-polishing device (EPAP) might benefit patients with initially deep pockets (probing pocket depth of 5.5 mm) [61]. Both treatment methods significantly reduced periodontitis-related bacterial species, as well as BoP, PPD, and the relative attachment level. No significant differences were found between the various treatment methods [61].

Another argument supporting the effectiveness of less traumatic air-polishing technology with new, less abrasive powders is presented by Moëne et al. [62]. However, they noted that there is limited short-term research on this topic. In contrast, Mensi et al. [63] found no significant additional advantage for patients with periodontitis at stages 3–4. According to Flemmig et al., subgingival biofilm in periodontal pockets with an APD $\leq$ 3 mm can be effectively removed by GPAP for 5 s per surface [15]. Hu et al. suggest that subgingival air-polishing and conventional manual scaling can improve supportive periodontal therapy in teeth with probing depths of 3 to 6 mm, but there is no discernible difference between the two modes [64].

Air-polishing with erythritol may cause a slight loss of dentin, influenced by the environment, as indicated by Kröger et al. [65]. Applying erythritol powder with an air-polishing tool seems to be a promising method for repeatedly instrumenting residual pockets during SPT, according to Hägi et al. [66]. Ulvik et al. suggest that both erythritol air-polishing and traditional mechanical debridement contribute to therapeutic improvements in mandibular furcations [67]. However, at the 6-month follow-up, traditional debridement was found to be more effective in terms of the clinical attachment level. Nonetheless, patients reported that they found the erythritol air-polishing device to be the most comfortable treatment [67].

Zhang et al. found that full-mouth SRP with or without GPAP had comparable effects on clinical, inflammatory, and microbiological outcomes in treating untreated periodontitis [68]. Similarly, Hägi et al. reported that subgingival EPAP is safe and provides similar clinical and microbiological results to SRP [69]. On the other hand, Simon et al. demonstrated that GPAP causes less gingival erosion than SBAP or ultrasonic instruments and improves plaque and gingival index scores [70].

In vitro studies have shown that subgingival air-polishing powders can affect wound healing, cell viability, morphology, and proliferation. The cytotoxicity of erythritol/clorhexidine (CHX) powder is primarily caused by the CHX component and can directly affect gingival fibroblasts [71]. Different polyols have varying impacts on dental health, with erythritol showing more effectiveness than sorbitol and xylitol in enhancing oral health [72]. Recurrent subgingival debridement using APDs during SPT produced similar clinical outcomes, but better patient comfort compared to traditional therapies, though there is insufficient evidence to support their superiority for implant maintenance [73]. An in vitro study [74] revealed comparable root surface loss with glycine powders, but spray patterns and tip apertures can influence the powder performance between units. Cementum loss may be higher than that with traditional biofilm removal techniques, but more research is needed. Finally, according to Bains et al. [75], GPAP causes less gingival erosion than manual instrumentation or sodium bicarbonate air-polishing, but selective polishing data for teeth remain convincing despite advancements in the polishing technology.

According to Schulz et al., all therapeutic treatments tested, including full-mouth scaling (FMS), full-mouth disinfection (FMD), and adjuvant erythritol air-polishing (FM-DAP), were effective in reducing harmful bacteria in the short term [76]. However, after six months, there was a decline in the microbiological profile, and clinical outcomes either improved or remained stable. Studying subgingival bacteria may aid in evaluating periodontal treatment and implementing personalized therapy. Air-polishing therapy is the most effective treatment for cleaning implant surfaces during biofilm removal, and a 45 s treatment period significantly improves its performance, as stated by Mensi et al. [77].

3.2.3. Cellular and Tissular Impact

A systematic review conducted by Nascimento et al. found that air-polishing and hand or ultrasonic instruments have similar effectiveness in controlling biofilm formation and reducing periodontal inflammation [78]. This suggests that air-polishing can be considered an alternative for biofilm control [79]. Another systematic review suggests that there is no significant difference in the clinical outcomes of subgingival air-polishing and ultrasonic debridement [80]. However, the review acknowledges the limited evidence and calls for further long-term studies 80]. Moene et al. found that while a new subgingival air-polishing device was more time-saving and acceptable for patients, it did not have any microbiological advantages over traditional scaling and root planing (SRP) treatment [62].

Cannabidiol (CBD)-supplemented polishing powder, according to Stahl et al., can assist in the efficient removal and death of dental plaque bacteria during the polishing procedure and can be added as an enhancing supplement to currently available polishing powders [81]. Di Tinco et al. found that both powders are suitable for boosting the biocompatibility of titanium implants, since they exhibit excellent in vitro cleaning potential in the early stages and have no detrimental effects on human dental pulp stem cells' osteogenic differentiation process [82].

In vitro research by Weusmann et al. suggests that powders for air-polishing tools that can be applied subgingivally may control cytokine expression, cell survival, and proliferation [83]. The study indicates that these powders may affect growth factors through direct cell actions, and trehalose seems to be more inert than glycine powder. Even though some patients with periodontitis can regain their periodontal health, the majority of them will always be at risk of developing the condition [84]. Accurately assessing a patient's periodontal risk will allow for the proper monitoring of those who have undergone appropriate periodontal disease treatment.

Air-polishing was found to be superior to ultrasonic scalers in preserving cementum, while hand curettes were the most effective at removing cementum [85]. In a randomized controlled trial, periodontal therapy with adjunctive photodynamic therapy (aPDT) showed improved clinical outcomes and decreased levels of pathogenic bacteria in the subgingival biofilm when compared to scaling and root planing alone [86]. The effect was noted to be more pronounced in patients with deeper pockets and higher levels of initial bacterial colonization [86]. According to Dalvi et al., photobiomodulation therapy (PBMT) has shown promise as an adjunctive therapy for periodontitis. PBMT can reduce inflammation, promote tissue healing, and decrease the levels of harmful bacteria [87]. However, more high-quality clinical studies are required to confirm its effectiveness and determine the optimal parameters for treatment [87].

In a study by Persson et al., the air-abrasive group showed a reduction in *P. aeruginosa*, *S. aureus*, and *S. anaerobius*, while the laser group saw a decrease in *Fusobacterium* spp. after 1 month of treatment [88]. However, neither approach resulted in a significant decrease in bacterial numbers over a 6-month period, and there were no substantial clinical improvements observed [88]. McCollum et al. used a digitizer and software to calculate the percentage of the total abutment surface area covered by plaque, distinguishing between subgingival and supragingival plaque [89]. The study found that the air-powder abrasive had a total mean percent plaque surface area of 52.06%, while the plastic scalers had 55.29% [89,90].

4. Future Perspectives

While the current body of research provides valuable insights, there remain areas that warrant further exploration. Long-term studies, standardized protocols, and investigations into patient-centered outcomes are crucial to establishing the sustained efficacy and patient preference for air-polishing. Additionally, research into the effects of air-polishing on the oral microbiome, implant maintenance, and its potential combination with other therapies will contribute to a comprehensive understanding of its applications and benefits (Table 2).

As the dental community seeks innovative and patient-friendly approaches to periodontal care, air-polishing emerges as a promising tool that aligns with these goals. With continued research, the refinement of techniques, and collaboration among researchers, practitioners, and regulatory bodies, the future of air-polishing in periodontal therapy holds the potential to enhance patient outcomes and contribute to the advancement of modern periodontology. This could be achieved through the following:

1. Long-term comparative studies: conducting more long-term comparative studies to evaluate the sustained effects of air-polishing versus traditional methods, like ultrasonic scaling or hand instrumentation. This can provide a better understanding of the extended benefits and potential drawbacks of air-polishing over time.
2. Optimal parameters and techniques: further investigation into optimal air-polishing parameters, such as powder types, particle sizes, pressure, and angles, to maximize biofilm removal efficacy while minimizing any potential adverse effects on tooth surfaces or soft tissues.
3. Standardization of protocols: development of standardized protocols and guidelines for incorporating air-polishing into periodontal therapy, considering factors, like patient-specific conditions, disease severity, and treatment intervals. This can ensure consistency and reproducibility across different clinical settings.
4. Patient-centered outcomes: exploration of patient-centered outcomes beyond clinical parameters, such as patient comfort, satisfaction, and quality of life, to assess the overall acceptability and preference for air-polishing compared to traditional methods (such as the Dental Visit Satisfaction Scale, Dental Satisfaction Questionnaire or Patient Assessment Questionnaire) [91].
5. Subgingival applications: continued research into the safety, efficacy, and long-term effects of subgingival air-polishing, especially in deeper pockets and challenging-to-reach areas. This may involve investigating different nozzle designs, powder formulations, and application techniques.
6. Combination therapies: investigating the potential synergistic effects of combining air-polishing with other adjunctive therapies, such as photodynamic therapy, laser therapy, or antimicrobial agents, to enhance biofilm removal and overall treatment outcomes.

7. Impact on the microbiome: further studies on the impact of air-polishing on the oral microbiome, both short-term and long-term, to better understand how it influences the balance of beneficial and pathogenic microorganisms in the periodontal environment.
8. Implant maintenance: exploring the application of air-polishing for implant maintenance, including its effects on peri-implant health, biofilm removal from implant surfaces, and its potential role in preventing peri-implant diseases.
9. Personalized treatment approaches: Research into the development of personalized treatment approaches that consider individual patient characteristics, genetics, and the microbiome composition to tailor air-polishing techniques and protocols for optimized outcomes.
10. Education and training: enhanced education and training for dental professionals on the proper use of air-polishing equipment, techniques, and patient selection, ensuring its safe and effective integration into clinical practice.
11. Economic considerations: investigating the cost-effectiveness of air-polishing compared to traditional methods, considering factors, such as reduced chair time, patient satisfaction, and long-term maintenance requirements.
12. Regulatory approval and guidelines: collaborating with regulatory bodies and dental associations to establish clear guidelines and recommendations for the use of air-polishing in periodontal therapy, ensuring patient safety and standardized practices.

As research and technology continue to advance, these perspectives can help shape the future of air-polishing in periodontal therapy, leading to improved patient care and enhanced treatment outcomes [92,93].

Table 2. Synopsis of reviewed papers in alphabetical order (GPAP = glycine powder air-polishing, EPAP = erythritol powder air-polishing, TPAP = trehalose powder air-polishing).

Study	Air-Polishing Powder	Air-Polishing Device	On Teeth/On Implants	Findings
(Bains, et al., 2009) Review, India [75]	GPAP	-	Teeth	GPAP, which has recently been shown to remove subgingival biofilm, causes less gingival erosion than manual instrumentation or NaHCO(3) air-polishing. Despite the development of recent polishing advancements, data supporting the selective polishing of teeth remains persuasive.
(Bozbay, et al., 2018) Randomized Controlled Trial, Italy [85]	-	-	Teeth	Air-polishing was superior than ultrasonic scaler devices in cementum preservation, whereas hand curettes were the most efficient cementum-removal tools.
(Bühler, et al., 2016) Systematic Review, Switzerland [48]	GPAP	Electro Medical Systems (EMS)® Nyon, Switzerland	Teeth	When performing supra- and subgingival air-polishing as part of non-surgical periodontal therapy, using powders containing glycine, there seems to be less discomfort.
(Caygur, et al., 2017) Randomized Controlled Trial, Turkey [56]	GPAP	Air-Flow Perio® Powder; Electro Medical Systems® Nyon, Switzerland	Teeth	Treatment of halitosis and periodontitis with SRP is successful. However, employing GPAP in conjunction with mechanical instruments does not improve periodontal or halitosis characteristics.
(de Cock, et al., 2016) Review, Belgium [72]	EPAP	-	Teeth	The evidence in the research shows that erythritol is more effective in preserving and enhancing oral health than sorbitol and xylitol.
(Di Tinco, et al., 2021) In vitro, Italy [82]	GPAP TPAP	-	Implant	Both powders are suitable for boosting the biocompatibility of titanium implants since they both exhibit excellent in vitro cleaning potential in the early stages and have no detrimental impacts on hDPSCs' osteogenic differentiation process.
(Divnic-Resnik, et al., 2022) Randomized Controlled Trial, Australia [61]	EPAP	Air-flow Plus®, EMS, Electro Medical Systems, Nyon, Switzerland	Teeth	Initially deep pockets (PPD 5.5 mm) may benefit from subgingival airflow therapy combined with EPAP during the first phase of non-surgical periodontal therapy.
(Flemmig, et al., 2012) Randomized Controlled Trial, USA [59]	GPAP	EMS Air-Flow®, Electro Medical Systems EMS SA, Nyon, Switzerland	Teeth	Most of the subgingival biofilm in periodontal pockets with an APD ≤3 mm can be effectively removed by GPAP for 5 s per surface.

Table 2. Cont.

Study	Air-Polishing Powder	Air-Polishing Device	On Teeth/On Implants	Findings
(Flemmig, et al., 2015) Randomized Controlled Trial, USA [15]	GPAP	AIR-FLOW PERIO Powder®, E.M.S. Electro Medical Systems, Nyon, Switzerland. AIR-FLOW Master®, E.M.S. Electro Medical Systems. AIR-FLOW PERIO®, E.M.S. Electro Medical Systems.	Teeth	SubGPAP is more effective than SRP at removing subgingival biofilm in moderate-to-deep periodontal pockets. Furthermore, full-mouth GPAP seems to be well tolerated and may lead to a positive change in the oral microbiota.
(Hägi, et al., 2013) Randomized Controlled Trial, Switzerland [66]	EPAP	-	Teeth	A promising method for repeatedly instrumenting leftover pockets during SPT is the erythritol powder applied with an air-polishing tool.
(Hägi, et al., 2015) Randomized Controlled Trial, Switzerland [69]	EPAP GPAP	Air-Flow Master Piezon®, EMS, Nyon, Switzerland Air-Flow Master Piezon®, EMS; Air-Flow Powder Plus® 0.3% CHX, EMS, Nyon, Switzerland	Teeth	Applied ultrasonication and air-polishing with erythritol, as opposed to hand instrumentation, reduce material loss and produce a smooth surface with almost little residual biofilm, which encourages the reattachment of PDL fibroblasts. The subgingival application of EPAP using air-polishing equipment may be considered secure and may provide clinical and microbiologic results that are similar to those of SRP.
(Herr, et al., 2017) In vitro, USA [74]	GPAP	In vitro	Teeth	An evaluation of glycine powders revealed comparable root surface loss. Spray patterns and tip apertures may play a role in variations in powder performance between units. Cementum loss may be larger than that experienced with traditional biofilm-removal techniques, such as curets and ultrasonic scalers, although further investigation is required to confirm this.
(Hu, et al., 2015) Randomized Controlled Trial, China [64]	-	-	Teeth	In teeth with probing depths of 3 to 6 mm, supportive periodontal therapy can be improved clinically with subgingival air-polishing and conventional manual scaling.
(Jentsch, et al., 2020) Randomized Controlled Trial, Germany [60]	EPAP	Hu-Friedy® Manufacturing Co., Chicago, IL, USA and Dentsply Sirona, Bensheim, Germany	Teeth	Compared to subgingival instrumentation alone, decreasing the probing depth, as indicated by the frequency of residual periodontal pockets with PD 5 mm.
(Jiang & Tong, 2019) Clinical Trial, Chi [42]	GPAP	-	Implant	Treatment with air-polishing can be effective, although the improvement is short-term.

Table 2. Cont.

Study	Air-Polishing Powder	Air-Polishing Device	On Teeth/On Implants	Findings
(Jing, et al., 2017) Randomized Controlled Trial, China [43]	GPAP	-	Implant	Based on patients with early peri-implant diseases, the effectiveness of subgingival glycine air-polishing, ultrasonic scaling, and 0.12% chlorhexidine rinsing is similar. The early peri-implant inflammation may be more effectively controlled by the earlier treatment.
(Kargas, et al., 2015) Randomized Controlled Trial, Greece [53]	GPAP	-	Teeth	The study does not demonstrate the superiority of GPAP over SRP or subgingival ultrasonic scaling when used as the sole treatment, based on clinical or microbiological data.
(Kröger, et al., 2020) In vitro, Germany [65]	EPAP	-	Teeth	Depending on the distance, pressure, and angulation of the spray jet to the surface, a slight loss of dentin may occur after air-polishing with erythritol. The quantity of dentin loss is influenced by the environment.
(Kruse, et al., 2019) Randomized Controlled Trial, Germany [38]	TPAP	(1) Lunos® Prophylaxis Powder Perio Combi, DÜRR DENTAL, Bietigheim-Bissingen Germany (2) Perio-Flow® handpiece with Perio-Flow® Nozzle EMS, Nyon, Switzerland (3) Sonic Flex, KaVo, Charlotte, NC, USA	Teeth	Air-polishing to sonic scalers appear to provide an equivalent clinical result, with air-polishing causing less discomfort and less risk of damaging the tooth.
(Laleman, et al., 2017) Review, Belgium [47]	GPAP	-	Teeth	Regarding the therapeutic advantages or microbiological variations, none of these treatments appear to be preferable to any other. However, when compared to hand- and/or (ultra)sonic instrumentation, less treatment discomfort is recorded when employing laser, photodynamic therapy, or air-polishing.
(Lu, et al., 2018) Randomized Controlled Trial, China [50]	GPAP	Air-Flow Polishing Soft®; Air-Flow handy2® Air-Flow Masters® (EMS, Nyon, Switzerland)	Teeth	The removal of subgingival dental plaque biofilm via supragingival glycine air-polishing was consistently effective during the maintenance phase, and three months may be an appropriate maintenance interval for pockets that are no deeper than 5 mm.

Table 2. *Cont.*

Study	Air-Polishing Powder	Air-Polishing Device	On Teeth/On Implants	Findings
(Lu, et al., 2019) Randomized Controlled Trial, China [58]	-	-	Teeth	By reducing microbial diversity, the proportion of microbiota associated with periodontitis, and pathogenic metabolism, treatment with US or AP successfully lowered the pathogenicity of the subgingival microbiome. Over a single maintenance period of three months, it assisted in maintaining a balanced subgingival community and stable periodontal state.
(McCollum, et al., 1992) Comparative Study, USA [89]	flour of pumice	-	Teeth	The percentage of the total abutment surface area that the plaque covered was calculated using a digitizer and software. Subgingival and supragingival plaque were clearly distinguished from one another. Between 52.06% for the air-powder abrasive and 55.29% for the plastic scalers, the total mean percent plaque surface area was measured
(Mensi, et al., 2020) In vitro, Italy [77]	EPAP GPAP	-	Implant	The best treatment for cleaning the implant surface in the ink removal among the four options is air-polishing therapy. Furthermore, air-polishing performed significantly better when the treatment period was increased to 45 s
(Mensi, et al., 2020) Randomized Controlled Trial, Italy [63]	EPAP	Airflow prophylaxis Master®, EMS, Nyon, Switzerland	Teeth	There is no significant additional advantage for periodontitis patients at stages 3–4.
(Mensi, et al., 2017) Clinical Trial, Italy [79]	-	-	Teeth	Clinical outcomes produced by the OSFMI treatment were comparable to those attained with conventional SRP. It is advised for researchers to explore this approach in randomized clinical trials with longer observation times.
(Moene, et al., 2010) Randomized Controlled Trial, Switzerland [62]	GPAP	EMS®, Nyon, Switzerland	Teeth	The use of a new device for subgingival air-polishing was time-saving for patients and also more acceptable. Even so, it was not microbiologically superior to traditional SRP.
(Nascimento, et al., 2021) Review, Denmark [78]	GPAP (10) EPAP (2) TPAP (1)	EMS® Air Flow S1, Nyon, Switzerland	Teeth	Air-polishing is an alternative for biofilm control. The comparation between air-polishing and hand or ultrasonic instruments can be equal in controlling biofilm formation and also reducing periodontal inflammation.

Table 2. Cont.

Study	Air-Polishing Powder	Air-Polishing Device	On Teeth/On Implants	Findings
(Persson, et al., 2011) Randomized Controlled Trial, Sweden [88]	-	-	Teeth	At 1 month, the air-abrasive group had a decrease in P. aeruginosa, S. aureus, and S. anaerobius, whereas the laser group saw a decrease in Fusobacterium spp. Data collected over a six-month period showed that neither approach reduced bacterial numbers. Clinical advancements were not substantial.
(Petersilka, 2011) Review, Germany [92]	GPAP	EMS Airflow S1® and Easy Jet Pro®, Mectron, Munich, Germany	Teeth and implants	For biofilm removal, in periodontal patients with pockets up to 5 mm, low-abrasive glycine powder can be effective but is also needed a hand instrument or scaler. It is considered a comfortable and safe choice for the treatment of both periodontitis and peri-implantitis and it can be useful in operative dentistry, as well as in orthodontics.
(Petersilka, et al., 2003) Clinical Trial, Germany [39]	low-abrasive air-polishing powders	EMS Air Flow S1®, EMS, Nyon, Switzerland.	Teeth	When it comes to removing subgingival plaque at interdental locations with up to 5 mm of probing depth in PMT, the innovative low-abrasive air-polishing powder is superior to curets.
(Petersilka, et al., 2003) Clinical Trial, Germany [40]	Sodium bicarbonate Powder D	EMS Air Flow S1®, EMS, Nyon, Switzerland	Teeth	The innovative low-abrasive air-polishing powder provides higher patient comfort and is more effective than curettes in removing subgingival plaque from pockets that are 3–5 mm deep during supportive periodontal therapy.
(Petersilka, et al., 2008) Randomized Controlled Trial, Germany [54]	GPAP	EMS AirFlow® Powder, EMS, Nyon, Switzerland	Teeth	The research supported the safety of this debridement method by showing that GPAP causes less gingival erosion than SBAP or hand instrumentation.
(Petersilka, et al., 2020) Clinical Trial, Germany [45]	GPAP	-	Teeth Furcation defects	The use of GPAP alone to address furcation defects is contraindicated.
(Poornima, et al., 2019) Comparative Study, India [57]	GPAP	In vitro	Teeth	In this in vitro investigation, hand root surface smoothing with curettes was more effective than ultrasonic root smoothing. During periodontal maintenance therapy, the addition of GPAP for 5 s to hand scaling or ultrasonic scaling increased the smoothness of the root surface.
(Schlagenhauf, et al., 2021) Randomized Controlled Trial, Germany [44]	EPAP	AIRFLOW Prophylaxis Master®, EMS, Nyon, Switzerland	Teeth	In cases with a probing depth ≥ 6 mm, the results are successful only for the short-term gain of CAL.

Table 2. Cont.

Study	Air-Polishing Powder	Air-Polishing Device	On Teeth/On Implants	Findings
(Schulz, et al., 2022) Randomized Controlled Trial, Germany [76]	EPAP	E.M.S.® Electro Medical Systems, Nyon/Switzerland	Teeth	The reduction in harmful germs in the FMS, FMD, and FMDAP groups was linked to the effectiveness of all therapeutic therapies tested three months later. But after six months, they noticed a decline in the microbiological profile and either more improvement or some standstill in the clinical outcomes. A good periodontal treatment evaluation and personalized therapy implementation may be aided by research into the subgingival bacteria.
(Seidel, et al., 2021) Clinical Trial, Germany [51]	GPAP EPAP	PERIOFLOW® handpiece, EMS, Nyon, Switzerland Proxeo ultra®, W&H, Bürmoos, Austria AIR-FLOW PLUS® powder, EMS, Nyon, Switzerland	Teeth	Powered scalers used in conventional mechanical debridement were most efficient, but air-polishing was faster.
(Sekino, et al., 2020) Randomized Controlled Trial, Japan [41]	GPAP	Perio-Flow® Nozzle, EMS, Nyon, Switzerland	Teeth	Inflammation can be present in cases of supportive periodontal therapy, using un special nozzle for subgingival applications with air-polishing.
(Simon, et al., 2015) Randomized Controlled Trial, India [70]	GPAP	EMS—Air Flow classic Powder® Nyon, Switzerland; Dentsply ProphyJet®, Dentsply, York, PA, USA	Teeth	GPAP induces histologically less gingival erosion than SBAP or ultrasonic instruments and leads to clinically substantial improvements in plaque and gingival index scores.
(Stahl, et al., 2020) Clinical Trial, Belgium [81]	+CBD	In vitro	Teeth	In addition to being added as an enhancing supplement to the currently available polishing powders, the CBD (cannabidiol)-supplemented polishing powder can assist in the efficient removal and death of dental plaque bacteria during the polishing procedure.
(Tan, et al., 2022) Meta-analysis, Malaysia [73]	APDs in SPT	-	Implant	There is insufficient evidence to conclude that APDs are superior to conventional therapies for implant maintenance when they are applied repeatedly.

Table 2. Cont.

Study	Air-Polishing Powder	Air-Polishing Device	On Teeth/On Implants	Findings
(Ulvik, et al., 2021) Randomized Controlled Trial, Norway [67]	EPAP	Air-flow powder plus®, EMS, Nyon, Switzerland Air-Flow Master®, EMS, Nyon, Switzerland	Teeth Furcation defects	Erythritol air-polishing and traditional mechanical debridement both assist in therapeutic advancements to the of mandibular furcations. However, a significant difference in the clinical attachment level across treatments was found at 6 months, favoring traditional debridement. The patients thought that the erythritol air-polishing device was the most comfortable treatment.
(Wennström, et al., 2011) Randomized Controlled Trial, Sweden [49]	GPAP	Air-Flows Perio Powder®, EMS, Nyon, Switzerland Air-Flow Masters®, EMS Perio-Flows Nozzle®, EMS EMS Piezon Masters® 400, PerioSlim® tip, EMS, Nyon, Switzerland	Teeth	Both treatment methods significantly decreased the number of periodontitis-related bacterial species both immediately and two days after treatment, in addition to significantly lowering the BoP, PPD, and relative attachment level at two months. At any of the examination periods, there were no statistically significant differences between the various treatment methods. Compared to ultrasonic debridement, air-polishing was perceived as less uncomfortable during treatment.
(Wenzler, et al., 2021) In vitro, Germany [37]	GPAP TPAP	Air-Flow Perio® EMS, Nyon, Switzerland	Teeth	The subgingival air-polishing powders (glycine and trehalose) can, on the one hand, reduce periopathogenic bacteria, such as *Porphyromonas gingivalis* and *Tannerella forsythia*, and also provide an antimicrobial therapy approach.
(Weusmann, et al., 2021) In vitro, Germany [83]	GPAP TPAP	In vitro	Teeth	Powders for air-polishing tools that can be applied subgingivally can control cytokine expression, cell survival, and proliferation. This in vitro research indicates that the aforementioned powders may affect HGF through direct cell actions. When compared to glycine powder, trehalose seems to be more inert.
(Weusmann, et al., 2022) In vitro, Germany [71]	EPAP+CHX	In vitro	Teeth	The cytotoxic effect of erythritol/CHX powder is highly evident and primarily caused by the CHX component. These effects on fibroblasts are apparent and imply that powders applied subgingival have the ability to influence gingival fibroblasts directly.
(Zhang, et al., 2019) Review, China [80]	GPAP EPAP TPAP Sodium Bicarb.	-	Teeth	Neither subgingival air-polishing nor ultrasonic debridement seemed to have superior clinical results.

Table 2. Cont.

Study	Air-Polishing Powder	Air-Polishing Device	On Teeth/On Implants	Findings
(Zhang, et al., 2021) Randomized Controlled Trial, China [55]	GPAP	Air-Flow Polishing® Soft; EMS, Nyon, Switzerland Perio-Flow® Nozzle®, EMS, Switzerland	Teeth	The microbiological effects of full-mouth SRP with and without GPAP in the treatment of untreated periodontitis were substantially comparable.
(Zhang, et al., 2021) Randomized Controlled Trial, China [68]	GPAP	Air-Flow® Polishing Soft Powder; EMS, Nyon, Switzerland Perio-Flow®, Nozzle®, EMS, Switzerland	Teeth	The short-term effects of local periodontal therapy just disturb the stability of the blood microbiota. A possible method to minimize the entrance of bacteria into the bloodstream during the procedure is full-mouth SRP followed by adjunctive GPAP in the treatment of periodontitis.
(Zhao, et al., 2017) Randomized Controlled Trial, China [46]	GPAP	-	Teeth	Air-polishing with 65 μm glycine powder provides clinical effects that are comparable to those of ultrasonic scaling combined with polishing paste. Clinical indications should, however, only be used on patients who have shallow pockets and no visible tooth calculus.
(Zhu, et al., 2021) Meta-analysis, China [52]	GPAP	-	Teeth	The results of this study point to GPAP as a potential replacement for conventional treatments for gingival inflammation since it may do so more quickly and with less discomfort. Studies of a higher caliber are still required to evaluate the effects of GPAP.

5. Conclusions

In conclusion, the evolving field of air-polishing in periodontal therapy holds promise as an effective and less invasive approach for biofilm removal and periodontal health maintenance. A comprehensive review of the literature reveals a growing body of evidence supporting the efficacy of air-polishing in controlling biofilm formation, reducing periodontal inflammation, and contributing to overall periodontal health. Various studies have explored the use of different powders, equipment, and techniques, shedding light on the potential benefits and limitations of this innovative method.

Subgingival air-polishing has been shown to be comparable to traditional methods, such as ultrasonic scaling and hand instrumentation, in terms of clinical outcomes, suggesting that it can be considered a viable alternative or adjunctive therapy for managing periodontal conditions. Furthermore, advancements in powder formulations, nozzle designs, and application protocols continue to refine the practice of air-polishing, contributing to improved patient comfort and satisfaction during treatment.

Author Contributions: Conceptualization, D.N.G. and P.S.; methodology, D.-M.P., M.B. and P.S.; software, G.-A.M.; validation, F.B., D.-M.P. and P.S.; formal analysis, D.N.G. and M.S.; investigation, M.S.; resources, M.B. and G.-A.M.; data curation, D.N.G., M.S. and F.B.; writing—original draft preparation, D.N.G. and M.S.; writing—review and editing, M.B., D.-M.P., F.B., G.-A.M. and P.S.; visualization, D.-M.P. and P.S.; supervision, M.B. and P.S. All authors have read and agreed to the published version of the manuscript.

Funding: This research received no external funding.

Institutional Review Board Statement: Not applicable.

Informed Consent Statement: Not applicable.

Data Availability Statement: Not applicable.

Conflicts of Interest: The authors declare no conflict of interest. There are no financial and commercial conflicts of interest to disclose.

References

1. Hajishengallis, G.; Chavakis, T. Local and Systemic Mechanisms Linking Periodontal Disease and Inflammatory Comorbidities. *Nat. Rev. Immunol.* **2021**, *21*, 426–440. [CrossRef] [PubMed]
2. Lang, N.P.; Bartold, P.M. Periodontal Health. *J. Periodontol.* **2018**, *89*, S9–S16. [CrossRef]
3. Tonetti, M.S.; Greenwell, H.; Kornman, K.S. Staging and Grading of Periodontitis: Framework and Proposal of a New Classification and Case Definition. *J. Periodontol.* **2018**, *89*, S159–S172. [CrossRef] [PubMed]
4. Papapanou, P.N.; Sanz, M.; Buduneli, N.; Dietrich, T.; Feres, M.; Fine, D.H. Periodontitis: Consensus Report of Workgroup 2 of the 2017 World Workshop on the Classification of Periodontal and Peri-Implant Diseases and Conditions. *J. Clin. Periodontol.* **2018**, *45*, S162–S170. [CrossRef]
5. Hajishengallis, G.; Lamont, R.J. Beyond the Red Complex and into More Complexity: The Polymicrobial Synergy and Dysbiosis (PSD) Model of Periodontal Disease Etiology. *Mol. Oral Microbiol.* **2012**, *27*, 409–419. [CrossRef] [PubMed]
6. Pihlstrom, B.L.; Michalowicz, B.S.; Johnson, N.W. Periodontal Diseases. *Lancet* **2005**, *366*, 1809–1820. [CrossRef] [PubMed]
7. Hanioka, T.; Tanaka, M.; Ojima, M.; Yuuki, K.; Mita, H.; Shizukuishi, S. Association of Serum Antibody to *Porphyromonas gingivalis* and Inflammatory Markers with Smoking. *J. Periodontol.* **2011**, *82*, 1597–1604.
8. Holtfreter, B.; Albandar, J.M.; Dietrich, T.; Dye, B.A.; Eaton, K.A.; Eke, P.I.; Tonetti, M.S. Standards for Reporting Chronic Periodontitis Prevalence and Severity in Epidemiologic Studies: Proposed Standards from the Joint EU/USA Periodontal Epidemiology Working Group. *J. Clin. Periodontol.* **2019**, *46*, 303–311. [CrossRef]
9. Leite, F.R.M.; Nascimento, G.G.; Scheutz, F.; López, R.; Dörfer, C.E. The Effect of Smoking on Periodontitis: A Systematic Review and Meta-Regression. *J. Dent.* **2019**, *79*, 1–7. [CrossRef]
10. Huang, R.; Li, M.; Gregory, R.L.; Bélanger, M. Effect of Cigarette Smoke Extract on Growth and Biofilm Formation of *Porphyromonas gingivalis*. *J. Oral Microbiol.* **2019**, *11*, 1608149.
11. Goyal, L.; Tewari, S.; Duhan, J. Air Polishing: A Review. *Int. J. Oral Health Sci.* **2020**, *10*, 1–5.
12. Quirynen, M.; Bollen, C.M.; Vandekerckhove, B.N. Full-Versus Partial-Mouth Disinfection in the Treatment of Periodontal Infections: Short-Term Clinical and Microbiological Observations. *Periodontology 2000* **2009**, *51*, 47–56.
13. Araújo, M.W.; Lopes, A.L.; Elias, C.N.; Ruellas, A.C. Influence of an Air Polishing Protocol with Erythritol on the Mechanical and Morphological Properties of the Root Surface. *J. Periodontol.* **2015**, *86*, 743–751.

14. Sener, B.C.; Ertan, S.; Yıldırım, S.; Türker, A.R. The Effect of Different Air-Polishing Powders on Surface Roughness of Enamel. *Niger. J. Clin. Pract.* **2021**, *24*, 494–501.
15. Flemmig, T.F.; Arushanov, D.; Daubert, D.; Rothen, M.; Mueller, G.; Leroux, B.; Könönen, E. Randomized Controlled Trial Assessing Efficacy and Safety of Glycine Powder Air Polishing Versus Ultrasonic Scaling in Patients with Moderate-to-Advanced Periodontitis. *J. Clin. Periodontol.* **2015**, *42*, 845–852.
16. Munro, I.C.; Berndt, W.O.; Borzelleca, J.F.; Flamm, G.; Lynch, B.S.; Kennepohl, E.; Modderman, J. Erythritol: An Interpretive Summary of Biochemical, Metabolic, Toxicological and Clinical Data. *Food Chem. Toxicol.* **1998**, *36*, 1139–1174. [CrossRef] [PubMed]
17. Reimer, R.A.; Hlywka, J.J. Satiety and Glycemic Response After Starch Consumption: Effects of Added Sugar, Protein, and Acid. *Nutr. Neurosci.* **2006**, *9*, 9–17.
18. Storey, D.; Lee, A.; Bornet, F.; Brouns, F. Gastrointestinal Tolerance of Erythritol and Xylitol Ingested in a Liquid. *Eur. J. Clin. Nutr.* **2007**, *61*, 349–354. [CrossRef]
19. Rastogi, S.; Varadarajan, S.; Sankarapandian, P. Effect of Erythritol and Xylitol on Dental Caries Prevention in Children. *J. Pharm. Bioallied Sci.* **2017**, *9*, S116–S118.
20. Ribeiro, A.P.D.; Ribeiro, R.C.L.; Leite, F.R.M.; Padovani, G.C. Impact of Erythritol and Xylitol on Dental Caries Prevention in Children. *J. Appl. Oral Sci.* **2019**, *27*, e20180232.
21. Georgakopoulou, E.A.; Drosou, A.; Kazakos, N.; Koidis, P.T. Non-Surgical Periodontal Treatment with Adjunctive Erythritol: A Randomized Clinical Trial. *Clin. Oral Investig.* **2019**, *23*, 1809–1817.
22. Vandekerckhove, B.; Quirynen, M.; Warren, P.R. The Use of a 1.5% Erythritol Spray as an Adjunct to Mechanical Debridement in Periodontitis Patients: A Randomized Clinical Trial. *J. Periodontol.* **2017**, *88*, 372–381.
23. Assev, S.; Rölla, G.; Söderling, E. Antimicrobial Effect of Erythritol on Plaque. *J. Dent. Res.* **2017**, *96*, 599–604.
24. Lang, N.P.; Tonetti, M.S.; Suvan, J.E.; Papapanou, P. A Tribute to the Oral Hygiene Research of the Late Professor Jørgen Slots (1942–2015). *J. Clin. Periodontol.* **2015**, *42*, 919–923.
25. Cobb, C.M.; MacNeill, S.R.; Satheesh, K.M.; Brown, A.T.; Kugel, A.; Koerber, A.; Derman, R. Two-Year Clinical Effectiveness of an Electric Rechargeable Toothbrush on Periodontal Health, Oral Hygiene, and Plaque Removal: A Randomized Controlled Trial. *J. Clin. Periodontol.* **2015**, *42*, 446–452.
26. Hujoel, P.P.; Cunha-Cruz, J.; Banting, D.W.; Loesche, W.J. Dental Flossing and Interproximal Caries: A Systematic Review. *J. Dent. Res.* **2013**, *92*, 359–365. [CrossRef] [PubMed]
27. Alcoforado, G.A.C.; Rams, T.E.; Feine, J.S.; de Albuquerque Junior, R.F. Home Oral Hygiene Interventions in Adults with Periodontitis: A Systematic Review. *J. Periodontol.* **2019**, *90*, 391–411.
28. Sanz, M.; Herrera, D.; Kebschull, M.; Chapple, I.; Jepsen, S.; Berglundh, T.; Sculean, A. Treatment of Stage I–III Periodontitis—The EFP S3 Level Clinical Practice Guideline. *J. Clin. Periodontol.* **2020**, *47*, 4–60. [CrossRef]
29. Carra, M.C.; Detzen, L.; Kitzmann, J.; Woelber, J.P.; Ramseier, C.A.; Bouchard, P. Promoting behavioural changes to improve oral hygiene in patients with periodontal diseases: A systematic review. *J. Clin. Periodontol.* **2020**, *47*, 72–89. [CrossRef]
30. Slot, D.E.; Valkenburg, C.; Van der Weijden, G.A.F. Mechanical plaque removal of periodontal maintenance patients: A systematic review and network meta-analysis. *J. Clin. Periodontol.* **2020**, *47*, 107–124. [CrossRef]
31. Sgolastra, F.; Petrucci, A.; Gatto, R.; Marzo, G.; Monaco, A. Effectiveness of Ultrasonic Instruments in the Treatment of Adult Periodontitis: A Systematic Review. *J. Am. Dent. Assoc.* **2013**, *144*, 524–538.
32. Salvi, G.E.; Mischler, D.C.; Schmidlin, K.; Matuliene, G.; Pjetursson, B.E.; Brägger, U.; Lang, N.P. Risk Factors Associated with the Longevity of Multi-Rooted Teeth. Long-Term Outcomes after Active and Supportive Periodontal Therapy. *J. Clin. Periodontol.* **2015**, *42*, 1037–1047. [CrossRef]
33. Sgolastra, F.; Petrucci, A.; Gatto, R.; Marzo, G.; Monaco, A. Systematic Review of Randomized Controlled Trials on Clinical Outcomes in Adults Treated with Surgical Periodontal Therapy with and without Antibiotics. *J. Clin. Periodontol.* **2016**, *43*, 934–947.
34. Herrera, D.; Sanz, M.; Jepsen, S.; Needleman, I.; Roldán, S. A Systematic Review on the Effect of Systemic Antimicrobials as an Adjunct to Scaling and Root Planing in Periodontitis Patients. *J. Clin. Periodontol.* **2012**, *39*, S136–S159. [CrossRef] [PubMed]
35. Slots, J.; Paster, B.J. Treatment of Periodontitis: The Role of Systemic Antimicrobials. *Periodontol. 2000* **2019**, *79*, 154–184.
36. Heitz-Mayfield, L.J.A.; Lang, N.P.; Salvi, G.E. Supportive Periodontal Therapy. *J. Clin. Periodontol.* **2018**, *45*, S112–S125.
37. Wenzler, J.-S.; Krause, F.; Böcher, S.; Falk, W.; Birkenmaier, A.; Conrads, G.; Braun, A. Antimicrobial Impact of Different Air-Polishing Powders in a Subgingival Biofilm Model. *Antibiotics* **2021**, *10*, 1464. [CrossRef] [PubMed]
38. Kruse, A.B.; Maamar, R.; Akakpo, D.L.; Woelber, J.P.; Wittmer, A.; Vach, K.; Ratka-Krüger, P.; Al-Ahmad, A. Effects of Subgingival Air-Polishing with Trehalose Powder on Oral Biofilm during Periodontal Maintenance Therapy: A Randomized-Controlled Pilot Study. *BMC Oral Health* **2020**, *20*, 123. [CrossRef] [PubMed]
39. Petersilka, G.J.; Steinmann, D.; Häberlein, I.; Heinecke, A.; Flemmig, T.F. Subgingival Plaque Removal in Buccal and Lingual Sites Using a Novel Low Abrasive Air-Polishing Powder. *J. Clin. Periodontol.* **2003**, *30*, 328–333. [CrossRef] [PubMed]
40. Petersilka, G.J.; Tunkel, J.; Barakos, K.; Heinecke, A.; Häberlein, I.; Flemmig, T.F. Subgingival Plaque Removal at Interdental Sites Using a Low-Abrasive Air Polishing Powder. *J. Periodontol.* **2003**, *74*, 307–311. [CrossRef]
41. Sekino, S.; Ogawa, T.; Murakashi, E.; Ito, H.; Numabe, Y. Clinical and Microbiological Effect of Frequent Subgingival Air Polishing on Periodontal Conditions: A Split-Mouth Randomized Controlled Trial. *Odontology* **2020**, *108*, 688–696. [CrossRef]

42. Jiang, Y.; Tong, X. Efficacy of Subgingival Glycine Air Polishing on the Treatment of Moderate-Mild Peri-Implantitis. *Shanghai Kou Qiang Yi Xue* **2019**, *28*, 93–96.
43. Jing, W.D.; Wang, X.E.; Xie, Y.S.; Han, J.; Xu, L. Efficacy of Subgingival Glycine Air Polishing on Patients with Early Peri-Implant Diseases. *Zhonghua Kou Qiang Yi Xue Za Zhi* **2017**, *9*, 480–485.
44. Schlagenhauf, U.; Hess, J.V.; Stölzel, P.; Haubitz, I.; Jockel-Schneider, Y. Impact of a Two-Stage Subgingival Instrumentation Scheme Involving Air Polishing on Attachment Gain after Active Periodontal Therapy. *J. Periodontol.* **2022**, *93*, 1500–1509. [CrossRef] [PubMed]
45. Petersilka, G.; Koch, R.; Vomhof, A.; Joda, T.; Harks, I.; Arweiler, N.; Ehmke, B. Retrospective Analysis of the Long-Term Effect of Subgingival Air Polishing in Supportive Periodontal Therapy. *J. Clin. Periodontol.* **2020**, *48*, 263–271. [CrossRef] [PubMed]
46. Zhao, Y.B.; Jin, D.S.S.; He, L.; Meng, H.X. Preliminary Study of Subgingival Microorganism Changes after Glycine Powder Air-Polishing Treatment during Periodontal Maintenance Phase. *Zhonghua Kou Qiang Yi Xue Za Zhi* **2017**, *9*, 410–414.
47. Laleman, I.; Cortellini, S.; De Winter, S.; Rodriguez Herrero, E.; Dekeyser, C.; Quirynen, M.; Teughels, W. Subgingival Debridement: End Point, Methods and How Often? *Periodontology 2000* **2017**, *75*, 189–204. [CrossRef]
48. Bühler, J.; Amato, M.; Weiger, R.; Walter, C. A Systematic Review on the Patient Perception of Periodontal Treatment Using Air Polishing Devices. *Int. J. Dent. Hyg.* **2015**, *14*, 4–14. [CrossRef]
49. Wennström, J.L.; Dahlén, G.; Ramberg, P. Subgingival Debridement of Periodontal Pockets by Air Polishing in Comparison with Ultrasonic Instrumentation during Maintenance Therapy. *J. Clin. Periodontol.* **2011**, *38*, 820–827. [CrossRef]
50. Lu, H.; He, L.; Zhao, Y.; Meng, H. The Effect of Supragingival Glycine Air Polishing on Periodontitis during Maintenance Therapy: A Randomized Controlled Trial. *PeerJ* **2018**, *6*, e4371. [CrossRef]
51. Seidel, M.; Borenius, H.; Schorr, S.; Christofzik, D.; Graetz, C. Results of an Experimental Study of Subgingival Cleaning Effectiveness in the Furcation Area. *BMC Oral Health* **2021**, *21*, 381. [CrossRef]
52. Zhu, M.; Zhao, M.; Hu, B.; Wang, Y.; Li, Y.; Song, J. Efficacy of Glycine Powder Air Polishing in Supportive Periodontal Therapy: A Systematic Review and Meta-Analysis. *J. Periodontal Implant. Sci.* **2021**, *51*, 147. [CrossRef] [PubMed]
53. Kargas, K.; Tsalikis, L.; Sakellari, D.; Menexes, G.; Konstantinidis, A. Pilot Study on the Clinical and Microbiological Effect of Subgingival Glycine Powder Air Polishing Using a Cannula-Like Jet. *Int. J. Dent. Hyg.* **2014**, *13*, 161–169. [CrossRef]
54. Petersilka, G.; Faggion, C.M.; Stratmann, U.; Gerss, J.; Ehmke, B.; Haeberlein, I.; Flemmig, T.F. Effect of Glycine Powder Air Polishing on the Gingiva. *J. Clin. Periodontol.* **2008**, *35*, 324–332. [CrossRef] [PubMed]
55. Zhang, W.; Wang, W.; Chu, C.; Jing, J.; Yao, N.A.; Sun, Q.; Li, S. Clinical, Inflammatory and Microbiological Outcomes of Full-Mouth Scaling with Adjunctive Glycine Powder Air Polishing: A Randomized Trial. *J. Clin. Periodontol.* **2021**, *48*, 389–399. [CrossRef]
56. Caygur, A.; Albaba, M.R.; Berberoglu, A.; Yilmaz, H.G. Efficacy of Glycine Powder Air Polishing Combined with Scaling and Root Planing in the Treatment of Periodontitis and Halitosis: A Randomised Clinical Study. *J. Int. Med. Res.* **2017**, *45*, 1168–1174. [CrossRef] [PubMed]
57. Poornima, R.; Meena, A.K.; Pratibha, G. Comparison of Root Surface Roughness Produced by Air Polishing Combined with Hand Instrumentation or Ultrasonic Instrumentation: An In Vitro Study. *Gen. Dent.* **2019**, *67*, 75–77.
58. Lu, H.; Zhao, Y.; Feng, X.; He, L.; Meng, H. Microbiome in Maintained Periodontitis and Its Shift over a Single Maintenance Interval of 3 Months. *J. Clin. Periodontol.* **2019**, *46*, 1094–1104. [CrossRef] [PubMed]
59. Flemmig, T.F.; Arushanov, D.; Daubert, D.; Rothen, M.; Mueller, G.; Leroux, B.G. Randomized Controlled Trial Assessing Efficacy and Safety of Glycine Powder Air Polishing in Moderate-to-Deep Periodontal Pockets. *J. Periodontol.* **2012**, *83*, 444–452. [CrossRef]
60. Jentsch, H.F.; Flechsig, C.; Kette, B.; Eick, S. Adjunctive air-polishing with erythritol in nonsurgical periodontal therapy: A randomized clinical trial. *BMC Oral Health* **2020**, *20*, 364. [CrossRef]
61. Divnic-Resnik, T.; Pradhan, H.; Spahr, A. The efficacy of the adjunct use of subgingival air-polishing therapy with erythritol powder compared to conventional debridement alone during initial non-surgical periodontal therapy. *J. Clin. Periodontol.* **2022**, *49*, 547–555. [CrossRef] [PubMed]
62. Moëne, R.; Décaillet, F.; Andersen, E.; Mombelli, A. Subgingival plaque removal using a new air-polishing device. *J. Periodontol.* **2010**, *81*, 79–88. [CrossRef]
63. Mensi, M.; Scotti, E.; Sordillo, A.; Calza, S.; Guarnelli, M.E.; Fabbri, C.; Farina, R.; Trombelli, L. Efficacy of the additional use of subgingival air polishing with erythritol powder in the treatment of periodontitis patients: A randomized controlled clinical trial. *Clin. Oral Investig.* **2021**, *25*, 729–736. [CrossRef]
64. Hu, C.J.; Yin, Y.Z.; Guan, D.P. Comparison of subgingival debridement efficacy of air polishing and manual scaling. *Shanghai Kou Qiang Yi Xue* **2015**, *24*, 602–606. [PubMed]
65. Kröger, J.C.; Haribyan, M.; Nergiz, I.; Schmage, P. Air polishing with erythritol powder—In vitro effects on dentin loss. *J. Indian Soc. Periodontol.* **2020**, *24*, 433–440. [CrossRef] [PubMed]
66. Hägi, T.T.; Hofmänner, P.; Salvi, G.E.; Ramseier, C.A.; Sculean, A. Clinical outcomes following subgingival application of a novel erythritol powder by means of air polishing in supportive periodontal therapy: A randomized, controlled clinical study. *Quintessence Int. (Berl. Ger. 1985)* **2013**, *44*, 753–761.
67. Ulvik, I.M.; Sæthre, T.; Bunæs, D.F.; Lie, S.A.; Enersen, M.; Leknes, K.N. A 12-month randomized controlled trial evaluating erythritol air-polishing versus Curette/ultrasonic debridement of mandibular furcations in supportive periodontal therapy. *BMC Oral Health* **2021**, *21*, 38. [CrossRef]

68. Zhang, W.; Meng, Y.; Jing, J.; Wu, Y.; Li, S. Influence of periodontal treatment on Blood Microbiotas: A clinical trial. *PeerJ* **2021**, *9*, e10846. [CrossRef]
69. Hägi, T.T.; Hofmänner, P.; Eick, S.; Donnet, M.; Salvi, G.E.; Sculean, A.; Ramseier, C.A. The effects of erythritol air-polishing powder on microbiologic and clinical outcomes during supportive periodontal therapy: Six-month results of a randomized controlled clinical trial. *Quintessence Int. (Berl. Ger. 1985)* **2015**, *46*, 31–41.
70. Simon, C.J.; Munivenkatappa Lakshmaiah Venkatesh, P.; Chickanna, R. Efficacy of glycine powder air polishing in comparison with sodium bicarbonate air polishing and ultrasonic scaling—A double-blind Clinico-histopathologic study. *Int. J. Dent. Hyg.* **2015**, *13*, 177–183. [CrossRef]
71. Weusmann, J.; Deschner, J.; Imber, J.-C.; Damanaki, A.; Cerri, P.S.; Leguizamón, N.; Beisel-Memmert, S.; Nogueira, A.V. Impact of glycine and erythritol/chlorhexidine air-polishing powders on human gingival fibroblasts: An in vitro study. *Ann. Anat.—Anat. Anz.* **2022**, *243*, 151949. [CrossRef]
72. de Cock, P.; Mäkinen, K.; Honkala, E.; Saag, M.; Kennepohl, E.; Eapen, A. Erythritol is more effective than xylitol and sorbitol in managing oral health endpoints. *Int. J. Dent.* **2016**, *2016*, 9868421. [CrossRef] [PubMed]
73. Tan, S.L.; Grewal, G.K.; Mohamed Nazari, N.S.; Mohd-Dom, T.N.; Baharuddin, N.A. Efficacy of air polishing in comparison with hand instruments and/or power-driven instruments in supportive periodontal therapy and Implant Maintenance: A systematic review and meta-analysis. *BMC Oral Health* **2022**, *22*, 85. [CrossRef]
74. Herr, M.L.; DeLong, R.; Li, Y.; Lunos, S.A.; Stoltenberg, J.L. Use of a continual sweep motion to compare air polishing devices, powders and exposure time on unexposed root cementum. *Odontology* **2017**, *105*, 311–319. [CrossRef] [PubMed]
75. Bains, V.K.; Madan, C.; Bains, R. Tooth polishing: Relevance in present day periodontal practice. *J. Indian Soc. Periodontol.* **2009**, *13*, 58. [CrossRef] [PubMed]
76. Schulz, S.; Stein, J.M.; Schumacher, A.; Kupietz, D.; Yekta-Michael, S.S.; Schittenhelm, F.; Conrads, G.; Schaller, H.-G.; Reichert, S. Nonsurgical periodontal treatment options and their impact on subgingival microbiota. *J. Clin. Med.* **2022**, *11*, 1187. [CrossRef] [PubMed]
77. Mensi, M.; Viviani, L.; Agosti, R.; Scotti, E.; Garzetti, G.; Calza, S. Comparison between four different implant surface debridement methods: An in-vitro experimental study. *Minerva Stomatol.* **2020**, *69*, 286–294. [CrossRef]
78. Nascimento, G.G.; Leite, F.R.; Pennisi, P.R.; López, R.; Paranhos, L.R. Use of air polishing for supra- and subgingival biofilm removal for treatment of residual periodontal pockets and supportive periodontal care: A systematic review. *Clin. Oral Investig.* **2021**, *25*, 779–795. [CrossRef] [PubMed]
79. Mensi, M.; Scotti, E.; Calza, S.; Pilloni, A.; Grusovin, M.G.; Mongardini, C. A new multiple anti-infective non-surgical therapy in the treatment of peri-implantitis: A case series. *Minerva Dent. Oral Sci.* **2017**, *66*, 255–266. [CrossRef]
80. Zhang, J.; Liu, J.; Li, J.; Chen, B.; Li, H.; Yan, F. The clinical efficacy of subgingival debridement by ultrasonic instrumentation compared with subgingival air polishing during periodontal maintenance: A systematic review. *J. Evid. Based Dent. Pract.* **2019**, *19*, 101314. [CrossRef]
81. Stahl, V.; Vasudevan, K. CBD-supplemented polishing powder enhances tooth polishing by inhibiting dental plaque bacteria. *J. Int. Soc. Prev. Community Dent.* **2020**, *10*, 766–770. [CrossRef]
82. Di Tinco, R.; Bertani, G.; Pisciotta, A.; Bertoni, L.; Bertacchini, J.; Colombari, B.; Conserva, E.; Blasi, E.; Consolo, U.; Carnevale, G. Evaluation of antimicrobial effect of air-polishing treatments and their influence on human dental pulp stem cells seeded on titanium disks. *Int. J. Mol. Sci.* **2021**, *22*, 865. [CrossRef]
83. Weusmann, J.; Deschner, J.; Imber, J.-C.; Damanaki, A.; Leguizamón, N.D.; Nogueira, A.V. Cellular effects of glycine and trehalose air-polishing powders on human gingival fibroblasts in vitro. *Clin. Oral Investig.* **2021**, *26*, 1569–1578. [CrossRef] [PubMed]
84. Vinel, A.; Al Halabi, A.; Roumi, S.; Le Neindre, H.; Millavet, P.; Simon, M.; Cuny, C.; Barthet, J.-S.; Barthet, P.; Laurencin-Dalicieux, S. Non-surgical periodontal treatment: SRP and Innovative Therapeutic Approaches. *Adv. Exp. Med. Biol.* **2022**, *1373*, 303–327.
85. Bozbay, E.; Dominici, F.; Gokbuget, A.Y.; Cintan, S.; Guida, L.; Aydin, M.S.; Mariotti, A.; Pilloni, A. Preservation of root cementum: A comparative evaluation of power-driven versus hand instruments. *Int. J. Dent. Hyg.* **2016**, *16*, 202–209. [CrossRef]
86. Alwaeli, H.A.; Al-Khateeb, S.N.; Al-Sadi, A. Long-term clinical effect of adjunctive antimicrobial photodynamic therapy in periodontal treatment: A randomized clinical trial. *Lasers Med. Sci.* **2015**, *30*, 801–807. [CrossRef]
87. Dalvi, S.; Benedicenti, S.; Hanna, R. Effectiveness of Photobiomodulation as an Adjunct to Nonsurgical Periodontal Therapy in the Management of Periodontitis—A Systematic Review of in vivo Human Studies. *Photochem. Photobiol.* **2021**, *97*, 223–242. [CrossRef] [PubMed]
88. Persson, G.R.; Roos-Jansåker, A.-M.; Lindahl, C.; Renvert, S. Microbiologic results after non-surgical erbium-doped:yttrium, aluminum, and garnet laser or air-abrasive treatment of peri-implantitis: A randomized clinical trial. *J. Periodontol.* **2011**, *82*, 1267–1278. [CrossRef] [PubMed]
89. McCollum, J.; O'Neal, R.B.; Brennan, W.A.; Van Dyke, T.E.; Horner, J.A. The effect of titanium implant abutment surface irregularities on plaque accumulation in vivo. *J. Periodontol.* **1992**, *63*, 802–805. [CrossRef]
90. Kruse, A.B.; Akakpo, D.L.; Maamar, R.; Woelber, J.P.; Al-Ahmad, A.; Vach, K.; Ratka-Krueger, P. Trehalose powder for subgingival air-polishing during periodontal maintenance therapy: A randomized controlled trial. *J. Periodontol.* **2018**, *90*, 263–270. [CrossRef]
91. Luo, J.Y.N.; Liu, P.P.; Wong, M.C.M. Patients' satisfaction with dental care: A qualitative study to develop a satisfaction instrument. *BMC Oral Health* **2018**, *18*, 15. [CrossRef] [PubMed]

92. Bennardo, F.; Barone, S.; Vocaturo, C.; Gheorghe, D.N.; Cosentini, G.; Antonelli, A.; Giudice, A. Comparison between Magneto-Dynamic, Piezoelectric, and Conventional Surgery for Dental Extractions: A Pilot Study. *Dent. J.* **2023**, *11*, 60. [CrossRef] [PubMed]
93. Petersilka, G.J. Subgingival air-polishing in the treatment of periodontal biofilm infections. *Periodontology 2000* **2010**, *55*, 124–142. [CrossRef] [PubMed]

Disclaimer/Publisher's Note: The statements, opinions and data contained in all publications are solely those of the individual author(s) and contributor(s) and not of MDPI and/or the editor(s). MDPI and/or the editor(s) disclaim responsibility for any injury to people or property resulting from any ideas, methods, instructions or products referred to in the content.

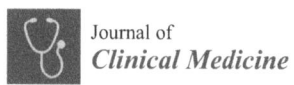

Article

Detection of Periodontal Bone Loss on Periapical Radiographs—A Diagnostic Study Using Different Convolutional Neural Networks

Patrick Hoss [1], Ole Meyer [2], Uta Christine Wölfle [1], Annika Wülk [1], Theresa Meusburger [1], Leon Meier [1], Reinhard Hickel [1], Volker Gruhn [2], Marc Hesenius [2], Jan Kühnisch [1,*] and Helena Dujic [1]

[1] Department of Conservative Dentistry and Periodontology, LMU University Hospital, LMU Munich, 80336 Munich, Germany; patrick.hoss@t-online.de (P.H.); uta.woelfle@med.uni-muenchen.de (U.C.W.); annika.wuelk@gmx.de (A.W.); theresa.meusburger@hotmail.com (T.M.); meierl.leon@gmail.com (L.M.); hickel@dent.med.uni-muenchen.de (R.H.); h.dujic@med.uni-muenchen.de (H.D.)

[2] Institute for Software Engineering, University of Duisburg-Essen, 45127 Essen, Germany; ole.meyer@uni-due.de (O.M.); volker.gruhn@paluno.uni-due.de (V.G.); marc.hesenius@uni-due.de (M.H.)

* Correspondence: jkuehn@dent.med.uni-muenchen.de; Tel.: +49-89-4400-59343 (ext. 59301)

Abstract: Interest in machine learning models and convolutional neural networks (CNNs) for diagnostic purposes is steadily increasing in dentistry. Here, CNNs can potentially help in the classification of periodontal bone loss (PBL). In this study, the diagnostic performance of five CNNs in detecting PBL on periapical radiographs was analyzed. A set of anonymized periapical radiographs (N = 21,819) was evaluated by a group of trained and calibrated dentists and classified into radiographs without PBL or with mild, moderate, or severe PBL. Five CNNs were trained over five epochs. Statistically, diagnostic performance was analyzed using accuracy (ACC), sensitivity (SE), specificity (SP), and area under the receiver operating curve (AUC). Here, overall ACC ranged from 82.0% to 84.8%, SE 88.8–90.7%, SP 66.2–71.2%, and AUC 0.884–0.913, indicating similar diagnostic performance of the five CNNs. Furthermore, performance differences were evident in the individual sextant groups. Here, the highest values were found for the mandibular anterior teeth (ACC 94.9–96.0%) and the lowest values for the maxillary posterior teeth (78.0–80.7%). It can be concluded that automatic assessment of PBL seems to be possible, but that diagnostic accuracy varies depending on the location in the dentition. Future research is needed to improve performance for all tooth groups.

Keywords: artificial intelligence; bone loss; convolutional neural networks; deep learning; dental radiography; machine learning; periodontitis

Citation: Hoss, P.; Meyer, O.; Wölfle, U.C.; Wülk, A.; Meusburger, T.; Meier, L.; Hickel, R.; Gruhn, V.; Hesenius, M.; Kühnisch, J.; et al. Detection of Periodontal Bone Loss on Periapical Radiographs—A Diagnostic Study Using Different Convolutional Neural Networks. *J. Clin. Med.* **2023**, *12*, 7189. https://doi.org/10.3390/jcm12227189

Academic Editor: Agostino Guida

Received: 3 November 2023
Revised: 14 November 2023
Accepted: 18 November 2023
Published: 20 November 2023

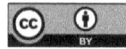

Copyright: © 2023 by the authors. Licensee MDPI, Basel, Switzerland. This article is an open access article distributed under the terms and conditions of the Creative Commons Attribution (CC BY) license (https://creativecommons.org/licenses/by/4.0/).

1. Introduction

Periodontitis is a prevalent dental health problem and can be classified as a major global challenge that affects developed and developing countries [1–3]. Triggered by bacterial colonization of the root surface, the host's immune system reacts with inflammatory processes to the microbial transition from a symbiotic bacterial environment to that of dysbiotic pathogens, leading to loss of supporting tooth tissue, pocket formation, and ulceration of the pocket epithelium [4,5]. If the condition advances, periodontal bone loss (PBL) can occur as the principal pathological characteristic of periodontitis [6]. Moreover, severe periodontitis is a major cause of missing teeth in adults, leading to reduced oral functioning and ultimately having an adverse effect on general health [7,8]. In this context, the link between periodontal disease and various systemic diseases such as cardiovascular diseases [9], diabetes [10], and respiratory diseases [11] should be emphasized. Considering the mostly irreversible consequences of periodontal disease, frequent periodontal screening is essential for the treatment of all patients and should be part of routine oral inspection [12]. According to the new guidelines introduced by the workshop on the classification of periodontal and peri-implant diseases and conditions [13,14], the evaluation of clinical attachment loss as well as the radiographic assessment of PBL has become critical in categorizing periodontitis into specific stages and subsequently in indicating optimal disease management. Nevertheless, both the clinical measurements and the radiographic assessment of PBL remain controversial in terms of their reliability. The measurement of clinical attachment loss by periodontal probing varies due to individual probing force, probe angulation, and varying probe tip diameter [15,16]. In addition, radiographic PBL evaluation represents a challenging task for a clinician due to possible variations in contrast and exposure angle as well as structural overlap, so that the interpretation of dental radiographs may lead to inconsistencies among dentists [17–19]. Here, the use of artificial intelligence (AI)-based diagnostics could reduce these diagnostic discrepancies. Consequently, several work groups have investigated the use of AI-based methods for automatized PBL detection on periapical radiographs [19–29] and panoramic X-rays [18,30–40]. In these studies, on the one hand, convolutional neural networks (CNNs) have shown potential in accurately detecting PBL on radiographs. However, due to differing CNNs and varying data sets, the existing studies show significant heterogeneity and, therefore, are difficult to compare [41–43]. In addition, little is known about whether different CNNs or anatomical regions influence diagnostic performance. Therefore, the aim of this study was to evaluate the diagnostic performance of five commonly used CNNs for automated PBL detection on periapical radiographs representing all sextants (upper and lower posterior teeth and upper and lower anterior teeth) and to statistically report their diagnostic performance with standardized variables, avoiding non-comparable results. In detail, it was first hypothesized that the diagnostic performance of the tested CNNs would have an accuracy of at least 90%. Secondly, diagnostic accuracy was hypothesized to be the same between all CNNs and anatomical regions.

2. Materials and Methods

2.1. Study Design

The Ethics Committee of the Medical Faculty of the Ludwig-Maximilians University of Munich approved this study protocol with project number 020-798. The recommendations of the Standard for Reporting of Diagnostic Accuracy Studies (STARD) steering committee [44] and the recommendations for the reporting of AI studies in dentistry [45] were followed in the study report.

2.2. Periapical Radiographs

For this study, anonymized periapical radiographs taken at the Department of Conservative Dentistry and Periodontology (Dental School of the LMU) and other dental practices were used. A high-quality image sample was secured by excluding inadequate X-rays, e.g., distorted images, images with incomplete teeth, or radiographs with implants. Following these exclusion criteria, a data set with 21,819 periapical radiographs stored in jpg format was assembled.

2.3. Categorization of Periodontal Bone Loss (Reference Standard)

Prior to the start of the study, a two-day workshop was held by the principal investigator (J.K.), during which the group of participating dentists ($N = 7$) was trained. In addition, the efficiency of the training was determined during a calibration course. Reproducibility of PBL within and between investigators was assessed using 150 periapical radiographs, and the corresponding inter- and intra-examiner reliability showed substantial kappa values [17]. The detailed kappa values are specified in Table 1. A group of graduated dentists (P.H., T.M., A.W., L.M.) then pre-categorized all X-rays by differentiating between healthy periodontium and mild, moderate, or severe PBL [13,14]. Following this, more clinically experienced examiners (H.D., U.W., J.K.) independently counterchecked each diagnostic decision. More specifically, these diagnostic criteria and ratings were applied: 0—healthy periodontium, PBL not detectable, 1—mild radiographic PBL up to 15% in the coronal third of the tooth, 2—moderate radiographic PBL between 15% and 33% of the root length, and 3—severe radiographic PBL beyond the coronal third of the tooth (Figure 1). In case of differing diagnostic opinions, each image was subject to continued discussion until consensus was achieved. The use of anonymized periapical radiographs meant that no further clinical information could have been acquired to make a diagnostic decision. One dichotomized diagnosis decision (0 vs. 1–3) was made for each X-ray, which consequently became the reference standard for the cyclic training and the repeated evaluation of the AI-based CNN.

Table 1. Cohen's kappa values for inter- and intra-examiner reliability for the detection of PBL, calculated among participating dentists ($N = 7$) in relation to the reference standard.

Examiner	Inter-Examiner	Intra-Examiner
P.H.	0.601–0.650	0.889
T.M.	0.620–0.658	0.554
A.W.	0.762–0.796	0.779
L.M.	0.516–0.565	0.797
U.W.	0.658–0.699	0.455
J.K.	0.706–0.748	0.579
H.D.	0.529–0.534	0.767

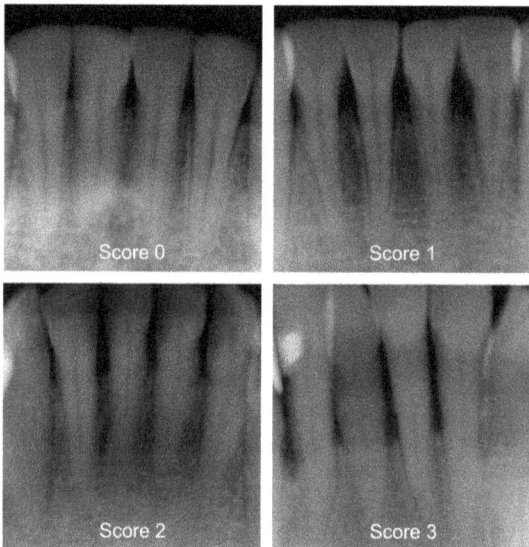

Figure 1. Examples of periapical radiographs for all categories: healthy periodontium, periodontal bone loss (PBL) not detectable (Score 0), mild radiographic PBL up to 15% in the coronal third of the tooth (Score 1), moderate radiographic PBL between 15% and 33% of the root length (Score 2), and severe radiographic PBL beyond the coronal third of the tooth (Score 3).

2.4. Training of the Deep-Learning-Based CNNs (Test Method)

Hereafter, the utilized pipeline of well-established methods for developing the AI-based algorithm is explained. Initially, the whole image set of 21,819 periapical radiographs was subdivided into a training set ($N = 18,819$) and a test set ($N = 3000$). The latter was randomly selected from the entire data set, ensuring that all sextants were equally represented. This served as an independent test set for evaluation purposes only and was not included in the model training.

By using Python (version 3.8.5, https://www.python.org accessed on 17 November 2023) in conjunction with the PyTorch library (version 1.12.0, https://pytorch.org accessed on 17 November 2023), the training set was augmented so that the variability of the included radiographs could be improved. Therefore, images were modified using different transformations: random rotation up to 180 degrees, random changes in brightness, contrast, and saturation up to 20% with color jitter, and random affine transformation (translation up to 30% of the image size and zooming out up to 70%). As a result, a new, unique, and virtual grayscale image (RGB format) was created.

The augmented images were used to train the following pretrained CNNs: ResNet-18 [46], MobileNet V2 [47], ConvNeXT/small, ConvNeXT/base, and ConvNeXT/large [48]. The batch size amounted to 16 randomly selected images. The random selection of the respective images into batches was done using PyTorch's built-in DataLoader class. The learning performance was repeatedly verified with the test set after 30 training steps. All CNNs were trained using backpropagation to determine the gradient for learning. Furthermore, the training was accelerated using Floating Point 16 and a university-based computer (i9 10850K 10 × 3.60 GHz, Intel Corp., Santa Clara, CA, USA) equipped with 48 GB RAM and a professional graphic card (GeForce RTX 3060, Nvidia, Santa Clara, CA, USA). Each CNN was trained over 5 epochs, with cross entropy loss as an error function and an application of the Adam optimizer (Betas 0.9 and 0.999, Epsilon $\times 10^{-8}$).

2.5. Statistical Analysis

The data were analyzed using Python (version 3.8.5). By computing the number of true positives (TPs), false positives (FPs), true negatives (TNs) and false negatives (FNs), the diagnostic accuracy (ACC = (TN + TP)/(TN + TP + FN + FP)) was identified. The sensitivity (SE), specificity (SP), positive predictive values (PPVs), negative predictive values (NPVs), and the area under the receiver operating characteristic (ROC) curve (AUC) were calculated with respect to the utilized CNN [49].

3. Results

For the purpose of this study, a total of 21,819 periapical radiographs were selected and divided into sextants (upper and lower posterior teeth as well as upper and lower anterior teeth). The image distribution in relation to the anatomical region and the PBL can be taken from Table 2. While the number of radiographs from the upper jaw was found to be comparable to that from the lower jaw, the overwhelming majority of images originated from posterior teeth compared to anterior teeth. Moreover, most included periapical radiographs showing teeth affected by mild PBL (42.6%). In contrast, radiographs with severe PBL had a notably lower proportion (6.9%) in the total data set.

Table 2. Overview of the included periapical radiographs (N = 21,819) in relation to the corresponding sextants and periodontal diagnosis.

	Expert Classification	Healthy Periodontium (Score 0)		Mild PBL (Score 1)		Moderate PBL (Score 2)		Severe PBL (Score 3)		Total	
		N	%	N	%	N	%	N	%	N	%
Upper jaw	Anteriors	653	3.0	661	3.0	433	2.0	197	0.9	1944	8.9
	1st Quadrant	1701	7.8	1826	8.4	851	3.9	367	1.7	4745	21.8
	2nd Quadrant	1231	5.6	2080	9.5	1093	5.0	312	1.5	4716	21.6
Lower jaw	Anteriors	202	0.9	676	3.1	786	3.6	325	1.5	1989	9.1
	3rd Quadrant	1477	6.8	2033	9.3	593	2.7	157	0.7	4260	19.5
	4th Quadrant	1282	5.9	2027	9.3	713	3.3	143	0.6	4165	19.1
	Total	6546	30.0	9303	42.6	4469	20.5	1501	6.9	21,819	100

The overall diagnostic performance for automatized detection of PBL on periapical radiographs in relation to the CNNs used are specified in Tables 3 and 4. The CNNs achieved an overall ACC between 82.0% and 84.8%. The associated AUC values ranged from 0.884 to 0.913. Moreover, all tested CNNs showed consistently higher SE values varying between 88.8% and 90.7% compared to the SP values, which ranged from 66.2% to 71.2%.

Table 3. Overview of the true positive (TP), true negative (TN), false positive (FP), and false negative (FN) distribution for the independent test set (N = 3000 radiographs), which was evaluated by the AI-based algorithm for the assessment of periodontal bone loss.

CNN	True Positive (TP)		True Negative (TN)		False Positive (FP)		False Negative (FN)	
	N	%	N	%	N	%	N	%
ResNet-18	1876	62.5	609	20.3	294	9.8	221	7.4
MobileNetV2	1863	62.1	598	19.9	305	10.2	234	7.8
ConvNeXT/s [1]	1877	62.6	639	21.3	264	8.8	220	7.3
ConvNeXT/b [2]	1901	63.4	643	21.4	260	8.7	196	6.5
ConvNeXT/l [3]	1890	63.0	637	21.2	266	8.9	207	6.9

[1] small, [2] base, [3] large.

Table 4. Overview of the overall diagnostic performance of the developed convolutional neural network (CNN), where the independent test set (N = 3000 radiographs) was evaluated by the AI-based algorithm for the assessment of periodontal bone loss. The overall diagnostic accuracy (ACC), sensitivity (SE), specificity (SP), negative predictive value (NPV), positive predictive value (PPV), and area under the receiver operating characteristic curve (AUC) were predicted.

CNN	Diagnostic Performance					
	ACC	SE	SP	NPV	PPV	AUC
ResNet-18	82.8	89.5	67.4	73.4	86.5	0.884
MobileNetV2	82.0	88.8	66.2	71.9	85.9	0.884
ConvNeXT/s [1]	83.9	89.5	70.8	74.4	87.7	0.903
ConvNeXT/b [2]	84.8	90.7	71.2	76.6	88.0	0.911
ConvNeXT/l [3]	84.2	90.1	70.5	75.5	87.7	0.913

[1] small, [2] base, [3] large.

When investigating the diagnostic performance of the CNNs depending on the anatomical region (Tables 5 and 6), better results were mainly documented for mandibular teeth compared to maxillary teeth. In the anterior region, ACC values from 94.9% to 96.0% were observed for mandibular teeth and from 86.0% to 88.6% for maxillary teeth. When considering posterior teeth only, the ACC ranged from 82.2% to 86.1% for mandibular teeth and varied between 78.0% and 80.7% for maxillary teeth. In principle, the same tendency was also observed for the AUC values (Table 6).

Table 5. Overview of the true positive (TP), true negative (TN), false positive (FP), and false negative (FN) distribution for the independent test set (N = 3000 radiographs) in different sextants, which was evaluated by the AI-based algorithm for the assessment of periodontal bone loss.

CNN	True Positive (TP)		True Negative (TN)		False Positive (FP)		False Negative (FN)	
	N	%	N	%	N	%	N	%
Radiographs with maxillary anterior teeth								
ResNet-18	155	58.7	72	27.3	27	10.2	10	3.8
MobileNetV2	154	58.3	79	29.9	20	7.6	11	4.2
ConvNeXT/s [1]	155	58.7	79	29.9	20	7.6	10	3.8
ConvNeXT/b [2]	157	59.5	77	29.2	22	8.3	8	3.0
ConvNeXT/l [3]	158	59.8	74	28.0	25	9.5	7	2.7
Radiographs with maxillary posterior teeth								
ResNet-18	786	59.1	263	19.8	151	11.4	129	9.7
MobileNetV2	798	60.0	239	18.0	175	13.2	117	8.8
ConvNeXT/s [1]	783	58.9	275	20.7	139	10.5	132	9.9
ConvNeXT/b [2]	794	59.7	278	20.9	136	10.2	121	9.1
ConvNeXT/l [3]	794	59.8	266	20.0	148	11.1	121	9.1

Table 5. Cont.

CNN	True Positive (TP)		True Negative (TN)		False Positive (FP)		False Negative (FN)	
	N	%	N	%	N	%	N	%
Radiographs with mandibular anterior teeth								
ResNet-18	244	89.7	14	5.2	11	4.0	3	1.1
MobileNetV2	239	87.9	19	7.0	6	2.2	8	2.9
ConvNeXT/s [1]	242	89.0	19	7.0	6	2.2	5	1.8
ConvNeXT/b [2]	244	89.7	17	6.3	8	2.9	3	1.1
ConvNeXT/l [3]	243	89.3	18	6.6	7	2.6	4	1.5
Radiographs with mandibular posterior teeth								
ResNet-18	691	60.9	260	22.9	105	9.3	79	6.9
MobileNetV2	672	59.2	261	23.0	104	9.2	98	8.6
ConvNeXT/s [1]	697	61.4	266	23.4	99	8.7	73	6.4
ConvNeXT/b [2]	706	62.2	271	23.9	94	8.3	64	5.6
ConvNeXT/l [3]	695	61.2	279	24.6	86	7.6	75	6.6

[1] small, [2] base, [3] large.

Table 6. Overview of the diagnostic performance of the developed convolutional neural networks (CNNs) for different sextants, where the independent test set (N = 3000 radiographs) was evaluated by the AI-based algorithm for the assessment of periodontal bone loss. The overall diagnostic accuracy (ACC), sensitivity (SE), specificity (SP), negative predictive value (NPV), positive predictive value (PPV), and area under the receiver operating characteristic curve (AUC) were predicted.

	Diagnostic Performance					
	ACC	SE	SP	NPV	PPV	AUC
Radiographs with maxillary anterior teeth						
ResNet-18	86.0	93.9	72.7	87.8	85.2	0.925
MobileNetV2	88.3	93.3	79.8	87.8	88.5	0.935
ConvNeXT/s [1]	88.6	93.9	79.8	88.8	88.6	0.951
ConvNeXT/b [2]	88.6	95.2	77.8	90.6	87.7	0.959
ConvNeXT/l [3]	87.9	95.8	74.7	91.4	86.3	0.950
Radiographs with maxillary posterior teeth						
ResNet-18	78.9	85.9	63.5	67.1	83.9	0.844
MobileNetV2	78.0	87.2	57.7	67.1	82.0	0.839
ConvNeXT/s [1]	79.6	85.6	66.4	67.6	84.9	0.858
ConvNeXT/b [2]	80.7	86.8	67.1	69.7	85.4	0.868
ConvNeXT/l [3]	79.8	86.8	64.3	68.7	84.3	0.866
Radiographs with mandibular anterior teeth						
ResNet-18	94.9	98.8	56.0	82.4	95.7	0.942
MobileNetV2	94.9	96.8	76.0	70.4	97.6	0.960
ConvNeXT/s [1]	96.0	98.0	76.0	79.2	97.6	0.969
ConvNeXT/b [2]	96.0	98.8	68.0	85.0	96.8	0.978
ConvNeXT/l [3]	96.0	98.4	72.0	81.8	97.2	0.980
Radiographs with mandibular posterior teeth						
ResNet-18	83.8	89.7	71.2	76.7	86.8	0.895
MobileNetV2	82.2	87.3	71.5	72.7	86.6	0.893
ConvNeXT/s [1]	84.8	90.5	72.9	78.5	87.6	0.916
ConvNeXT/b [2]	86.1	91.7	74.2	80.9	88.3	0.921
ConvNeXT/l [3]	85.8	90.3	76.4	78.8	89.0	0.930

[1] small, [2] base, [3] large.

All five CNNs, ResNet-18 (ACC 82.8%; AUC 0.884), MobileNetV2 (82.0%; 0.884), ConvNeXT/s (83.9%; 0.903), ConvNeXT/b (84.8%; 0.911) and ConvNeXT/l (84.2%; 0.913), tended to show similar performance data (Table 4). Furthermore, the hierarchy of results is evident in the receiver operating characteristic (ROC) curves of the five CNNs used to graphically compare diagnostic performance in detecting PBL (Figure 2).

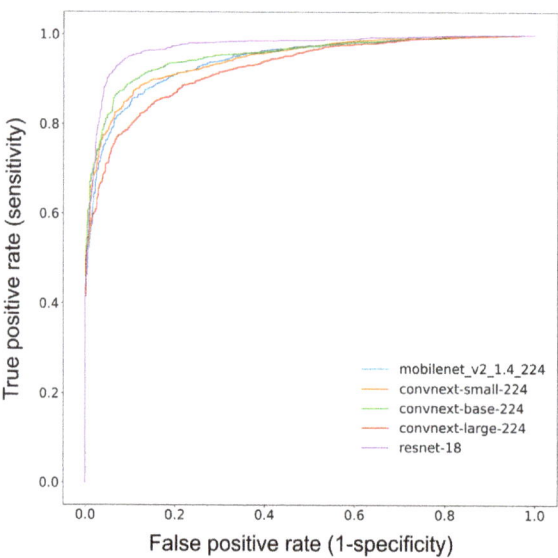

Figure 2. The receiver operating characteristic (ROC) curves graphically visualize the diagnostic performance of the developed convolutional neural networks (CNNs) in detecting PBL.

4. Discussion

The present study was able to demonstrate that different CNN architectures are able to detect PBL on periapical radiographs. However, with an overall accuracy between 82.0% and 84.8%, none of the CNNs tested were able to achieve the primary expected accuracy of 90%. Although the CNNs achieved similar diagnostic performance compared to one another, there were differences for the various sextants. This led to the rejection of the originally formulated hypothesis. Nevertheless, the results obtained provide important information for the discussion.

When considering the ability of the tested CNNs to detect PBL in relation to sextants on periapical radiographs, differences between teeth in the lower and upper jaw were observed (Table 6). Here, the projection technique and overlaying anatomical structures such as the maxillary sinuses or the nasal cavities may have negatively affected the diagnostic performance in the upper jaw. In contrast to the maxilla, mandibular sextants can be captured more accurately by use of the right-angle technique, which results in less distorted images and better diagnostic performance data (Table 6). The previously mentioned factors most likely explain the documented differences in the model performance among sextants, which were found to be similar throughout all included CNNs (Table 6). Such differences are of methodological importance. For example, Tsoromokos et al. [24] included only periapical radiographs with mandibular teeth in their pilot study to avoid data inconsistencies. Additionally, other author groups excluded radiographs from some sextants [20] or vertically rotated maxillary to mandibular teeth [26]. Such procedures may have resulted in biased and/or noncomparable results. Consequently, aiming at increasing the comparability of future studies, it is suggested to provide data for each sextant based on a well-powered image sample.

The diagnostic performance between the included CNNs was found to be similar. In general, our study results are basically in line with recently published studies of similar methodologies for evaluating PBL on periapical radiographs [19–24,26,29]. For example, Lee et al. [26] presented a model that could detect periodontally compromised premolars and molars with a diagnostic accuracy of 82.8% and 73.5%, respectively. As part of the PBL assessment, Chen et al. [25] compared so-called fast and faster R-CNNs and then determined the severity of PBL. Unfortunately, no detailed accuracy values were provided [25]. Lee et al. [23] trained a machine learning model with precisely annotated periapical radiographs, which also classified PBL according to the latest classification [13]. In this context, high AUC values of 0.89, 0.90, and 0.90 were obtained for stages I, II, and III, respectively [23]. Another study with an accurate annotation process was introduced by Chen et al. [29]. Here, the model based on deep CNN algorithms provided an accuracy of 97% for the detection of PBL on periapical radiographs and showed superior performance compared to dentists. To the best of our knowledge, no study has compared multiple CNNs for PBL detection on periapical radiographs. In the literature, there is only one similarly designed study available that tested different CNNs to identify implant characteristics on periapical radiographs [50]. When also considering studies that analyzed panoramic X-rays for the presence of PBL, it can be concluded that the model metrics were found to be similar [18,30–34,36–40]. For instance, Krois et al. [38] presented a deep feed-forward CNN to detect PBL on image segments from panoramic radiographs. They chose binary decision making to distinguish between the presence or absence of PBL by introducing a cut-off value (20%, 25%, and 30%). A mean accuracy of 81% for PBL detection was achieved by the utilized CNN. In addition, the panoramic radiographs were manually cropped, focusing on a single tooth, and the images were flipped vertically by 180 degrees during pre-processing. Subsequently, it can be seen from the results that the diagnostic performance was validated in certain subgroups of teeth, with the highest accuracy value being reported for molars (86%). The deep learning model proposed in the study of Jiang et al. [30] was also applied to detect PBL on panoramic radiographs. The diagnostic performance of the model varied between 71% and 81% for different tooth groups. Interestingly, lower accuracy values were obtained not only for maxillary molars but also for mandibular anterior teeth, suggesting that overlapping anatomical structures may negatively impact the diagnostic performance for the anterior region in panoramic radiographs. Furthermore, the diagnostic performance for each periodontal stage was compared between the model and dentists. At all stages, the model achieved higher accuracy and sensitivity values compared to the dentists. Considering the reported results, it is worth noting that the author groups that accurately annotated PBL or features of PBL on panoramic radiographs generally published more favorable results [29,32,34,37].

This study has strengths and limitations. In view of the significant heterogeneity that previous studies have shown not only in their data sets (e.g., excluding certain tooth groups, the number of radiographs) but also in the evaluation method of diagnostic performance, then the training of commonly used CNNs with a data set representative of all sextants and the representation of their diagnostic performance with standardized variables can be considered a strength of this study [24,41–43]. Establishing a representative image data set for a particular finding with a relevant number of images can be considered a crucial factor. When comparing studies in terms of the total number of periapical radiographs, our study revealed a large data set ($N = 21,819$). Only Kearney et al. [51] utilized a larger data set, with over 100,000 radiographs; however, this study differed from our study methodologically by determining the clinical attachment level instead of PBL. Additionally, studies with panoramic radiographs should be mentioned in this context. With the exception of Kim et al. with more than 12,000 radiographs [37], almost all identified studies reported data sets with less than 2000 panoramic radiographs [18,30–36,38–40]. Moreover, our study allows the comparison of different CNNs for detecting PBL for each sextant. In addition, the data set included periapical radiographs with a broad spectrum of dental pathologies or restorations.

As a limiting factor of our study, the unbalanced image distribution across all sextants should be discussed. Although the number of radiographs from the maxilla was found to be similar to that of the mandible, less than half of the images were available from anterior teeth compared to posterior teeth (Table 2), which possibly indicates an imbalance in the data set. The main reason leading to this unequal image distribution might be that under clinical conditions, the justification of an indication for radiography varies between the different sextants. In addition, moderate and severe PBL were also underrepresented. Such imbalances may negatively influence the diagnostic performance of CNNs. Therefore, it is crucial to safeguard a representative and well-balanced number of images for each sextant and severity score in order to improve the metrics of the models. Furthermore, this study utilized periapical radiographs only. However, both panoramic and periapical radiographs are considered relevant for PBL assessment. As for the aspect of comparing the diagnostic performance within different sextants, panoramic radiographs might be considered less applicable, since overlapping anatomical structures could potentially limit the diagnostic performance for the anterior region. Moreover, our data set was compiled from anonymized periapical X-rays; thus, no conclusions can be drawn about further, patient-specific diagnostic information. Additional diagnostic information, such as clinical attachment loss and pocket depths, would be particularly helpful for the initial diagnosis of periodontal disease, considering that the radiographic assessment of periodontal bone defects of low depth and buccolingual width might be restricted [52]. Here, the radiographic assessment of PBL becomes more relevant with further disease progression when the extent of osseous lesions can be visualized more accurately [53]. Another limitation to be mentioned is that we made a diagnosis for each image by distinguishing between a healthy periodontium and teeth affected with PBL (score 0 vs. 1–3). Considering that none of the five CNNs showed the hypothesized accuracy of 90%, this binary decision-making has to be understood as a limitation, which also negatively influenced the metrics of the models. It can be assumed that the precise annotation of PBL-related structures may increase the performance of the CNNs [23,29]. However, exact image labelling is time-consuming and requires extensive resources, especially with such large data sets. Nevertheless, it can be expected that precisely annotated radiographs representing a large and balanced data set would probably increase the precision of machine-based PBL detection.

5. Conclusions

In summary, the CNNs used showed nearly identical diagnostic performance in detecting PBL on periapical radiographs. However, different outcomes were documented among sextants, which can be primarily explained by the radiographic anatomy. With regard to comparable projects in the future, it is expected that the diagnostic performance can be further increased by precise annotations.

Author Contributions: Conceptualization, project administration, and supervision, J.K. and H.D.; study design, J.K., H.D. and O.M.; visualization, R.H. and V.G.; investigation, P.H., H.D., L.M., T.M., A.W., U.C.W. and J.K.; transformer network training and statistical analysis, O.M. and M.H.; writing—original draft preparation, P.H., J.K. and H.D. All authors have read and agreed to the published version of the manuscript.

Funding: This research received no external funding.

Institutional Review Board Statement: This study was approved by the Ethics Committee of the Medical Faculty of the LMU Munich (project number 020-798, approved on 8 October 2020).

Informed Consent Statement: The procedures used in studies with human participants were all in accordance with the ethical standards of the institutional and/or national research committee and the 1964 Helsinki Declaration and its subsequent amendments or comparable ethical standards.

Data Availability Statement: The data that support the findings of this study are available from the corresponding author upon reasonable request.

Conflicts of Interest: The authors declare no conflict of interest.

References

1. Kassebaum, N.J.; Bernabe, E.; Dahiya, M.; Bhandari, B.; Murray, C.J.; Marcenes, W. Global burden of severe periodontitis in 1990–2010: A systematic review and meta-regression. *J. Dent. Res.* **2014**, *93*, 1045–1053. [CrossRef] [PubMed]
2. Frencken, J.E.; Sharma, P.; Stenhouse, L.; Green, D.; Laverty, D.; Dietrich, T. Global epidemiology of dental caries and severe periodontitis—A comprehensive review. *J. Clin. Periodontol.* **2017**, *44* (Suppl. S18), S94–S105. [CrossRef] [PubMed]
3. Nazir, M.A. Prevalence of periodontal disease, its association with systemic diseases and prevention. *Int. J. Health Sci.* **2017**, *11*, 72–80.
4. Damgaard, C.; Holmstrup, P.; Van Dyke, T.E.; Nielsen, C.H. The complement system and its role in the pathogenesis of periodontitis: Current concepts. *J. Periodontal. Res.* **2015**, *50*, 283–293. [CrossRef]
5. Abdulkareem, A.A.; Al-Taweel, F.B.; Al-Sharqi, A.J.B.; Gul, S.S.; Sha, A.; Chapple, I.L.C. Current concepts in the pathogenesis of periodontitis: From symbiosis to dysbiosis. *J. Oral Microbiol.* **2023**, *15*, 2197779. [CrossRef]
6. Könönen, E.; Gursoy, M.; Gursoy, U.K. Periodontitis: A Multifaceted Disease of Tooth-Supporting Tissues. *J. Clin. Med.* **2019**, *8*, 1135. [CrossRef]
7. Kandelman, D.; Petersen, P.E.; Ueda, H. Oral health, general health, and quality of life in older people. *Spec. Care Dent.* **2008**, *28*, 224–236. [CrossRef]
8. Tonetti, M.S.; Jepsen, S.; Jin, L.; Otomo-Corgel, J. Impact of the global burden of periodontal diseases on health, nutrition and wellbeing of mankind: A call for global action. *J. Clin. Periodontol.* **2017**, *44*, 456–462. [CrossRef]
9. Chistiakov, D.A.; Orekhov, A.N.; Bobryshev, Y.V. Links between atherosclerotic and periodontal disease. *Exp. Mol. Pathol.* **2016**, *100*, 220–235. [CrossRef]
10. Borgnakke, W.S.; Ylöstalo, P.V.; Taylor, G.W.; Genco, R.J. Effect of periodontal disease on diabetes: Systematic review of epidemiologic observational evidence. *J. Periodontol.* **2013**, *84* (Suppl. S4), S135–S152. [CrossRef]
11. Gomes-Filho, I.S.; Cruz, S.S.D.; Trindade, S.C.; Passos-Soares, J.S.; Carvalho-Filho, P.C.; Figueiredo, A.; Lyrio, A.O.; Hintz, A.M.; Pereira, M.G.; Scannapieco, F. Periodontitis and respiratory diseases: A systematic review with meta-analysis. *Oral Dis.* **2020**, *26*, 439–446. [CrossRef]
12. Preshaw, P.M. Detection and diagnosis of periodontal conditions amenable to prevention. *BMC Oral Health* **2015**, *15* (Suppl. S1), S5. [CrossRef]
13. Papapanou, P.N.; Sanz, M.; Buduneli, N.; Dietrich, T.; Feres, M.; Fine, D.H.; Flemmig, T.F.; Garcia, R.; Giannobile, W.V.; Graziani, F.; et al. Periodontitis: Consensus report of workgroup 2 of the 2017 World Workshop on the Classification of Periodontal and Peri-Implant Diseases and Conditions. *J. Periodontol.* **2018**, *89* (Suppl. S1), S173–S182. [CrossRef]
14. Tonetti, M.S.; Greenwell, H.; Kornman, K.S. Staging and grading of periodontitis: Framework and proposal of a new classification and case definition. *J. Periodontol.* **2018**, *89* (Suppl. S1), S159–S172. [CrossRef] [PubMed]
15. Garnick, J.J.; Silverstein, L. Periodontal probing: Probe tip diameter. *J. Periodontol.* **2000**, *71*, 96–103. [CrossRef] [PubMed]
16. Leroy, R.; Eaton, K.A.; Savage, A. Methodological issues in epidemiological studies of periodontitis—How can it be improved? *BMC Oral Health* **2010**, *10*, 8. [CrossRef]
17. Meusburger, T.; Wulk, A.; Kessler, A.; Heck, K.; Hickel, R.; Dujic, H.; Kuhnisch, J. The Detection of Dental Pathologies on Periapical Radiographs-Results from a Reliability Study. *J. Clin. Med.* **2023**, *12*, 2224. [CrossRef] [PubMed]
18. Kong, Z.; Ouyang, H.; Cao, Y.; Huang, T.; Ahn, E.; Zhang, M.; Liu, H. Automated periodontitis bone loss diagnosis in panoramic radiographs using a bespoke two-stage detector. *Comput. Biol. Med.* **2023**, *152*, 106374. [CrossRef]
19. Danks, R.P.; Bano, S.; Orishko, A.; Tan, H.J.; Moreno Sancho, F.; D'Aiuto, F.; Stoyanov, D. Automating Periodontal bone loss measurement via dental landmark localization. *Int. J. Comput. Assist. Radiol. Surg.* **2021**, *16*, 1189–1199. [CrossRef]
20. Alotaibi, G.; Awawdeh, M.; Farook, F.F.; Aljohani, M.; Aldhafiri, R.M.; Aldhoayan, M. Artificial intelligence (AI) diagnostic tools: Utilizing a convolutional neural network (CNN) to assess periodontal bone level radiographically a retrospective study. *BMC Oral Health* **2022**, *22*, 399. [CrossRef]
21. Chang, J.; Chang, M.F.; Angelov, N.; Hsu, C.Y.; Meng, H.W.; Sheng, S.; Glick, A.; Chang, K.; He, Y.R.; Lin, Y.B.; et al. Application of deep machine learning for the radiographic diagnosis of periodontitis. *Clin. Oral Investig.* **2022**, *26*, 6629–6637. [CrossRef] [PubMed]
22. Kabir, T.; Lee, C.T.; Chen, L.; Jiang, X.; Shams, S. A comprehensive artificial intelligence framework for dental diagnosis and charting. *BMC Oral Health* **2022**, *22*, 480. [CrossRef] [PubMed]
23. Lee, C.T.; Kabir, T.; Nelson, J.; Sheng, S.; Meng, H.W.; Van Dyke, T.E.; Walji, M.F.; Jiang, X.; Shams, S. Use of the deep learning approach to measure alveolar bone level. *J. Clin. Periodontol.* **2022**, *49*, 260–269. [CrossRef]
24. Tsoromokos, N.; Parinussa, S.; Claessen, F.; Moin, D.A.; Loos, B.G. Estimation of Alveolar Bone Loss in Periodontitis Using Machine Learning. *Int. Dent. J.* **2022**, *72*, 621–627. [CrossRef] [PubMed]
25. Chen, H.; Li, H.; Zhao, Y.; Zhao, J.; Wang, Y. Dental disease detection on periapical radiographs based on deep convolutional neural networks. *Int. J. Comput. Assist. Radiol. Surg.* **2021**, *16*, 649–661. [CrossRef] [PubMed]
26. Lee, J.-H.; Kim, D.-h.; Jeong, S.-N.; Choi, S.-H. Diagnosis and prediction of periodontally compromised teeth using a deep learning-based convolutional neural network algorithm. *J. Periodontal Implant Sci.* **2018**, *48*. [CrossRef] [PubMed]
27. Lin, P.L.; Huang, P.Y.; Huang, P.W. Automatic methods for alveolar bone loss degree measurement in periodontitis periapical radiographs. *Comput. Methods Programs Biomed.* **2017**, *148*, 1–11. [CrossRef]
28. Lin, P.L.; Huang, P.W.; Huang, P.Y.; Hsu, H.C. Alveolar bone-loss area localization in periodontitis radiographs based on threshold segmentation with a hybrid feature fused of intensity and the H-value of fractional Brownian motion model. *Comput. Methods Programs Biomed.* **2015**, *121*, 117–126. [CrossRef]

29. Chen, C.C.; Wu, Y.F.; Aung, L.M.; Lin, J.C.; Ngo, S.T.; Su, J.N.; Lin, Y.M.; Chang, W.J. Automatic recognition of teeth and periodontal bone loss measurement in digital radiographs using deep-learning artificial intelligence. *J. Dent. Sci.* **2023**, *18*, 1301–1309. [CrossRef]
30. Jiang, L.; Chen, D.; Cao, Z.; Wu, F.; Zhu, H.; Zhu, F. A two-stage deep learning architecture for radiographic staging of periodontal bone loss. *BMC Oral Health* **2022**, *22*, 106. [CrossRef]
31. Ertas, K.; Pence, I.; Cesmeli, M.S.; Ay, Z.Y. Determination of the stage and grade of periodontitis according to the current classification of periodontal and peri-implant diseases and conditions (2018) using machine learning algorithms. *J. Periodontal. Implant Sci.* **2023**, *53*, 38. [CrossRef] [PubMed]
32. Widyaningrum, R.; Candradewi, I.; Aji, N.; Aulianisa, R. Comparison of Multi-Label U-Net and Mask R-CNN for panoramic radiograph segmentation to detect periodontitis. *Imaging Sci. Dent.* **2022**, *52*, 383–391. [CrossRef] [PubMed]
33. Zadrozny, L.; Regulski, P.; Brus-Sawczuk, K.; Czajkowska, M.; Parkanyi, L.; Ganz, S.; Mijiritsky, E. Artificial Intelligence Application in Assessment of Panoramic Radiographs. *Diagnostics* **2022**, *12*, 224. [CrossRef] [PubMed]
34. Li, H.; Zhou, J.; Zhou, Y.; Chen, Q.; She, Y.; Gao, F.; Xu, Y.; Chen, J.; Gao, X. An Interpretable Computer-Aided Diagnosis Method for Periodontitis from Panoramic Radiographs. *Front. Physiol.* **2021**, *12*, 655556. [CrossRef]
35. Chang, H.J.; Lee, S.J.; Yong, T.H.; Shin, N.Y.; Jang, B.G.; Kim, J.E.; Huh, K.H.; Lee, S.S.; Heo, M.S.; Choi, S.C.; et al. Deep Learning Hybrid Method to Automatically Diagnose Periodontal Bone Loss and Stage Periodontitis. *Sci. Rep.* **2020**, *10*, 7531. [CrossRef]
36. Thanathornwong, B.; Suebnukarn, S. Automatic detection of periodontal compromised teeth in digital panoramic radiographs using faster regional convolutional neural networks. *Imaging Sci. Dent.* **2020**, *50*, 169–174. [CrossRef]
37. Kim, J.; Lee, H.S.; Song, I.S.; Jung, K.H. DeNTNet: Deep Neural Transfer Network for the detection of periodontal bone loss using panoramic dental radiographs. *Sci. Rep.* **2019**, *9*, 17615. [CrossRef]
38. Krois, J.; Ekert, T.; Meinhold, L.; Golla, T.; Kharbot, B.; Wittemeier, A.; Dorfer, C.; Schwendicke, F. Deep Learning for the Radiographic Detection of Periodontal Bone Loss. *Sci. Rep.* **2019**, *9*, 8495. [CrossRef]
39. Liu, Q.; Dai, F.; Zhu, H.; Yang, H.; Huang, Y.; Jiang, L.; Tang, X.; Deng, L.; Song, L. Deep learning for the early identification of periodontitis: A retrospective, multicentre study. *Clin. Radiol.* **2023**, *78*, e985–e992. [CrossRef]
40. Orhan, K.; Aktuna Belgin, C.; Manulis, D.; Golitsyna, M.; Bayrak, S.; Aksoy, S.; Sanders, A.; Onder, M.; Ezhov, M.; Shamshiev, M.; et al. Determining the reliability of diagnosis and treatment using artificial intelligence software with panoramic radiographs. *Imaging Sci. Dent.* **2023**, *53*, 199–208. [CrossRef]
41. Scott, J.; Biancardi, A.M.; Jones, O.; Andrew, D. Artificial Intelligence in Periodontology: A Scoping Review. *Dent. J.* **2023**, *11*, 43. [CrossRef] [PubMed]
42. Patil, S.; Joda, T.; Soffe, B.; Awan, K.H.; Fageeh, H.N.; Tovani-Palone, M.R.; Licari, F.W. Efficacy of artificial intelligence in the detection of periodontal bone loss and classification of periodontal diseases: A systematic review. *J. Am. Dent. Assoc.* **2023**, *154*, 795–804.e1. [CrossRef] [PubMed]
43. Turosz, N.; Checinska, K.; Checinski, M.; Brzozowska, A.; Nowak, Z.; Sikora, M. Applications of artificial intelligence in the analysis of dental panoramic radiographs: An overview of systematic reviews. *Dentomaxillofac. Radiol.* **2023**, *52*, 20230284. [CrossRef] [PubMed]
44. Bossuyt, P.M.; Reitsma, J.B.; Bruns, D.E.; Gatsonis, C.A.; Glasziou, P.P.; Irwig, L.; Lijmer, J.G.; Moher, D.; Rennie, D.; de Vet, H.C.; et al. STARD 2015: An updated list of essential items for reporting diagnostic accuracy studies. *BMJ* **2015**, *351*, h5527. [CrossRef]
45. Schwendicke, F.; Singh, T.; Lee, J.H.; Gaudin, R.; Chaurasia, A.; Wiegand, T.; Uribe, S.; Krois, J.; on behalf of the IADR E-oral Health Network and the ITU WHO Focus Group AI for Health. Artificial intelligence in dental research: Checklist for authors, reviewers, readers. *J. Dent.* **2021**, *107*, 103610. [CrossRef]
46. He, K.; Zhang, X.; Ren, S.; Sun, J. Deep Residual Learning for Image Recognition. *arXiv* **2015**, arXiv:1512.03385.
47. Sandler, M.; Howard, A.; Zhu, M.; Zhmoginov, A.; Chen, L.-C. MobileNetV2: Inverted Residuals and Linear Bottlenecks. *arXiv* **2019**, arXiv:1801.04381.
48. Liu, Z.; Mao, H.; Wu, C.-Y.; Feichtenhofer, C.; Darrell, T.; Xie, S. A ConvNet for the 2020s. *arXiv* **2022**, arXiv:2201.03545.
49. Matthews, D.E.; Farewell, V.T. *Using and Understanding Medical Statistics*; S.Karger AG: Basel, Switzerland, 2015.
50. Kim, J.E.; Nam, N.E.; Shim, J.S.; Jung, Y.H.; Cho, B.H.; Hwang, J.J. Transfer Learning via Deep Neural Networks for Implant Fixture System Classification Using Periapical Radiographs. *J. Clin. Med.* **2020**, *9*, 1117. [CrossRef]
51. Kearney, V.P.; Yansane, A.M.; Brandon, R.G.; Vaderhobli, R.; Lin, G.H.; Hekmatian, H.; Deng, W.; Joshi, N.; Bhandari, H.; Sadat, A.S.; et al. A generative adversarial inpainting network to enhance prediction of periodontal clinical attachment level. *J. Dent.* **2022**, *123*, 104211. [CrossRef]
52. Pepelassi, E.A.; Tsiklakis, K.; Diamanti-Kipioti, A. Radiographic detection and assessment of the periodontal endosseous defects. *J. Clin. Periodontol.* **2000**, *27*, 224–230. [CrossRef] [PubMed]
53. Fiorellini, J.P.; Sourvanos, D.; Sarimento, H.; Karimbux, N.; Luan, K.W. Periodontal and Implant Radiology. *Dent. Clin. N. Am.* **2021**, *65*, 447–473. [CrossRef] [PubMed]

Disclaimer/Publisher's Note: The statements, opinions and data contained in all publications are solely those of the individual author(s) and contributor(s) and not of MDPI and/or the editor(s). MDPI and/or the editor(s) disclaim responsibility for any injury to people or property resulting from any ideas, methods, instructions or products referred to in the content.

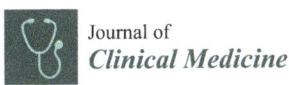 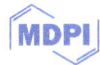

Article

The Follow-Up Necessity in Human Papilloma Virus-Positive vs. Human Papilloma Virus-Negative Oral Mucosal Lesions: A Retrospective Study

Armina Rushiti [1], Chiara Castellani [2], Alessia Cerrato [1], Marny Fedrigo [2], Luca Sbricoli [1], Eriberto Bressan [1], Annalisa Angelini [1] and Christian Bacci [1,*]

[1] Unit of Oral Pathology and Medicine and Odontostomatological Diagnostics, Section of Clinical Dentistry, Department of Neurosciences, University of Padova, 35122 Padova, Italy; arminarushiti@gmail.com (A.R.); cerrato.alessia92@gmail.com (A.C.); luca.sbricoli@unipd.it (L.S.); eriberto.bressan@unidp.it (E.B.); annalisa.angelini@unipd.it (A.A.)

[2] Cardiovascular Pathology, University of Padova Medical School, University of Padova, 35122 Padova, Italy; chiara.castellani@unipd.it (C.C.); marny.fedrigo@unipd.it (M.F.)

* Correspondence: christian.bacci@unipd.it

Abstract: Human papilloma virus (HPV) is known as the main cause of cervical cancer. Data also indicate its role in head–neck cancer, especially oropharyngeal cancer. The correlation between high-risk HPV and oral cancer is still controversial. HPV-related lesions of the oral cavity are frequent and, in most cases, benign. The primary aim of this study was to establish if there is a different follow-up necessity between HPV-positive compared to HPV-negative oral lesions. The secondary aim was to evaluate the recurrence of HPV-related lesions. All patients who underwent a surgical procedure of oral biopsy between 2018 and 2022, with ulterior histopathological examination and HPV typing, were examined. A total of 230 patients were included: 75 received traumatic fibroma as diagnosis, 131 HPV-related lesions, 9 proliferative verrucous leukoplakia, and 15 leukoplakia. The frequency and period of follow-up varied in relation to HPV positivity and diagnosis. This study confirms what has already been reported by other authors regarding the absence of recommendations of follow-up necessity in patients with oral mucosal lesions. However, the data demonstrate that there was a statistically significant difference in the sample analyzed regarding the follow-up of HPV-positive vs. HPV-negative patients. It also confirms the low recurrence frequency of HPV-related oral lesions.

Keywords: oral HPV; oral pathology; follow-up

1. Introduction

Human papilloma viruses or HPVs (an acronym for "human papilloma virus") are non-enveloped DNA viruses belonging to the papillomaviridae family. They can infect not only humans but also different animal species in a species-specific way [1].

HPVs are epitheliotropic viruses that can cause a variety of lesions at cutaneous and mucosal sites; they can only replicate within epithelial cells. While on the skin, they are generally associated with the development of benign hyperplastic lesions (warts); for some HPVs with mucosal tropism, it has been widely demonstrated that they increase the risk of neoplastic transformation of the infected site [2]. Indeed, it has been estimated that high-risk HPV is present in 100% of cervical cancers worldwide [3]. In recent years, data on the association between HPV and oropharyngeal cancer have emerged, with an estimated 80% of oropharyngeal cancers in the United States and Western Europe being attributed to HPV [4].

Human papilloma viruses are divided into five genera, based on the analysis of their DNA: alpha-papillomavirus, beta-papillomavirus, gamma-papillomavirus, nu-papillomavirus, and mu-papillomavirus [5]. Due to their association with cancer, scientific research has mainly focused on the study of HPVs of the genus alpha. The biological mechanisms underlying neoplastic development are widely known [2]; the role of HPV16 in the development of cervical cancer has been demonstrated [3,6]. HPVs belonging to the genus alpha are classified according to the risk of malignant transformation of the infected site into low risk and high risk.

The HPV genome has about 8000 base pairs that code for seven or eight early viral proteins (E1, E2, E3, E4, E5, E6, E7, and E8), two late proteins (L1 and L2), and a "long control region" (LCR) [2]. Since the virus does not code for its own DNA polymerase, it needs the replicative mechanisms of the host cell in order to replicate. For this reason, viral replication occurs only in cells undergoing mitosis [7].

In a healthy epithelium, basal cells exit the cell cycle soon after migrating to the next layer, initiating a process of terminal differentiation. In the case of papilloma virus infection, E6 and E7 stimulate cell cycle progression, and the normal differentiation process is delayed [8]. Keratinocytes normally undergo terminal differentiation, but in the case of HPV infection, E7 stimulates the progression from G1-phase to S-phase of the cell cycle (the phase in which the cell's genome replication occurs). The cell is stimulated to enter the S-phase even in the absence of mitogenic signals [9].

E7 associates with pRb, p107, and p130 proteins, tumor suppressors belonging to the retinoblastoma (Rb) family, which is involved in controlling cell cycle restriction. Since E7 alters their function, the cell is then stimulated to progress through the cell cycle [10]; E7 also causes accumulation of the tumor suppressor p16 in cells infected with HPV. For this reason, p16 is considered a marker of HPV infection in some head and neck cancers [11].

In a healthy epithelium, in case of uncontrolled cell proliferation, p53 induces cell apoptosis. p53 is a tumor suppressor with a dual function: it is involved in DNA repair or triggers apoptosis in cells with irreversible genome damage. Since E6 has the ability to induce the degradation of p53, keratinocytes infected with HPV are predisposed to accumulate gene mutations, which increase the possibility of malignant transformation. The ability to degrade p53, however, is a peculiarity of high-risk HPV and plays a key role in carcinogenesis. The role of E6 and E7 in the carcinogenesis process is evident in [6] and [12–15].

Studies in the literature report differing data on the prevalence of oral HPV in healthy subjects, with a median of 11% [16–18]. Several studies have tried to study the clearance of oral HPV infections, but the comparison is difficult due to the different follow-ups used by the various studies. Generally, the virus is completely eliminated over a period of 1–2 years [19]. However, in certain cases, high-risk HPV infection persists in basal layer cells (for about 10 years) and causes squamous cell carcinomas of the oropharynx [20].

Several authors have analyzed the possible association between HPV and squamous cell carcinoma of the oral cavity, as well as numerous oral potentially malignant disorders, including lichen planus, leukoplakia, and erythroplakia. A recent meta-review of the literature conducted on 52 studies, for a total of 2677 subjects with oral potentially malignant disorders of the oral cavity, reports a prevalence of oral HPV of 22.5%, significantly higher than the percentages reported for the healthy population [21]. In a systematic review of the literature published in 2011, it was reported that patients with oral lichen planus are five times more likely to have a HPV infection than healthy subjects [22]. In patients with leukoplakia, the prevalence of HPV ranges from 20.2% to 24.7% in the proliferative form [21]. Although the presence of HPV in leukoplasic lesions is frequent, several authors suggest that the data available are simply not enough to demonstrate the causal role of the virus in the development of leukoplakia nor the progression of this lesion to carcinoma [23].

In 2011, the IARC (International Agency for Research on Cancer) concluded that there was sufficient evidence for a causal role of HPV16 in oral cancer, while the role of HPV18 was considered possible [24].

A meta-analysis that included more than 2500 patients with oral cancer reports a prevalence of 23.5% of HPV-positive cancers, with a predominance of HPV16 (16% of cases) and HPV18 (8% of cases) [25]. A 2021 study reports that HPV16 infection may increase the risk of developing cancer in all oral cavity sites [26]. Lately, some authors have been recommending the use of narrow-band imaging for the early detection of oral squamous cell carcinoma, which showed high reliability, but it seems that oral lichen planus may lead to false positives [27].

A total of 82% of HPV-positive oropharyngeal carcinomas are due to HPV16 [28]. The prevalence of HPV infection in oral cancer is significantly lower than in oropharyngeal cancer. The reason for this different anatomical predisposition is not clear [29].

2. Materials and Methods

This study used a retrospective design. The primary aim of this study was to establish if there is a different follow-up necessity between HPV-positive compared to HPV-negative oral lesions. The secondary aim was to evaluate the recurrence of HPV-related lesions.

The population of this study was all the patients referred to the Dental Clinic of the University of Padova for the presence of lesions in the oral cavity from 1 January 2018 to 31 December 2022 who received an excisional or incisional biopsy.

The inclusion criteria were patients with the following clinical–histological diagnoses:

- Traumatic fibroma;
- HPV-related lesions (squamous papilloma, condyloma acuminatum, and verruca vulgaris);
- Proliferative verrucous leukoplakia (PVL);
- Leukoplakia.

Patients who received a clinical–histological diagnosis different from the above-mentioned ones were excluded.

Patients who did not respect the follow-up program were excluded.

Patients' data were obtained from dental records. Age, sex, anatomical site of the lesion, positivity or negativity to the high-risk HPV group, positivity or negativity to the generic-risk HPV group, the frequency of follow-ups (e.g., follow-up at 4 months, 6 months, 12 months, etc.), and recurrence were recorded.

The molecular investigation for the search of HPV DNA was performed via a polymerase chain reaction (PCR) using a CE-IVD certified kit (Papilloma Virus Nested Kit, Experteam s.r.l., Venice, Italy) following the user manual by the Cardiovascular Pathological Anatomy Unit, followed by gel electrophoresis on agarose gel (Ultrapure Agarose, Thermo Fischer Scientific, Rome, Italy) and visualized using the fluorescence imaging system Alliance 2.7 (UVITEC, Eppendorf, Milan, Italy).

The genomes identified were divided into two groups, as follows:

1. Human papilloma virus generic-risk genotypes (HPV gr): 6, 11, 16, 18, 31, 33, 35, 39, 40, 42, 43, 45, 51, 52, 53, 54, 56, 58, 59, 66, 67, 68, 70, 71, 72, 73, 81, 82, 84, and 85;
2. Human papilloma virus high-risk genotypes (HPV hr): 16, 18, 31, 33, 35, 52, and 58.

Patients were identified with a code, and the data concerning them, collected during the study, were recorded, processed, and stored with this code only and not with the patient's name, in accordance with EU regulation 2016/679, known as GDPR (General Data Protection Regulation), approved by the Institutional Review Board of Azienda Ospedaliera di Padova (CESC CODE 162n/AO/21 date 23 September 2021).

Informed consent was obtained from all subjects involved in the study.

A database was created using Microsoft Excel 2023©. Patients were inserted into the database in a completely anonymous form and were numbered with increasing prime numbers. The database was organized in a way that included some key items (Table 1).

The first entry corresponds to the patient's code, entered anonymously. The second entry, "age", indicates the age of the patient. The third entry, "sex", indicates the sex of the patient (M/F). The fourth entry, "exam date", indicates the date on which the bioptic examination was performed. The fifth entry, "diagnosis", indicates the clinical–histological diagnosis, indicated with capital letters of the alphabet, and each letter represents a specific diagnosis; for example, the letter "A" indicates "traumatic fibroma of the oral mucosa", the letter "B" indicates "HPV-related lesion", the letter "C" indicates "proliferative verrucous leukoplakia (PVL)", and the letter "D" indicates "leukoplakia" (Table 2).

Table 1. The database created for the management of patients' data.

Patient	Age	Sex	Biopsy Date	Histological Exam	Anatomical Site	HPV hr	HPV gr	Follow Up 4 w	2 Months	3 Months	4 Months
Patient 122	61	M	11/01/21	D	b	0	0	1	0	0	0
Patient 123	56	M	12/01/21	B	b	0	0	1	0	0	0
Patient 124	47	F	15/01/21	A	a	0	0	1	0	0	0
Patient 125	62	M	19/01/21	B	d	0	1	1	0	0	0
Patient 126	23	F	04/02/21	B	a	1	1	1	0	0	0
Patient 127	70	M	09/02/21	A	k	0	0	1	0	0	0
Patient 128	64	F	09/02/21	B	e	0	0	1	0	0	0
Patient 129	49	M	09/02/21	B	h	0	1	1	0	0	0
Patient 130	65	F	09/02/21	A	e	0	0	1	0	0	0
Patient 131	30	F	10/02/21	B	g	1	1	1	0	0	0
Patient 132	18	M	23/02/21	B	b	0	1	1	0	0	0
Patient 133	47	F	23/02/21	B	f	1	1	1	0	0	0
Patient 134	48	M	02/03/21	B	i	1	1	1	0	0	0
Patient 135	32	M	09/03/21	C	a	1	0	1	1	0	0
Patient 136	59	F	15/03/21	B	a	0	0	1	0	0	0
Patient 137	39	M	15/03/21	B	c	0	0	1	0	0	0
Patient 138	16	M	16/03/21	B	d	0	1	1	0	0	0

Table 2. The four clinical–histological diagnoses and the respective codes with which they were reported in the database.

	Code	Diagnosis
1	A	Clinical–histological picture compatible with traumatic fibroma of the oral mucosa
2	B	Clinical–histological picture compatible with HPV-related lesions [1] [Morphological findings compatible with viral cytopathic alterations (HPV) of the oral mucosa: fragments of oral mucosa with epithelial hyperplasia and focal hyperkeratosis and koilocytosis]
3	C	Clinical–histological picture compatible with proliferative verrucous leukoplakia of the oral mucosa (PVL, proliferative verrucous leukoplakia)
4	D	Clinical–histological picture compatible with leukoplakia

[1] To simplify the statistical analysis, all cases of squamous papilloma, verruca vulgaris, and condyloma acuminatum have been grouped under the heading "HPV-related lesions" (B).

The sixth entry, "anatomical site", indicates the site where the sample was taken and in the database, it is marked with lowercase letters of the alphabet, and each letter represents a specific site; for example, the letter "a" indicates "lateral margin of the tongue", the letter "b" indicates "retromolar trigon", and so on, as can be seen in Table 3.

Table 3. The anatomical sites of the lesions and the respective code under which they were reported in the database.

	Code	Anatomical Site
1	a	Lateral margin of the tongue
2	b	Retromolar trigone
3	c	Hard palate mucosa
4	d	Soft palate mucosa
5	e	Buccal mucosa
6	f	Vestibular gingiva of the upper maxilla
7	g	Vestibular gingiva of the inferior jaw
8	h	Tongue tip
9	i	Dorsal surface of the tongue
10	j	Ventral surface of the tongue
11	k	Retrocommissure of lower lip
12	l	Lingual gingiva of the upper maxilla
13	m	Upper lip mucosa
14	n	Lower lip mucosa

The seventh entry, "HPV hr", indicates high-risk HPV positivity or negativity; positive cases were marked with 1, and negative cases were marked with 0. The eighth entry, "HPV gr", indicates positivity or negativity to generic-risk HPV; positivity was indicated as 1, and negativity was indicated as 0. The ninth entry, "4-week follow-up", indicates whether a follow-up visit at 4 weeks after the biopsy was performed. In case the visit took place, it was marked with 1; otherwise, it was marked with 0. The tenth entry, "2-month follow-up", indicates whether there was a follow-up visit 2 months after the biopsy, and so on up to 5 years of follow-up. In case the visit took place, it was marked with 1; otherwise, it was marked with 0.

Possible cases of recurrence of HPV-positive lesions were also evaluated. Cases of recurrence were marked as "1r" during the various check-ups.

The data were analyzed using the statistical software R version 4.3.1 (R Foundation for Statistical Computing, Vienna, Austria). The R software studied the periodicity of follow-up frequencies in HPV-positive and HPV-negative patients. Dependency between qualitative and quantitative variables under evaluation was also tested using a Z-Test. A p-value lower than 0.05 was considered statistically significant.

3. Results

3.1. Sample Analysis

The total number of patients who underwent oral biopsy between 1 January 2018 and 31 December 2022 was 988, while the total number of samples on which HPV typing was performed was 284. However, not all of them respected the inclusion criteria; therefore, 230 cases were included in this study (as stated in Section 2).

The data showed that the patients were mostly over 50 (median age): for both sexes, the distributions are uniform and are concentrated between 42 and 67 years for women and between 40 and 63 for men (Figure 1).

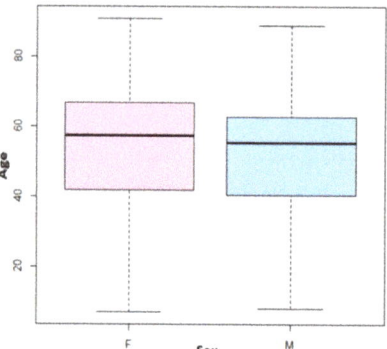

Figure 1. Age distribution for each sex.

Of the 230 cases considered, the most frequent diagnosis was type B (HPV-related lesions). Type C (PVL) and D (leukoplakia) were much rarer. Specifically, (Figure 2):

- A total of 75 cases of traumatic fibroma (A) (32.6% of total cases);
- A total of 131 cases of HPV-related lesions (B) (56.9% of total cases);
- A total of 9 cases of PVL (C) (3.9% of total cases);
- A total of 15 cases of leukoplakia (D) (6.5% of total cases).

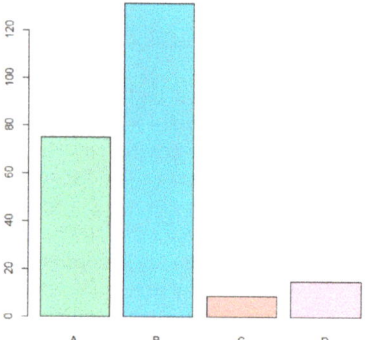

Figure 2. Distribution of each diagnosis type in the analyzed sample.

Figure 3 shows how each type of diagnosis has a different age distribution. In the case of "traumatic fibroma" (A), the age distribution is uniform; the median is around 55 years, which is slightly higher than the median age of "HPV-related lesions" (B). In this case, however, the ages are less uniform, especially between the first and second quartiles, indicating greater variability in younger patients. Precisely, 12 patients under the age of 20 were diagnosed with "HPV-related lesions". As for "PVL" (C) and "leukoplakia" (D), the distributions are much more concentrated on high values; both medians are positioned around 65 years of age with few younger outliers.

The outlier case with PVL was a 32-year-old patient, while the two outliers diagnosed with leukoplakia were 34 and 27 years old.

As can be seen from Figure 4, the most frequent anatomical sites for traumatic fibroma were, in order, buccal mucosa, lateral margin of the tongue, and labial retro-commissure.

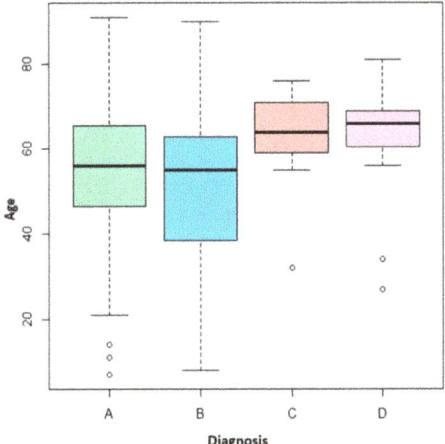

Figure 3. Age distribution by diagnosis: traumatic fibroid (**A**), HPV-related lesions (**B**), PVL (**C**), and leukoplakia (**D**).

		Hystological diagnosis			
		A	B	C	D
Anatomical site	a	26.67	13.74	11.11	13.33
	b	6.67	7.63	11.11	26.67
	c	1.33	11.45	22.22	0
	d	0	15.27	0	0
	e	36	4.58	22.22	0
	f	2.67	6.11	22.22	40
	g	1.33	6.87	11.11	6.67
	h	1.33	3.82	0	6.67
	i	2.67	16.03	0	0
	j	1.33	3.05	0	6.67
	k	14.67	2.29	0	0
	l	0	1.53	0	0
	m	2.67	0.76	0	0
	n	2.67	6.87	0	0
	Total	100	100	100	100

Figure 4. Distribution of the anatomical sites according to the diagnosis.

Regarding HPV-related lesions, the most frequent sites were the dorsal surface of the tongue, the mucosa of the soft palate, and the lateral margin of the tongue.

In PVL patients, the most affected sites were the hard palate mucosa, vestibular gingiva of the upper maxillary, and buccal mucosa.

In patients with leukoplakia, the most frequent site was the retromolar trigone.

3.2. Follow-Up Comparison

Analyzing the comparison of follow-ups between HPV-positive lesions compared to HPV-negative lesions, it emerges that:

- Patients diagnosed with traumatic fibroma (A) negative for both HPV hr and HPV gr were seen only after 1 month for a check-up visit. Patients with positive HPV hr received a further check-up after 6 months;
- Patients diagnosed with HPV-related (B) lesions negative for both HPV hr and HPV gr were seen on average only after 1 month; those who tested positive for HPV gr were seen after 1 and 6 months. The patients positive for HPV hr typing were generally seen at 1, 6, and 12 months for check-ups;

- Patients diagnosed with PVL (C) received, on average, periodic follow-ups every 4 months in case of HPV positivity and follow-up every 6 months in case of HPV negativity;
- Patients diagnosed with leukoplakia (D) received periodic follow-ups every 6 months regardless of the positivity or negativity of HPV.

A multinomial model was built, in which the database was divided between the 80% and 20% rules, and then the error was calculated on the smallest set of tests. The output showed that there is a statistically significant difference between the number of follow-up visits ("sum" variable) in all four groups. Positive and negative HPV cases have a statistically significant difference in the number of follow-ups ($p < 0.05$) but are related to histological types A, B, and C. There were no statistically significant data regarding sex and age ($p > 0.05$).

3.3. Recurrence Rate of HPV-Related Lesions

Recurrence of HPV-related lesions occurred in 4.6% of cases; 50% relapsed at 12 months, 33.3% at 6 months, and 16.7% at 16 months. On average, relapses occurred within the first year (Table 4).

Table 4. Recurrence cases of HPV-related lesions from 2018 to 2022.

	Cases	Age	Sex	Histological Diagnosis	Anatomical Site	HPV hr	HPV gr	Recurrence
1	Patient 22	58	F	B	a	+	+	12 months
2	Patient 23	84	M	B	c	+	+	16 months
3	Patient 168	81	F	B	b	+	+	12 months
4	Patient 176	41	M	B	c	−	+	12 months
5	Patient 179	63	F	B	g	+	+	6 months
6	Patient 194	20	M	B	c	+	+	6 months

4. Discussion

4.1. Oral Lesions Follow-Up

No data similar to those reported in this study are available in the literature: there are no comparison articles available on a follow-up basis of patients presenting HPV-positive or HPV-negative lesions. However, numerous studies [30–35] and systematic reviews recommend a certain follow-up of some oral lesions, considering only the diagnosis.

A study that included 1566 samples compared the histological and clinical diagnosis of oral lesions [36]. The study showed that in 31.5% of cases, the dentists' clinical diagnosis was wrong. Given the high error rate, good clinical practice should always consider the submission of excised samples for histologic examination, which is why we also decided to include recurrent benign lesions, such as traumatic fibromas [36].

There are no studies that report the follow-up necessity of traumatic fibromas, as surgical excision is resolutive and has a low recurrence rate [37,38]. For this reason, patients with traumatic fibromas were not included in a follow-up program but were seen after 4 weeks for a single check-up.

In a review published in 2021, Fiorillo et al. wanted to clarify the main features of HPV-related lesions of the oral cavity, the symptoms, the treatment, and the approach to be taken in HPV-positive patients. Given the high incidence rate of oropharyngeal carcinomas due to HPV (in particular HPV16) and given the still controversial correlation between HPV and oral cancer, the authors conclude not to underestimate HPV oral infections and suggest a multidisciplinary approach in the treatment plan and the follow-up program. Therefore, they propose a follow-up program carried out by different specialists (dentist, ENT, and gynecologist); however, they do not provide any information on the timing within which it should be carried out [34].

The data from the current study show a statistically significant difference in follow-up between patients diagnosed with HPV-related lesions with negative typing and patients diagnosed with HPV-related lesions with HPV hr positive typing: particular attention was paid to the last ones, who underwent a higher number of check-ups (at 1, 6, and 12 months).

Another review with conclusions similar to Fiorillo's, published in 2019 by Orrù et al., reports that outpatient visits to the dentist often represent the "front line" of a diagnostic–therapeutic pathway based on the evaluation of HPV-related lesions in the oral cavity. This means that proper patient management can prevent the degeneration of viral lesions to neoplastic ones, with obvious benefits for the patient [39]. Narrow-band imaging is a tool that has the potential to discern a malignant transformation occurring in some lesions of the oral cavity undergoing long-term follow-up. However, studies are available regarding the use of narrow-band imaging on oral lichen planus or lichenoid lesions, but not HPV-related lesions [40].

As for leukoplakia, data available in the literature indicate that the majority of patients with leukoplakia are over 50 years of age, and only 1% of patients are under 30 [41,42]. Our data are consistent with what has been reported regarding the leukoplakia-age distribution (median age of 65).

In this review, Siracusa et al. (who used the keywords "follow-up", "oral", and "leukoplakia") found that there are no consistent data regarding the follow-up to apply to patients with leukoplakia. Therefore, they believe that it is necessary to standardize a protocol that establishes the frequency and duration of follow-ups and the parameters to consider at each check-up [31]. They also hypothesize that the low % of malignant transformation of leukoplakia that they found (13%) is because few studies analyze extended follow-up over time [31]. However, the % of malignant transformation was not evaluated by our study.

Another literature review that analyzed 24 studies, with a total of 12,703 cases of leukoplakia, reports that check-ups should be every 3 months [32]. Other authors recommend lifelong follow-ups, with a frequency of 6 to 12 months [35]. A recent meta-analysis in 2020 [43], which considered 24 articles for a total of 16,604 cases of leukoplakia, repeats the discrepancy between the follow-up of leukoplakia patients in the various studies, and their analysis seems to be indicative of a necessity for internationally accepted guidelines for the diagnosis and follow-up of leukoplakia cases.

From the data that emerged from this study, patients with leukoplakia had semestral check-ups every 6 months, in line with the suggestions of some studies in the literature.

In a meta-analysis published in 2021 [33], 12 articles were considered, with 397 patients diagnosed with PVL. The median age was 62.34 ± 0.12 years, consistent with the median age of patients in this study, as can be seen from Figure 4. The median follow-up time for the various studies was 79.3 months, with a range of 6–171 months, and 14.6% of cases were HPV positive. Haro and his colleagues report that there is no univocity regarding the treatment, definition of recurrence, and follow-up of patients diagnosed with PVL [33]. They recommend check-ups every 3 to 6 months with photographic documentation to more easily detect clinical changes in the lesion and strongly advise motivating patients to eliminate possible risk factors for the development of oral cancer, such as alcohol and smoking. They conclude that further randomized, controlled, longitudinal, multicenter trials are needed, with a longer follow-up period and a larger patient sample [33].

The mean follow-up of the patients considered by our study was every 4 months for PVL and HPV-positive patients and every 6 months for PVL and HPV-negative patients. The timing of our follow-up (4–6 months) is in line with some evidence in the literature.

An increasing number of epidemiological and molecular studies have demonstrated a strong association between HPV and a large proportion of oral cancers of the oral cavity, tongue, oropharynx, palate, tongue, and tonsils. The prevalence of HPV infection in cancer varies widely based on the geographic region, the HPV DNA detection method used, demographics, the type of clinical specimen used, and the anatomical location of the tumor. Surprisingly, the incidence of HPV-related oral cancer is increasing rapidly (42–70%) in younger populations, mainly in developed countries. High-risk HPV type 16 is the predominant type, accounting for more than 90% of HPV-related oral cancers. Therefore, early detection is currently very important [44].

4.2. Recurrence Rate of HPV-Related Oral Lesions

Data in the literature report a rare recurrence rate for HPV-related lesions (papilloma, warts, and condiloma) [45–47]. Likewise, a very low recurrence rate was found by our data: only 4.6% of HPV-positive lesions recurred, and on average, it happened within the first 12 months (50% of cases at 12 months, 33.3% at 6 months, and 16.7% at 16 months).

4.3. Limits of This Study

The main limitations of this study, as well as the reasons why it was not possible to fill the gap in the literature, are represented by the size of the sample examined and the time interval in which the follow-ups took place. In this study, the follow-ups of 230 patients were evaluated. The number of follow-ups and their frequencies were considered from the time of diagnosis (time 0) until 1 June 2023; therefore, not all cases could have the same follow-up period. The maximum possible follow-up window for 2018 cases was 66 months. However, 2022 patients had a maximum possible follow-up window of 18 months (Table 5).

Table 5. Maximum possible follow-up window.

Year	Maximum Follow-Up Period (Starting from the Date of Diagnosis until 1 June 2023)
2018	66
2019	54
2020	42
2021	30
2022	18

5. Conclusions

The literature is full of studies that analyze HPV-related lesions, leukoplakia, and proliferative verrucous leukoplakia on several levels, but there is a lack of parameters and time indications regarding the management of a follow-up program. Therefore, a standardized protocol that sets follow-up parameters and allows the interface of several professional figures is needed to ensure the most effective therapeutic pathway.

In conclusion, although this study confirms what has already been reported by other authors regarding the criticalities present in the follow-up of these patients, it shows that there was a statistically significant difference in the sample under analysis regarding the follow-up of HPV-positive vs. HPV-negative patients. It also confirms the low frequency of recurrence of HPV-positive oral lesions and clarifies epidemiological aspects in accordance with data available in the literature.

Author Contributions: Conceptualization, A.R., C.C. and C.B.; methodology, M.F. and A.A.; software, A.R. and A.C.; validation, A.C., M.F., L.S. and E.B.; formal analysis, E.B. and A.C.; investigation C.C.; resources, C.B.; data curation, A.R.; writing—original draft preparation, A.R.; writing—review and editing, C.B., A.C. and A.R.; visualization, C.B.; supervision, C.B. and A.A.; project administration, L.S. and C.B. All authors have read and agreed to the published version of the manuscript.

Funding: This research received no external funding.

Institutional Review Board Statement: The study was conducted in accordance with the Declaration of Helsinki and approved by the Institutional Review Board of Azienda Ospedaliera di Padova(CESC CODE 162n/AO/21 date 23 September 2021).

Informed Consent Statement: Informed consent was obtained from all subjects involved in the study.

Data Availability Statement: Data are contained within the article.

Conflicts of Interest: The authors declare no conflict of interest.

References

1. Gupta, S.; Kumar, P.; Das, B.C. HPV: Molecular pathways and targets. *Curr. Probl. Cancer* **2018**, *42*, 161–174. [CrossRef] [PubMed]
2. Doorbar, J.; Egawa, N.; Griffin, H.; Kranjec, C.; Murakami, I. Human papillomavirus molecular biology and disease association. *Rev. Med. Virol.* **2015**, *25*, 2–23. [CrossRef] [PubMed]
3. De Martel, C.; Ferlay, J.; Franceschi, S.; Vignat, J.; Bray, F.; Forman, D.; Plummer, M. Global burden of cancers attributable to infections in 2008: A review and synthetic analysis. *Lancet Oncol.* **2012**, *13*, 607–615. [CrossRef] [PubMed]
4. Berman, T.A.; Schiller, J.T. Human papillomavirus in cervical cancer and oropharyngeal cancer: One cause, two diseases. *Cancer* **2017**, *123*, 2219–2229. [CrossRef] [PubMed]
5. Bernard, H.-U.; Burk, R.D.; Chen, Z.; van Doorslaer, K.; zur Hausen, H.; de Villiers, E.-M. Classification of papillomaviruses (PVs) based on 189 PV types and proposal of taxonomic amendments. *Virology* **2010**, *401*, 70–79. [CrossRef] [PubMed]
6. Lucchese, A.; Serpico, R.; Guida, A.; Crincoli, V.; Scully, C.; Kanduc, D. Interkeratin Peptide-Protein Interactions That Promote HPV16 E7 Gene Expression. *Int. J. Immunopathol. Pharmacol.* **2010**, *23*, 857–864. [CrossRef] [PubMed]
7. Pyeon, D.; Pearce, S.M.; Lank, S.M.; Ahlquist, P.; Lambert, P.F. Establishment of human papillomavirus infection requires cell cycle progression. *PLoS Pathog.* **2009**, *5*, e1000318. [CrossRef]
8. Stacey, S.N.; Jordan, D.; Williamson, A.J.K.; Brown, M.; Coote, J.H.; Arrand, J.R. Leaky Scanning Is the Predominant Mechanism for Translation of Human Papillomavirus Type 16 E7 Oncoprotein from E6/E7 Bicistronic mRNA. *J. Virol.* **2000**, *74*, 7284–7297. [CrossRef]
9. Graham, S.V. The human papillomavirus replication cycle, and its links to cancer progression: A comprehensive review. *Clin. Sci.* **2017**, *131*, 2201–2221. [CrossRef]
10. Giacinti, C.; Giordano, A. RB and cell cycle progression. *Oncogene* **2006**, *25*, 5220–5227. [CrossRef]
11. Sritippho, T.; Chotjumlong, P.; Iamaroon, A. Roles of human papillomaviruses and p16 in oral cancer. *Asian Pac. J. Cancer Prev.* **2015**, *16*, 6193–6200. [CrossRef] [PubMed]
12. Skelin, J.; Sabol, I.; Tomaić, V. Do or Die: HPV E5, E6 and E7 in Cell Death Evasion. *Pathogens* **2022**, *11*, 1027. [CrossRef] [PubMed]
13. Basukala, O.; Banks, L. The not-so-good, the bad and the ugly: HPV E5, E6 and E7 oncoproteins in the orchestration of carcinogenesis. *Viruses* **2021**, *13*, 1892. [CrossRef] [PubMed]
14. Estêvão, D.; Costa, N.R.; Gil da Costa, R.M.; Medeiros, R. Hallmarks of HPV carcinogenesis: The role of E6, E7 and E5 oncoproteins in cellular malignancy. *Biochim. Biophys. Acta (BBA)—Gene Regul. Mech.* **2019**, *1862*, 153–162. [CrossRef] [PubMed]
15. Vats, A.; Trejo-Cerro, O.; Thomas, M.; Banks, L. Human papillomavirus E6 and E7: What remains? *Tumour Virus Res.* **2021**, *11*, 200213. [CrossRef] [PubMed]
16. Kreimer, A.R.; Campbell, C.M.P.; Lin, H.-Y.; Fulp, W.; Papenfuss, M.R.; Abrahamsen, M.; Hildesheim, A.; Villa, L.L.; Salmerón, J.J.; Lazcano-Ponce, E.; et al. Incidence and clearance of oral human papillomavirus infection in men: The HIM cohort study. *Lancet* **2013**, *382*, 877–887. [CrossRef]
17. Kreimer, A.R.; Bhatia, R.K.; Messeguer, A.L.; González, P.; Herrero, R.; Giuliano, A.R. Oral Human Papillomavirus in Healthy Individuals: A Systematic Review of the Literature. *Sex. Transm. Dis.* **2010**, *37*, 386–391. Available online: https://journals.lww.com/stdjournal/Fulltext/2010/06000/Oral_Human_Papillomavirus_in_Healthy_Individuals_.10.aspx (accessed on 6 July 2023). [CrossRef]
18. Esquenazi, D.; Filho, I.B.; Carvalho, M.d.G.d.C.; de Barros, F.S. The frequency of human papillomavirus findings in normal oral mucosa of healthy people by PCR. *Braz. J. Otorhinolaryngol.* **2010**, *76*, 78–84. [CrossRef]
19. Tam, S.; Fu, S.; Xu, L.; Krause, K.J.; Lairson, D.R.; Miao, H.; Sturgis, E.M.; Dahlstrom, K.R. The epidemiology of oral human papillomavirus infection in healthy populations: A systematic review and meta-analysis. *Oral Oncol.* **2018**, *82*, 91–99. [CrossRef]
20. Taberna, M.; Mena, M.; Pavón, M.A.; Alemany, L.; Gillison, M.L.; Mesía, R. Human papillomavirus-related oropharyngeal cancer. *Ann. Oncol.* **2017**, *28*, 2386–2398. [CrossRef]
21. de la Cour, C.D.; Sperling, C.D.; Belmonte, F.; Syrjänen, S.; Kjaer, S.K. Human papillomavirus prevalence in oral potentially malignant disorders: Systematic review and meta-analysis. *Oral Dis.* **2021**, *27*, 431–438. [CrossRef] [PubMed]
22. Syrjänen, S.; Lodi, G.; von Bültzingslöwen, I.; Aliko, A.; Arduino, P.; Campisi, G.; Challacombe, S.; Ficarra, G.; Flaitz, C.; Zhou, H.; et al. Human papillomaviruses in oral carcinoma and oral potentially malignant disorders: A systematic review. *Oral Dis.* **2011**, *17*, 58–72. [CrossRef]
23. Feller, L.; Lemmer, J. Oral Leukoplakia as It Relates to HPV Infection: A Review. *Int. J. Dent.* **2012**, *2012*, 540561. [CrossRef] [PubMed]
24. Bouvard, V.; Baan, R.; Straif, K.; Grosse, Y.; Secretan, B.; El Ghissassi, F.; Benbrahim-Tallaa, L.; Guha, N.; Freeman, C.; Galichet, L.; et al. A review of human carcinogens—Part B: Biological agents. *Lancet Oncol.* **2009**, *10*, 321–322. [CrossRef] [PubMed]
25. Kreimer, A.R.; Clifford, G.M.; Boyle, P.; Franceschi, S. Human papillomavirus types in head and neck squamous cell carcinomas worldwide: A systematic review. *Cancer Epidemiol. Biomark. Prev.* **2005**, *14*, 467–475. [CrossRef] [PubMed]
26. Giraldi, L.; Collatuzzo, G.; Hashim, D.; Franceschi, S.; Herrero, R.; Chen, C.; Schwartz, S.M.; Smith, E.; Kelsey, K.; McClean, M.; et al. Infection with Human Papilloma Virus (HPV) and risk of subsites within the oral cancer. *Cancer Epidemiol.* **2021**, *75*, 102020. [CrossRef]

27. Guida, A.; Maglione, M.; Crispo, A.; Perri, F.; Villano, S.; Pavone, E.; Aversa, C.; Longo, F.; Feroce, F.; Botti, G.; et al. Oral lichen planus and other confounding factors in narrow band imaging (NBI) during routine inspection of oral cavity for early detection of oral squamous cell carcinoma: A retrospective pilot study. *BMC Oral Health* **2019**, *19*, 70. [CrossRef]
28. Ndiaye, C.; Mena, M.; Alemany, L.; Arbyn, M.; Castellsagué, X.; Laporte, L.; Bosch, F.X.; de Sanjosé, S.; Trottier, H. HPV DNA, E6/E7 mRNA, and p16INK4a detection in head and neck cancers: A systematic review and meta-analysis. *Lancet Oncol.* **2014**, *15*, 1319–1331. [CrossRef]
29. Wierzbicka, M.; San Giorgi, M.R.M.; Dikkers, F.G. Transmission and clearance of human papillomavirus infection in the oral cavity and its role in oropharyngeal carcinoma—A review. *Rev. Med. Virol.* **2023**, *33*, e2337. [CrossRef]
30. Villa, A.; Bin Woo, S. Leukoplakia—A Diagnostic and Management Algorithm. *J. Oral Maxillofac. Surg.* **2017**, *75*, 723–734. [CrossRef]
31. Saldivia-Siracusa, C.; González-Arriagada, W.A. Difficulties in the Prognostic Study of Oral Leukoplakia: Standardisation Proposal of Follow-Up Parameters. *Front. Oral Health* **2021**, *2*, 614045. [CrossRef] [PubMed]
32. Warnakulasuriya, S.; Ariyawardana, A. Malignant transformation of oral leukoplakia: A systematic review of observational studies. *J. Oral Pathol. Med.* **2016**, *45*, 155–166. [CrossRef]
33. Proaño-Haro, A.; Bagan, L.; Bagan, J.V. Recurrences following treatment of proliferative verrucous leukoplakia: A systematic review and meta-analysis. *J. Oral Pathol. Med.* **2021**, *50*, 820–828. [CrossRef]
34. Fiorillo, L.; Cervino, G.; Surace, G.; De Stefano, R.; Laino, L.; D'amico, C.; Fiorillo, M.T.; Meto, A.; Herford, A.S.; Arzukanyan, A.V.; et al. Human Papilloma Virus: Current Knowledge and Focus on Oral Health. *BioMed Res. Int.* **2021**, *2021*, 6631757. [CrossRef] [PubMed]
35. Van Der Waal, I.; Schepman, K.P.; Van Der Meij, E.H.; Smeele, L.E. Oral Leukoplakia: A Clinicopathological Review. *Oral Oncol.* **1997**, *33*, 291–301. [CrossRef]
36. Bacci, C.; Donolato, L.; Stellini, E.; Berengo, M.; Valente, M. A comparison between histologic and clinical diagnoses of oral lesions. *Quintessence Int.* **2014**, *45*, 789–794. [CrossRef]
37. Suradi, D.; Abdullah, H.; Pang, P.; Yi, E.E. The Prevalence of Fibroma in Oral Mucosa Among Patient Attending USM Dental Clinic Year 2006–2010. *Indones. J. Dent. Res.* **2010**, *1*, 61–66. Available online: http://the-indonesian-jdr.fkg.ugm.ac.id (accessed on 6 July 2023).
38. Valério, R.A.; de Queiroz, A.M.; Romualdo, P.C.; Brentegani, L.G.; de Paula-Silva, F.W.G. Mucocele and Fibroma: Treatment and Clinical Features for Differential Diagnosis. *Braz. Dent. J.* **2013**, *24*, 537–541. [CrossRef]
39. Orrù, G.; Mameli, A.; Demontis, C.; Rossi, P.; Ratto, D.; Occhinegro, A.; Piras, V.; Kuqi, L.; Berretta, M.; Taibi, R.; et al. Oral human papilloma virus infection: An overview of clinical-laboratory diagnosis and treatment. *Eur. Rev. Med. Pharmacol. Sci.* **2019**, *23*, 8148–8157.
40. Guida, A.; Ionna, F.; Farah, C.S. Narrow-band imaging features of oral lichenoid conditions: A multicentre retrospective study. *Oral Dis.* **2023**, *29*, 764–771. [CrossRef]
41. Ries, J.; Agaimy, A.; Vairaktaris, E.; Kwon, Y.; Neukam, F.W.; Strassburg, L.H.; Nkenke, E. Evaluation of MAGE-A expression and grade of dysplasia for predicting malignant progression of oral leukoplakia. *Int. J. Oncol.* **2012**, *41*, 1085–1093. [CrossRef] [PubMed]
42. Gandara-Vila, P.; Sayáns, M.P.; Suarez-Penaranda, J.; Gallas-Torreira, M.; Martín, J.M.S.; Lopez, R.; Blanco-Carrion, A.; Garcia-Garcia, A. Survival study of leukoplakia malignant transformation in a region of northern Spain. *Med. Oral Patol. Oral Cir. Bucal* **2018**, *23*, e413–e420. [CrossRef] [PubMed]
43. Aguirre-Urizar, J.M.; Lafuente-Ibáñez de Mendoza, I.; Warnakulasuriya, S. Malignant transformation of oral leukoplakia: Systematic review and meta-analysis of the last 5 years. *Oral Dis.* **2021**, *27*, 1881–1895. [CrossRef] [PubMed]
44. Carneiro, T.E.; Marinho, S.A.; Verli, F.D.; Mesquita, A.T.M.; Lima, N.L.; Miranda, J.L. Oral squamous papilloma: Clinical, histologic and immunohistochemical analyses. *J. Oral Sci.* **2009**, *51*, 367–372. [CrossRef] [PubMed]
45. Abbey, L.M.; Page, D.G.; Sawyer, D.R. The clinical and histopathologic features of a series of 464 oral squamous cell papillomas. *Oral Surg. Oral Med. Oral Pathol.* **1980**, *49*, 419–428. [CrossRef]
46. Pringle, G.A. The Role of Human Papillomavirus in Oral Disease. *Dent. Clin. N. Am.* **2014**, *58*, 385–399. [CrossRef]
47. Kumar, P.; Gupta, S.; Das, B.C. Saliva as a potential non-invasive liquid biopsy for early and easy diagnosis/prognosis of head and neck cancer. *Transl. Oncol.* **2023**, *40*, 101827. [CrossRef]

Disclaimer/Publisher's Note: The statements, opinions and data contained in all publications are solely those of the individual author(s) and contributor(s) and not of MDPI and/or the editor(s). MDPI and/or the editor(s) disclaim responsibility for any injury to people or property resulting from any ideas, methods, instructions or products referred to in the content.

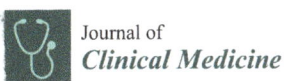

Article

Extracellular DNA and Markers of Neutrophil Extracellular Traps in Saliva from Patients with Periodontitis—A Case–Control Study

Alexandra Gaál Kovalčíková [1], Bohuslav Novák [2], Oksana Roshko [3], Eva Kovaľová [3], Michal Pastorek [4], Barbora Vlková [4] and Peter Celec [4,5,*]

1. Department of Pediatrics, National Institute of Children's Diseases and Faculty of Medicine, Comenius University in Bratislava, 83340 Bratislava, Slovakia; alexandra.kovalcikova114@gmail.com
2. Department of Stomatology and Maxillofacial Surgery, Faculty of Medicine, Comenius University, 81250 Bratislava, Slovakia; bohuslav.novak@fmed.uniba.sk
3. Department of Dental Hygiene, Faculty of Health Care, Prešov University, 08001 Prešov, Slovakia; oksana.roshko@unipo.sk (O.R.); kovalova@nextra.sk (E.K.)
4. Institute of Molecular Biomedicine, Faculty of Medicine, Comenius University, 81108 Bratislava, Slovakia; michal.pastorek@imbm.sk (M.P.); barbora.vlkova@imbm.sk (B.V.)
5. Institute of Pathophysiology, Faculty of Medicine, Comenius University, 81108 Bratislava, Slovakia
* Correspondence: petercelec@gmail.com

Abstract: Periodontitis is a chronic inflammatory disease. We have previously shown that salivary DNA is higher in patients with periodontitis. Neutrophil extracellular traps (NETs) are involved in the pathogenesis of chronic inflammatory diseases. The objective of this case–control study was to compare patients with periodontitis and healthy controls regarding the salivary concentrations of extracellular DNA and NET components. Unstimulated saliva samples were collected from 49 patients with periodontitis and 71 controls before an oral examination. Salivary extracellular DNA was isolated and quantified fluorometrically and using PCR. NET-associated markers were assessed using ELISA. We have found significantly higher concentrations of salivary extracellular DNA in samples from periodontitis patients (five-times higher for supernatant and three times for pellet). Our results show that patients also have three-times-higher salivary nucleosomes and NET-associated enzymes—myeloperoxidase and neutrophil elastase (both two-times higher). Neutrophil elastase and salivary DNA in the pellet correlated positively with the pocket depth/clinical attachment level in periodontitis patients (r = 0.31—weak correlation; p = 0.03 and r = 0.41—moderate correlation, p = 0.004). Correlations between salivary extracellular DNA and NET enzymes were positive and significant. Based on our results, the higher salivary extracellular DNA in periodontitis seems to be related to components of NETs, albeit with weak to moderate correlations indicating that NETs are produced in periodontitis and can play a role in its pathogenesis similarly to other inflammatory diseases. Further studies should prove this assumption with potential diagnostic and therapeutic consequences.

Keywords: inflammation; alarmins; cell-free nucleic acids; biomarkers; immunogenic cell death

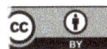

1. Introduction

Despite decades of research, the etiopathogenesis of periodontitis is incomplete. The consequence is the lack of a specific causal treatment, and so scaling and root planing are still used as the primary approach [1]. Periodontitis is a chronic inflammatory disease, and despite the undoubted role of periodontal microbial pathogens, it can potentially share some of the pathomechanisms that are involved in inflammatory diseases affecting other joints or tissues [2]. Neutrophils play an important role in innate immunity and in chronic inflammation, including periodontitis [3]. The neutrophilic inflammation that potentially starts as a response to pathogens is successfully targeted in several diseases [4], and it is likely that similar processes are ongoing in the periodontium. Proving this in a clinical study can pave the way for new therapeutic targets and interventions.

Neutrophils have several very different weapons to control infections. Neutrophil extracellular traps (NETs) have been described as an antimicrobial mechanism used in the fight against microorganisms [5]. However, it has become clear that NETs are also involved in the vicious cycle of sterile inflammation [6]. Especially, if not degraded completely and quickly, NETs and NET components are recognized by Toll-like receptors on immune cells. It is not completely clear which components are relevant, but NETs are not only produced as a consequence of inflammation, but are also able to induce inflammation, including NET formations [7]. This vicious cycle seems to be involved in the pathogenesis of various chronic inflammatory diseases [8] and can be partly responsible for the inflammation of the periodontium as well [9].

NETs are web-like structures composed of extracellular DNA, partially in the form of nucleosomes, but also neutrophil enzymes, including myeloperoxidase and neutrophil elastase [10,11]. These can be analyzed with immunohistochemistry and are observed in biopsies from periodontitis patients [12]. A common way to quantify NETs is the measurement of extracellular DNA. Whether any of these components are important for the pathogenesis of inflammatory diseases is not known. The most important proof of the role of NETs comes from a recent experimental study indicating that mice not able to produce NETs or mice treated to better cleave NETs have reduced symptoms of ligation-induced periodontitis [13]. The clinical part of their study analyzed NET-associated biomarkers in serum and gingival crevicular fluid, but not in saliva.

Saliva is a noninvasive diagnostic fluid that can easily be collected, even at home by patients, without the need for trained personnel. This is of importance for screening, but also for monitoring disease progression [14]. We and others have shown that salivary DNA is higher in periodontitis [15–17]. This increased DNA can originate from the necrosis or apoptosis of damaged mucosal tissue, but also from activated immune cells undergoing NETosis or NETs production [18]. This is not yet clear, based on the published literature on salivary extracellular DNA. Inside the cell, the DNA is protected in the nucleus and in the mitochondria. These types of DNA can be released by different mechanisms and can induce different immune responses [19]. It is, thus, important to quantify the subtypes of DNA in addition to the total extracellular DNA in saliva.

In plasma, the preparation of cell-free extracellular DNA requires a two-centrifugation protocol to remove cells and cell debris. The centrifugation force and proper handling of the supernatant after centrifugation affect the quality and quantity of the analyzed nucleic acids [20]. It has been shown that at least a part of the DNA is in extracellular vesicles that protect the DNA from degradation [21]. On the other hand, it is not completely clear what is in the pellet after the second spin. Whether these are large vesicles or organelles from damaged cells is not clear [22]. However, the further specificity contributed to by the analysis of the vesicles in addition to the DNA itself can be very helpful in the analysis of fetal or tumor DNA.

The aim of this case–control study is to compare patients with periodontitis and healthy controls regarding the salivary concentrations of extracellular DNA and NET components, including nucleosomes, neutrophil elastase, and myeloperoxidase. We hypothesize that salivary extracellular DNA in periodontitis originates from NETs and that periodontitis is associated with increased salivary extracellular DNA as well as the analyzed NET components.

2. Materials and Methods

2.1. Patients

This is a report from an observational single-center case–control study. Unstimulated saliva samples were collected at a dental clinic from consecutive patients with periodontitis (n = 49) and from healthy controls recruited from patients, healthcare personnel, and family members (n = 71). The diagnostic procedure leaned on the actual diagnostic criteria for chronic periodontitis [1] and were conducted by one examiner (OR) under the guidance of senior experts in periodontology (EK, BN). The clinical recruitment and examination took place at a single center—the Department of Dental Hygiene at the Prešov University in 2018–2019. The basic characteristics of the participants are shown in Table 1. The patients were instructed to abstain from eating and drinking at least one hour before sampling. Saliva was collected without any external stimulation by drooling and spitting into sterile tubes. The samples were processed immediately. Routine periodontal examinations, including papillary bleeding index (PBI), clinical attachment level (CAL), and probing pocket depth (PD), were conducted after saliva collection as already described [23]. The inclusion criteria included PD > 3 mm on at least 4 teeth with a BOP and CAL of 3 mm. The exclusion criteria were systemic diseases requiring pharmacological or surgical treatments or any other oral pathology. The study was approved by the ethics committee of the Institute of Molecular Biomedicine, Comenius University on 7 March 2018 (Registration number 2018-3-1). All participants signed an informed consent form.

Table 1. Patient characteristics included in the study.

Groups	Healthy Controls	Periodontitis
Number of subjects (n)	71	49
Age (years)	31.6 ± 9.5	48.5 ± 9.4
Papillary bleeding index	17.4 ± 11.8	41.0 ± 22.3
Probing depth (mm)	0.6 ± 0.4	6.2 ± 1.6
Clinical attachment level	-	3.2 ± 1.6
Bleeding on probing	-	1.4 ± 0.8

2.2. Salivary DNA

Fresh saliva was centrifuged at $1600\times g$ for 10 min at 4 °C to spin down the cells. The supernatant was transferred into clean tubes, frozen, and transported into the laboratory. Thawed samples were used for another centrifugation at $16,000\times g$ for 10 min at 4 °C to spin down the cell debris. From this processing step, both the supernatant and the pellet were used for DNA isolation with the protocol from the manufacturer (QIAmp DNA Mini kit, Qiagen, Hilden, Germany). The quantification of extracellular DNA was conducted using a fluorometric approach (Qubit high sensitivity dsDNA assay, Thermo Fisher Scientific, Waltham, MA, USA) and using quantitative PCR targeting unique nuclear and mitochondrial sequences as previously described [24]. PCR efficiency was between 90% and 110% based on the analyses of the standard dilutions. A melting curve analysis was conducted with the PCR products to confirm the specificity of the reaction. The coefficients of variation for the technical variability were 3% for fluorometry and 10% for PCR; the concentrations were expressed as ng/mL or genome equivalents (GE)/mL, respectively.

2.3. ELISA Assays

Nucleosomes were quantified using the cell death-detection ELISA kit (Roche, Basel, Switzerland). Arbitrary units (AUs) were used for the quantification since no consensus quantitative standard was available. The kit was based on the sandwich assay using antibodies against DNA and histones. Myeloperoxidase and neutrophil elastase were assessed using the corresponding DuoSet ELISA kits (R&D Systems, Minneapolis, MN, USA). Intra-assay and inter-assay coefficients of technical variation were below 5% and 10%, respectively.

2.4. Statistical Analysis

A comparison between the groups was conducted using a Student's *t*-test. The correlation analysis was performed using a Pearson correlation test. This was enabled by the lack of significant differences between the observed and normal distributions as tested using the goodness-of-fit test for normality. *p*-values less than 5% were considered significant.

The results are presented as the mean ± standard deviation. A statistical analysis was conducted using XLStatistics 5.71 (Rodney Carr, XLent Works, Deakin University, Warrnambool, Victoria, Australia). A multivariate analysis was conducted using the general liner model within SPSS version 21 (IBM, Armonk, NY, USA) taking into account age, sex, and the groups of patients.

3. Results

Patients with periodontitis and the healthy controls were not matched for age or gender, but were included in the study, consecutively explaining why there were significant differences in both factors. Healthy controls were younger and included more women (Table 1). PBI and PD were significantly higher in patients with periodontitis than in the healthy controls ($p < 0.001$). This was confirmed using a multivariate analysis with age and sex as covariates. Group (the classification into healthy controls and patients with periodontitis) was a highly significant factor affecting both the PBI (F = 17.4, eta = 0.33) and PD (F = 244.6, eta = 0.87).

Periodontitis is associated with higher total salivary extracellular DNA (Figure 1A,B). Despite the high variability, the difference in comparison to the healthy controls was statistically significant with an average of 582 ± 1023 ng/mL vs. 100 ± 259 ng/mL (t = 3.7, $p < 0.001$) for the supernatant. A similar significant difference was found in the pellet—272 ± 384 ng/mL vs. 81 ± 231 ng/mL (t = 3.3, $p < 0.01$). Nuclear DNA quantified using real-time PCR revealed similar outcomes. In comparison to the healthy controls, patients with periodontitis had a higher copy number of nuclear DNA in the saliva supernatant (Figure 2A, t = 3.2, $p < 0.01$) as well as in the pellet (Figure 2B, t = 2.4, $p < 0.05$). While the interindividual variability for mitochondrial DNA was even higher than for nuclear DNA, the average copy number of mitochondrial DNA was more than three-times higher in patients with periodontitis than in healthy controls (Figure 3A, t = 3, $p < 0.01$ for supernatant, Figure 3B, t = 2.9, $p < 0.01$ for pellet). The differences between the groups were all confirmed, even when controlled for the age and sex of the patients. The relevant eta-squared coefficients for the group factor in all types of analyzed DNA were between 0.10 and 0.19 with p-values lower than 0.001.

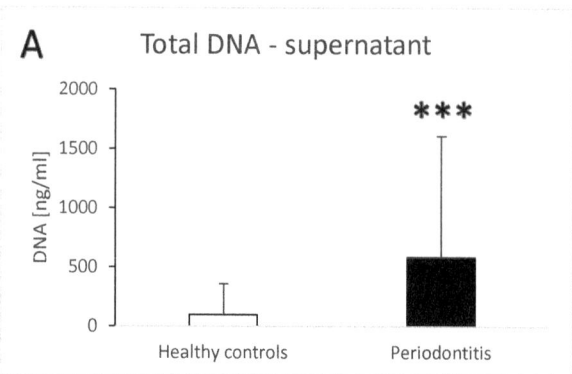

Figure 1. *Cont.*

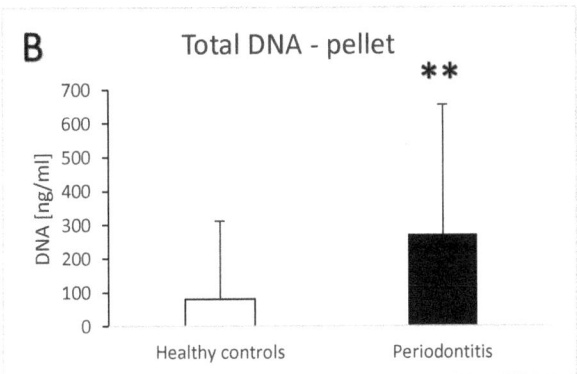

Figure 1. Total extracellular DNA in saliva supernatant (**A**) and pellet (**B**) samples from healthy controls and patients with periodontitis. **—$p < 0.01$, ***—$p < 0.001$.

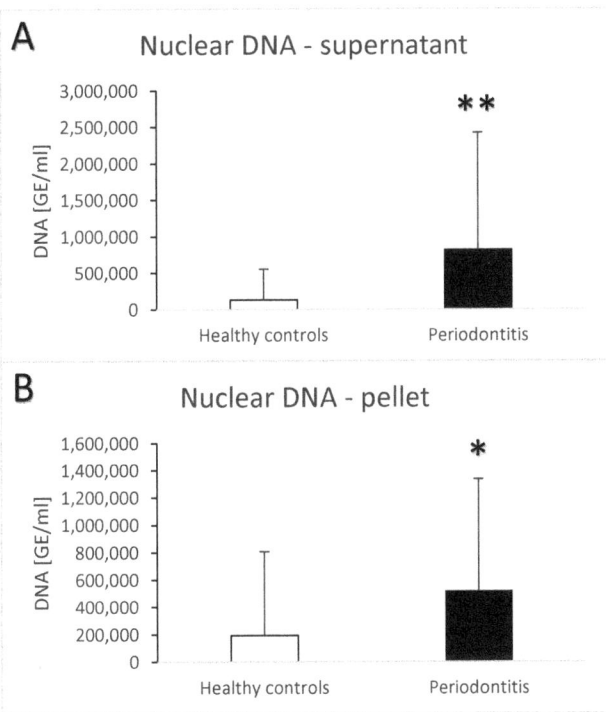

Figure 2. Nuclear extracellular DNA in saliva supernatant (**A**) and pellet (**B**) samples from healthy controls and patients with periodontitis. *—$p < 0.05$, **—$p < 0.01$.

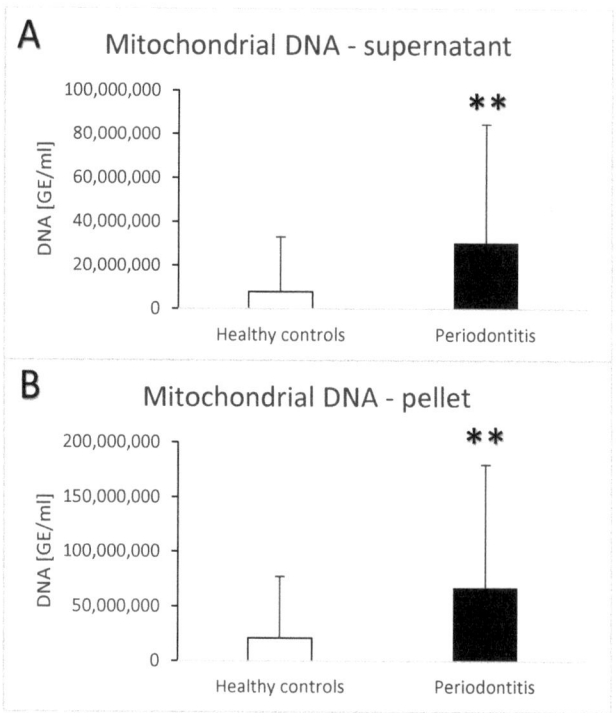

Figure 3. Mitochondrial extracellular DNA in saliva supernatant (**A**) and pellet (**B**) samples from healthy controls and patients with periodontitis. **—$p < 0.01$.

The semi-quantitative ELISA for nucleosomes showed that the saliva of patients with periodontitis contained more nucleosomes than the saliva from the healthy controls (Figure 4A, $t = 3.7$, $p < 0.001$). The quantitation was limited by the lack of a quantitative standard, but the final concentration was likely three-times higher in the periodontitis vs. healthy controls. Myeloperoxidase and neutrophil elastase as neutrophil enzymes were also higher in the saliva from patients vs. controls. On average, both enzymes were two-fold more abundant in the saliva from patients with periodontitis (Figure 4B, $t = 5.9$, $p < 0.001$ for myeloperoxidase; Figure 4C, $t = 6.4$, $p < 0.001$ for neutrophil elastase. When controlled for the age and sex of the participants, the differences between the groups remained the major significant contributor to the variability for nucleosomes ($F = 8$, eta $= 0.07$, $p < 0.01$), myeloperoxidase ($F = 15.5$, eta $= 0.0.13$, $p < 0.001$), and neutrophil elastase ($F = 19.1$, eta $= 0.15$, $p < 0.001$). Among all the measured biochemical parameters, age significantly affected only neutrophil elastase based on the multivariate analysis ($F = 6.2$, eta $= 0.05$, $p < 0.05$). The correlation between age and neutrophil elastase in the saliva was positive, weak, and significant ($r = 0.33$, $p < 0.05$).

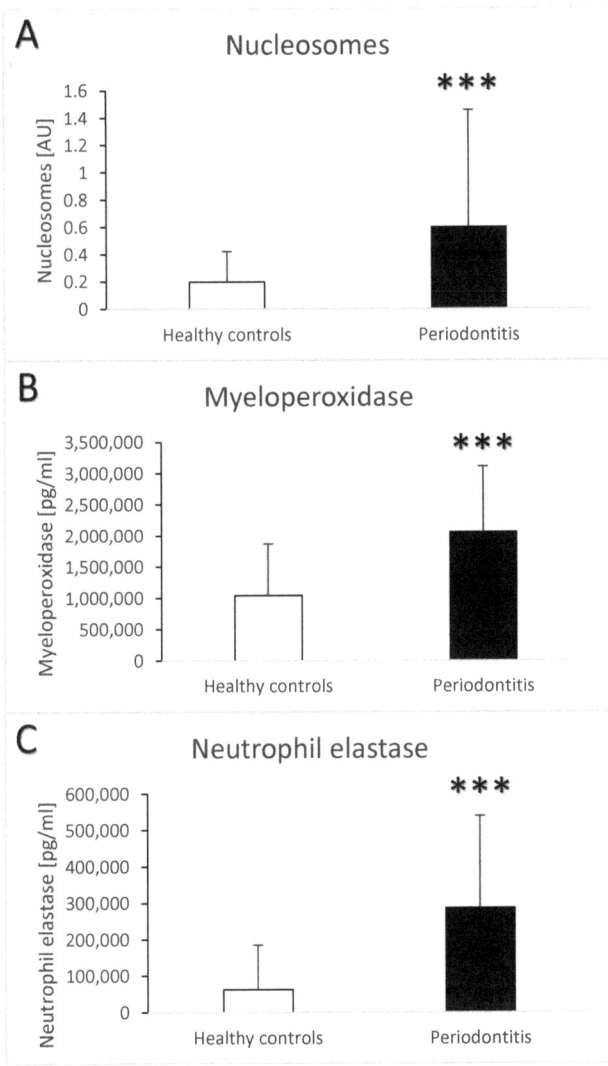

Figure 4. Salivary nucleosomes (**A**), myeloperoxidase (**B**), and neutrophil elastase (**C**) in saliva samples from healthy controls and patients with periodontitis. ***—$p < 0.001$.

The correlation matrix of the clinical and salivary parameters analyzed in this study in samples from patients with periodontitis is shown in Table 2. A moderate correlation can be observed between PD/CAL and total salivary DNA in the pellet ($r = 0.41$, $p < 0.01$). None of the NETs markers or DNA correlate with the PBI, except for a weak negative correlation with nucleosomes ($r = -0.32$, $p < 0.03$). Moderate positive correlations exist between salivary DNA and NET-associated markers (Table 3). Total DNA in the supernatant weakly positively correlates with myeloperoxidase ($r = 0.37$, $p < 0.001$) and neutrophil elastase ($r = 0.38$, $p < 0.001$). Similarly, the DNA in the pellet is moderately associated with the neutrophil enzymes ($r = 0.48$, $p < 0.001$ for myeloperoxidase and $r = 0.47$, $p < 0.001$ for neutrophil elastase). Regarding the subcellular origin of the DNA, nuclear DNA, similarly to total DNA, correlates weakly positively with myeloperoxidase ($r = 0.35$, $p < 0.001$ for the supernatant and $r = 0.39$, $p < 0.001$ for the pellet) and moderately with neutrophil elastase ($r = 0.45$, $p < 0.001$ for the supernatant and $r = 0.55$; $p < 0.001$ for the pellet). Mitochondrial

DNA correlates moderately positively with myeloperoxidase (r = 0.42, p < 0.01 for the supernatant and r = 0.45; p < 0.001 for the pellet), but not with neutrophil elastase. The associations with nucleosomes were statistically not significant.

Table 2. Correlation matrix between clinical and biochemical parameters. Bold correlations are statistically significant and weak or moderate. s—supernatant, p—pellet.

		Total ecDNA—s	Total ecDNA—p	Nc ecDNA—s	Nc ecDNA—p	Mt ecDNA—s	Mt ecDNA—p	Myeloperoxidase	Neutrophil Elastase	Nucleosomes
Age	r	0.02	0.02	0.09	0.12	−0.09	0.04	−0.06	**0.33**	−0.09
	p	0.91	0.92	0.53	0.43	0.55	0.77	0.69	0.02	0.53
PBI	r	−0.08	0.00	−0.12	−0.17	−0.02	0.04	0.10	0.07	**−0.32**
	p	0.58	0.98	0.40	0.24	0.92	0.78	0.48	0.61	0.03
Probing depth	r	0.26	**0.41**	0.24	0.28	0.28	0.28	0.26	**0.31**	−0.07
	p	0.08	0.00	0.10	0.06	0.05	0.05	0.07	0.03	0.64
Clinical attachment level	r	0.25	**0.41**	0.24	0.28	**0.29**	**0.29**	0.28	**0.31**	−0.08
	p	0.08	0.00	0.11	0.06	0.05	0.05	0.06	0.03	0.61

Table 3. Correlation matrix between salivary DNA and other components of neutrophil extracellular traps. Bold correlations are statistically significant. s—supernatant, p—pellet.

		Total ecDNA—s	Total ecDNA—p	Nc ecDNA—s	Nc ecDNA—p	Mt ecDNA—s	Mt ecDNA—p
Myeloperoxidase	r	**0.38**	**0.47**	**0.35**	**0.39**	**0.42**	**0.45**
	p	0.01	0.00	0.02	0.01	0.00	0.00
Neutrophil elastase	r	**0.37**	**0.48**	**0.45**	**0.55**	0.17	0.25
	p	0.01	0.00	0.00	0.00	0.24	0.08
Nucleosomes	r	0.13	0.04	0.17	0.13	−0.04	−0.09
	p	0.36	0.80	0.25	0.38	0.77	0.55

4. Discussion

Our results are in line with previous, published findings of higher salivary extracellular DNA in patients with periodontitis [15,16,23]. The outcomes of our case–control study were confirmed using a multivariate analysis controlling for age and sex as covariates. Despite the lack of ideal matching in this study, the differences in salivary DNA and other NET components between the groups were proved to be independent of these factors and remained highly significant. To better characterize the subcellular origin of the salivary extracellular DNA, PCR targeting nuclear and mitochondrial DNA was used. The outcome suggests that both nuclear and mitochondrial DNA contribute to the difference in total salivary DNA, although the majority of salivary extracellular DNA is of a nuclear origin and the quantity of copies is higher for mitochondrial DNA by orders of magnitude. The various types of DNA in saliva correlate with neutrophil enzymes. This is in line with the hypothesis that NETs are an important source of salivary extracellular DNA in periodontitis. Similarly, the findings of higher nucleosomes and neutrophil enzymes as components of NETs in saliva from patients with periodontitis further strengthen this hypothesis.

The extracellular or cell-free DNA in plasma is widely studied and there are already clear consensus protocols for the processing of blood and plasma samples [25,26]. No such widely accepted protocols exist for saliva and salivary extracellular DNA. We, thus, applied the EDTA blood plasma protocol for saliva. The extracellular DNA is usually isolated from the supernatant after the second centrifugation. We decided to also isolate the DNA from the pellet containing cell debris described by some as microparticle-associated DNA [27]. The direct comparison shows that the pellet DNA in periodontitis patients shows similar differences to the true cell-free or extracellular DNA in the supernatant. Further analyses of the microparticles are needed in the future to better characterize their origins, including tests analyzing the presence of NETs in this compartment. Whether they might play a direct role in the pathogenesis of periodontitis is not clear. This aspect of the study is novel and can be seen as preliminary, given the lack of any previous analyses of microparticle-associated DNA in saliva.

The findings of this study indicate that NETs are the likely source of higher salivary DNA in periodontitis. However, the proof is missing. An interventional study with the blocking of NET production in patients with periodontitis is needed. The recently published experiments using genetic models as well as pharmacological interventions are convincing [13], but are based on an animal model of ligature-induced periodontitis, which, despite being widely used, has a different pathogenesis than the human disease [28]. This does not have to be an issue for the evaluation of NETs and NET-associated extracellular DNA as biomarkers of periodontitis. Answering the research questions related to the etiopathogenesis of the disease with a model that does not recapitulate the relevant disease pathomechanisms is, however, cumbersome.

In the literature, there are several reviews published about the role of NETs in periodontitis [9,29,30]. At the same time, however, there are virtually no human studies on NETs in saliva. One exception could be the study that focused on rheumatoid arthritis associated with periodontitis [31]. However, looking into the methods, the authors rather measured the total salivary DNA, but presented the concentration as NETs. Other studies analyzed NETs, but in biopsies from mice or patients, and not in saliva [32,33]. Interestingly, some authors measured NETs in blood serum/plasma from patients with periodontitis and found that circulating NETs were higher in patients vs. controls suggesting the systemic effects of this presumably local oral disease [32,34,35]. On the contrary, in patients with rheumatoid arthritis, these complexes presented as serum NETs correlated positively with PD [35].

The current trend is to use a combined ELISA with antibodies against myeloperoxidase and DNA for the assessment of NETs [36]. However, there are several technical obstacles that likely lead to a low specificity of the assay, as previously described in detail [37]. In our study, the quantitative aspects of this assay, even if using in vitro-produced NETs, were very limited, and it seemed it was not a local laboratory issue. This can explain why this ELISA is still not commercially used, despite hundreds of laboratories around the world working on NETs' production, degradation, and their role in pathogenesis. In addition, the lack of a correlation between salivary nucleosomes and DNA or the negative correlation with PBI require further investigations, as any attempt to explain this based on the present results is pure speculation.

Based on our results, it is likely that increased salivary extracellular DNA in periodontitis stems from NETs. It is, however, not clear what should be the source of the NETs. It has been shown that some periodontal pathogens induce the formation of NETs when interacting with neutrophils [38]. Other pathogenic bacteria induce the formation of reactive oxygen species by neutrophils instead of NETs [39]. This is not mutually exclusive. Our previous research focused on oxidative stress markers in saliva in periodontitis [40,41]. This could be the consequence of bacteria- or NET-induced inflammation.

This study had several important limitations. The groups were not matched and, thus, a comparison could be biased. Dental plaque or oral hygiene indices were not included in the analysis as the study focused on the periodontal status. The changing classification of periodontitis was not reflected as staging and grading was not conducted. The observational nature of our study did not allow us to draw a conclusion regarding the causality of the identified associations. The concentrations of markers in saliva were neither normalized to salivation, which was not assessed, nor to total proteins, which could be biased, as well as shown for other biomarkers [42]. This study should test the practical applicability of the markers, which, if used in clinics, should be reported as the original concentrations. On the other hand, this study seems to be the first to study NET markers in saliva and not in serum or gingival crevicular fluid. A direct comparison of the different diagnostic fluids is needed to evaluate the specific advantages. The easy and non-invasive nature of saliva sampling makes saliva the most likely fluid to be used in the practice. The observed effects were convincing and consistent. A novel aspect is also the inclusion of total, nuclear, and mitochondrial DNA, which have divergent immune effects [43].

In conclusion, our results confirm that salivary extracellular DNA is high in periodontitis, regardless of its subcellular origin. In conjunction with the observed weak to moderate correlations of other analyzed NET components with the periodontal status, it is likely that NETs play a role as being a source of salivary extracellular DNA in periodontitis. Whether this association is causative and whether these NETs are involved in the pathogenesis of this chronic inflammatory disease is not clear. Future studies should test NET-targeting drugs for the treatment or prevention of periodontitis.

Author Contributions: Conceptualization, P.C. and E.K.; methodology, B.V.; investigation, A.G.K., B.N., M.P. and O.R.; resources, E.K. and P.C.; data curation, A.G.K.; writing—original draft preparation, P.C.; writing—review and editing, A.G.K. and E.K.; funding acquisition, P.C. All authors have read and agreed to the published version of the manuscript.

Funding: This study was supported by the Ministry of Education of the Slovak Republic (VEGA 1/0657/21).

Institutional Review Board Statement: The study was conducted in accordance with the Declaration of Helsinki and approved by the Ethics Committee of the Institute of Molecular Biomedicine on 7 March 2018 (2018-3-1).

Informed Consent Statement: Informed consent was obtained from all subjects involved in the study.

Data Availability Statement: The data obtained from this study are available from the authors upon reasonable request.

Acknowledgments: The authors would like to thank all the participating patients.

Conflicts of Interest: The authors declare no conflicts of interest.

References

1. Kinane, D.F.; Stathopoulou, P.G.; Papapanou, P.N. Periodontal diseases. *Nat. Rev. Dis. Primers* **2017**, *3*, 17038. [CrossRef]
2. Krutyhołowa, A.; Strzelec, K.; Dziedzic, A.; Bereta, G.P.; Łazarz-Bartyzel, K.; Potempa, J.; Gawron, K. Host and bacterial factors linking periodontitis and rheumatoid arthritis. *Front. Immunol.* **2022**, *13*, 980805. [CrossRef]
3. Scott, D.A.; Krauss, J. Neutrophils in Periodontal Inflammation. *Front. Oral Biol.* **2012**, *15*, 56–83. [CrossRef]
4. Filep, J.G. Targeting Neutrophils for Promoting the Resolution of Inflammation. *Front. Immunol.* **2022**, *13*, 866747. [CrossRef] [PubMed]
5. Brinkmann, V.; Reichard, U.; Goosmann, C.; Fauler, B.; Uhlemann, Y.; Weiss, D.S.; Weinrauch, Y.; Zychlinsky, A. Neutrophil extracellular traps kill bacteria. *Science* **2004**, *303*, 1532–1535. [CrossRef] [PubMed]
6. Kaplan, M.J.; Radic, M. Neutrophil extracellular traps: Double-edged swords of innate immunity. *J. Immunol.* **2012**, *189*, 2689–2695. [CrossRef] [PubMed]
7. Knight, J.S.; Carmona-Rivera, C.; Kaplan, M.J. Proteins derived from neutrophil extracellular traps may serve as self-antigens and mediate organ damage in autoimmune diseases. *Front. Immunol.* **2012**, *3*, 380. [CrossRef] [PubMed]
8. Wigerblad, G.; Kaplan, M.J. Neutrophil extracellular traps in systemic autoimmune and autoinflammatory diseases. *Nat. Rev. Immunol.* **2023**, *23*, 274–288. [CrossRef]
9. Magán-Fernández, A.; Rasheed Al-Bakri, S.M.; O'Valle, F.; Benavides-Reyes, C.; Abadía-Molina, F.; Mesa, F. Neutrophil Extracellular Traps in Periodontitis. *Cells* **2020**, *9*, 1494. [CrossRef]
10. Papayannopoulos, V.; Metzler, K.D.; Hakkim, A.; Zychlinsky, A. Neutrophil elastase and myeloperoxidase regulate the formation of neutrophil extracellular traps. *J. Cell Biol.* **2010**, *191*, 677–691. [CrossRef]
11. Pisareva, E.; Mihalovičová, L.; Pastor, B.; Kudriavtsev, A.; Mirandola, A.; Mazard, T.; Badiou, S.; Maus, U.; Ostermann, L.; Weinmann-Menke, J.; et al. Neutrophil extracellular traps have auto-catabolic activity and produce mononucleosome-associated circulating DNA. *Genome Med.* **2022**, *14*, 135. [CrossRef] [PubMed]
12. Vitkov, L.; Klappacher, M.; Hannig, M.; Krautgartner, W.D. Extracellular neutrophil traps in periodontitis. *J. Periodontal Res.* **2009**, *44*, 664–672. [CrossRef] [PubMed]
13. Kim, T.S.; Silva, L.M.; Theofilou, V.I.; Greenwell-Wild, T.; Li, L.; Williams, D.W.; Ikeuchi, T.; Brenchley, L.; Bugge, T.H.; Diaz, P.I.; et al. Neutrophil extracellular traps and extracellular histones potentiate IL-17 inflammation in periodontitis. *J. Exp. Med.* **2023**, *220*, e20221751. [CrossRef] [PubMed]
14. Nonaka, T.; Wong, D.T.W. Saliva Diagnostics. *Annu. Rev. Anal. Chem.* **2022**, *15*, 107–121. [CrossRef] [PubMed]
15. Baňasová, L.; Kamodyová, N.; Janšáková, K.; Tóthová, L'.; Stanko, P.; Turňa, J.; Celec, P. Salivary DNA and markers of oxidative stress in patients with chronic periodontitis. *Clin. Oral. Investig.* **2015**, *19*, 201–207. [CrossRef]

16. Su, H.; Gornitsky, M.; Velly, A.M.; Yu, H.; Benarroch, M.; Schipper, H.M. Salivary DNA, lipid, and protein oxidation in nonsmokers with periodontal disease. *Free Radic. Biol. Med.* **2009**, *46*, 914–921. [CrossRef]
17. Zhu, X.; Chu, C.J.; Pan, W.; Li, Y.; Huang, H.; Zhao, L. The Correlation between Periodontal Parameters and Cell-Free DNA in the Gingival Crevicular Fluid, Saliva, and Plasma in Chinese Patients: A Cross-Sectional Study. *J. Clin. Med.* **2022**, *11*, 6902. [CrossRef] [PubMed]
18. Pisetsky, D.S. The origin and properties of extracellular DNA: From PAMP to DAMP. *Clin. Immunol.* **2012**, *144*, 32–40. [CrossRef]
19. Stortz, J.A.; Hawkins, R.B.; Holden, D.C.; Raymond, S.L.; Wang, Z.; Brakenridge, S.C.; Cuschieri, J.; Moore, F.A.; Maier, R.V.; Moldawer, L.L.; et al. Cell-free nuclear, but not mitochondrial, DNA concentrations correlate with the early host inflammatory response after severe trauma. *Sci. Rep.* **2019**, *9*, 13648. [CrossRef]
20. Sorber, L.; Zwaenepoel, K.; Jacobs, J.; De Winne, K.; Goethals, S.; Reclusa, P.; Van Casteren, K.; Augustus, E.; Lardon, F.; Roeyen, G.; et al. Circulating Cell-Free DNA and RNA Analysis as Liquid Biopsy: Optimal Centrifugation Protocol. *Cancers* **2019**, *11*, 458. [CrossRef]
21. Jin, Y.; Chen, K.; Wang, Z.; Wang, Y.; Liu, J.; Lin, L.; Shao, Y.; Gao, L.; Yin, H.; Cui, C.; et al. DNA in serum extracellular vesicles is stable under different storage conditions. *BMC Cancer* **2016**, *16*, 753. [CrossRef] [PubMed]
22. Lapin, M.; Tjensvoll, K.; Nedrebø, K.; Taksdal, E.; Janssen, H.; Gilje, B.; Nordgård, O. Extracellular vesicles as a potential source of tumor-derived DNA in advanced pancreatic cancer. *PLoS ONE* **2023**, *18*, e0291623. [CrossRef] [PubMed]
23. Konečná, B.; Gaál Kovalčíková, A.; Pančíková, A.; Novák, B.; Kovaľová, E.; Celec, P.; Tóthová, Ľ. Salivary Extracellular DNA and DNase Activity in Periodontitis. *Appl. Sci.* **2020**, *10*, 7490. [CrossRef]
24. Janovičová, Ľ.; Konečná, B.; Vlková, B.; Celec, P. Isolation and Quantification of Extracellular DNA from Biofluids. *Bio-Protocol* **2020**, *10*, e3726. [CrossRef] [PubMed]
25. Bronkhorst, A.J.; Ungerer, V.; Diehl, F.; Anker, P.; Dor, Y.; Fleischhacker, M.; Gahan, P.B.; Hui, L.; Holdenrieder, S.; Thierry, A.R. Towards systematic nomenclature for cell-free DNA. *Hum. Genet.* **2021**, *140*, 565–578. [CrossRef]
26. Meddeb, R.; Dache, Z.A.A.; Thezenas, S.; Otandault, A.; Tanos, R.; Pastor, B.; Sanchez, C.; Azzi, J.; Tousch, G.; Azan, S.; et al. Quantifying circulating cell-free DNA in humans. *Sci. Rep.* **2019**, *9*, 5220. [CrossRef]
27. Pisetsky, D.S.; Gauley, J.; Ullal, A.J. Microparticles as a source of extracellular DNA. *Immunol. Res.* **2011**, *49*, 227–234. [CrossRef]
28. Li, D.; Feng, Y.; Tang, H.; Huang, L.; Tong, Z.; Hu, C.; Chen, X.; Tan, J. A Simplified and Effective Method for Generation of Experimental Murine Periodontitis Model. *Front. Bioeng. Biotechnol.* **2020**, *8*, 444. [CrossRef]
29. Vitkov, L.; Hartl, D.; Minnich, B.; Hannig, M. Janus-Faced Neutrophil Extracellular Traps in Periodontitis. *Front. Immunol.* **2017**, *8*, 1404. [CrossRef]
30. White, P.C.; Chicca, I.J.; Cooper, P.R.; Milward, M.R.; Chapple, I.L. Neutrophil Extracellular Traps in Periodontitis: A Web of Intrigue. *J. Dent. Res.* **2016**, *95*, 26–34. [CrossRef]
31. Oliveira, S.R.; de Arruda, J.A.A.; Schneider, A.H.; Carvalho, V.F.; Machado, C.C.; Corrêa, J.D.; Moura, M.F.; Duffles, L.F.; de Souza, F.F.L.; Ferreira, G.A.; et al. Are neutrophil extracellular traps the link for the cross-talk between periodontitis and rheumatoid arthritis physiopathology? *Rheumatology* **2021**, *61*, 174–184. [CrossRef] [PubMed]
32. Guilherme Neto, J.L.; Rodrigues Venturini, L.G.; Schneider, A.H.; Taira, T.M.; Duffles Rodrigues, L.F.; Veras, F.P.; Oliveira, S.R.; da Silva, T.A.; Cunha, F.Q.; Fukada, S.Y. Neutrophil Extracellular Traps Aggravate Apical Periodontitis by Stimulating Osteoclast Formation. *J. Endod.* **2023**, *49*, 1514–1521. [CrossRef] [PubMed]
33. Magán-Fernández, A.; O'Valle, F.; Abadía-Molina, F.; Muñoz, R.; Puga-Guil, P.; Mesa, F. Characterization and comparison of neutrophil extracellular traps in gingival samples of periodontitis and gingivitis: A pilot study. *J. Periodontal. Res.* **2019**, *54*, 218–224. [CrossRef]
34. White, P.; Sakellari, D.; Roberts, H.; Risafi, I.; Ling, M.; Cooper, P.; Milward, M.; Chapple, I. Peripheral blood neutrophil extracellular trap production and degradation in chronic periodontitis. *J. Clin. Periodontol.* **2016**, *43*, 1041–1049. [CrossRef] [PubMed]
35. Kaneko, C.; Kobayashi, T.; Ito, S.; Sugita, N.; Murasawa, A.; Nakazono, K.; Yoshie, H. Circulating levels of carbamylated protein and neutrophil extracellular traps are associated with periodontitis severity in patients with rheumatoid arthritis: A pilot case-control study. *PLoS ONE* **2018**, *13*, e0192365. [CrossRef] [PubMed]
36. Islam, M.M.; Salma, U.; Irahara, T.; Watanabe, E.; Takeyama, N. Quantifying Myeloperoxidase-DNA and Neutrophil Elastase-DNA Complexes from Neutrophil Extracellular Traps by Using a Modified Sandwich ELISA. *J. Vis. Exp.* **2023**, *195*, e64644. [CrossRef] [PubMed]
37. Hayden, H.; Ibrahim, N.; Klopf, J.; Zagrapan, B.; Mauracher, L.M.; Hell, L.; Hofbauer, T.M.; Ondracek, A.S.; Schoergenhofer, C.; Jilma, B.; et al. ELISA detection of MPO-DNA complexes in human plasma is error-prone and yields limited information on neutrophil extracellular traps formed in vivo. *PLoS ONE* **2021**, *16*, e0250265. [CrossRef]
38. Jayaprakash, K.; Demirel, I.; Khalaf, H.; Bengtsson, T. The role of phagocytosis, oxidative burst and neutrophil extracellular traps in the interaction between neutrophils and the periodontal pathogen Porphyromonas gingivalis. *Mol. Oral Microbiol.* **2015**, *30*, 361–375. [CrossRef]
39. White, P.; Cooper, P.; Milward, M.; Chapple, I. Differential activation of neutrophil extracellular traps by specific periodontal bacteria. *Free Radic. Biol. Med.* **2014**, *75* (Suppl. S1), S53. [CrossRef]
40. Celecová, V.; Kamodyová, N.; Tóthová, L.; Kúdela, M.; Celec, P. Salivary markers of oxidative stress are related to age and oral health in adult non-smokers. *J. Oral Pathol. Med.* **2013**, *42*, 263–266. [CrossRef]

41. Tóthová, L.; Celecová, V.; Celec, P. Salivary markers of oxidative stress and their relation to periodontal and dental status in children. *Dis. Markers* **2013**, *34*, 9–15. [CrossRef] [PubMed]
42. Contreras-Aguilar, M.D.; Escribano, D.; Martínez-Subiela, S.; Martínez-Miró, S.; Rubio, M.; Tvarijonaviciute, A.; Tecles, F.; Cerón, J.J. Influence of the way of reporting alpha-Amylase values in saliva in different naturalistic situations: A pilot study. *PLoS ONE* **2017**, *12*, e0180100. [CrossRef] [PubMed]
43. Riley, J.S.; Tait, S.W. Mitochondrial DNA in inflammation and immunity. *EMBO Rep.* **2020**, *21*, e49799. [CrossRef] [PubMed]

Disclaimer/Publisher's Note: The statements, opinions and data contained in all publications are solely those of the individual author(s) and contributor(s) and not of MDPI and/or the editor(s). MDPI and/or the editor(s) disclaim responsibility for any injury to people or property resulting from any ideas, methods, instructions or products referred to in the content.

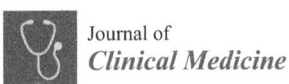

Review

Hepatitis C Virus (HCV) Infection: Pathogenesis, Oral Manifestations, and the Role of Direct-Acting Antiviral Therapy: A Narrative Review

Dario Di Stasio [1,†], Agostino Guida [2,*,†], Antonio Romano [1], Massimo Petruzzi [3], Aldo Marrone [1], Fausto Fiori [1] and Alberta Lucchese [1]

1. Multidisciplinary Department of Medical-Surgical and Dental Specialties, University of Campania "Luigi Vanvitelli", 81100 Naples, Italy; aldo.marrone@unicampania.it (A.M.); alberta.lucchese@unicampania.it (A.L.)
2. U.O.C. Odontostomatologia, A.O.R.N. "A. Cardarelli", 95123 Naples, Italy
3. Section of Dentistry, Interdisciplinary Department of Medicine (DIM), University "Aldo Moro" of Bari, Clinica Odontoiatrica del Policlinico di Bari, Piazza Giulio Cesare 11, 70124 Bari, Italy
* Correspondence: agostino.guida@aocardarelli.it; Tel.: +39-817472362
† These authors contributed equally to this work.

Abstract: Hepatitis C virus (HCV) infection is a global health concern with significant systemic implications, including a range of oral manifestations. This review aims to provide a comprehensive overview of the oral and dental pathologies related to HCV, the etiopathogenetic mechanisms linking such conditions to HCV and the impact of direct-acting antiviral (DAA) therapy. Common oral manifestations of HCV include oral lichen planus (OLP), periodontal disease, and xerostomia. The pathogenesis of these conditions involves both direct viral effects on oral tissues and indirect effects related to the immune response to HCV. Our literature analysis, using PubMed, Scopus, Web of Science, and Google Scholar, suggests that both the HCV infection and the immune response to HCV contribute to the increased prevalence of these oral diseases. The introduction of DAA therapy represents a significant advancement in HCV treatment, but its effects on oral manifestations, particularly OLP, are still under evaluation. Although a possible mechanism linking HCV to OSCC is yet to be determined, existing evidence encourages further investigation in this sense. Our findings highlight the need for established protocols for managing the oral health of patients with HCV, aiming to improve outcomes and quality of life.

Keywords: hepatitis C; extra-hepatic manifestations; oral mucosa; oral cavity

1. Introduction

Hepatitis C virus (HCV) infection is a critical public health issue, affecting millions worldwide. It is primarily known for its impact on liver function, but its systemic nature means that its effects can be far-reaching, including the oral cavity [1].

The global burden of HCV is substantial, with varying prevalence rates across different regions. The introduction of direct-acting antivirals (DAAs) has revolutionized the treatment landscape [2]. However, the oral implications of HCV, particularly in the context of oral lichen planus (OLP), xerostomia, and Sjögren's syndrome-like manifestations, periodontal diseases, and head and neck squamous cell carcinoma (HNSCC) require further exploration.

This narrative review seeks to elucidate the various oral manifestations of HCV, with a special focus on OLP [3]. Drawing from a range of sources, including a detailed cohort study on the impact of DAAs on HCV-related OLP, this review aims to provide a comprehensive overview of the current state of knowledge in this field [4].

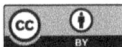

1.1. Pathophysiology

HCV is a small, enveloped RNA virus from the Flaviviridae family [5]. It primarily targets hepatocytes, leading to chronic inflammation, fibrosis, and potentially cirrhosis or hepatocellular carcinoma [6]. Beyond the liver, HCV affects various systems, including the oral cavity [7]. The virus's interaction with the immune system is critical for its persistence and the development of extrahepatic manifestations, such as OLP [8].

1.1.1. Viral Entry and Replication

HCV entry into liver cells involves interactions between viral envelope proteins (E1 and E2) and host cell receptors like CD81, SR-B1, CLDN1, and OCLN, facilitating endocytosis [9]. Once inside, the viral RNA genome is released and translated into a polyprotein, which is cleaved into structural and non-structural proteins. The non-structural proteins form a replicase complex that synthesizes new viral RNA, highlighting the virus's dependence on the host's lipid metabolism and VLDL synthesis pathway [10–12].

1.1.2. Immune Response and Liver Damage

HCV infection triggers the innate immune system via pattern recognition receptors, leading to the production of type I and III interferons (IFNs). These IFNs induce an antiviral state in hepatocytes and activate immune cells like NK cells and macrophages [13]. The adaptive immune response involves B-cells producing specific antibodies and T-cells targeting infected hepatocytes [14]. Chronic HCV infection often results in an insufficient T-cell response, leading to persistent inflammation, hepatocyte injury, and the activation of hepatic stellate cells, promoting fibrosis [15]. HCV evades the immune response through rapid mutation, the suppression of IFN pathways, and the induction of immune cell exhaustion, complicating viral clearance [16,17].

1.1.3. Chronic Infection and Fibrosis

Chronic HCV infection maintains liver inflammation, activating hepatic stellate cells (HSCs) to produce excessive extracellular matrix, leading to fibrosis and cirrhosis [18,19]. This process is mediated by cytokines like TGF-β and involves interactions between HSCs, immune cells, and liver epithelial cells. Chronic inflammation and oxidative stress perpetuate fibrosis, disrupting liver architecture and function [20,21]. Advanced fibrosis results in cirrhosis, impairing liver function and causing complications such as portal hypertension and liver failure [22].

1.1.4. Extrahepatic Manifestations

HCV's systemic effects include immune complex formation, cryoglobulinemia, and direct viral effects on various tissues. These mechanisms lead to conditions like mixed cryoglobulinemia syndrome, neuropsychiatric disorders, thyroid dysfunction, renal disease, pulmonary conditions, dermatological manifestations, and ocular diseases [23–26]. Cryoglobulinemia, involving immunoglobulins that precipitate in the cold, can cause organ damage through hyperviscosity syndrome or immune-mediated mechanisms [27]. Research shows HCV RNA in B-cells, indicating viral replication within these cells. This interaction with the immune system, particularly through the CD81 receptor on B-cells, plays a significant role in HCV pathogenesis and the development of cryoglobulinemia, which is closely linked to lymphoproliferative disorders and an increased risk of non-Hodgkin's lymphoma [28,29].

2. Oral Manifestations

OLP, xerostomia, and periodontal disease have been reported as oral manifestations in patients with HCV infection. These associations are thought to be mediated through both direct viral effects on oral tissues and indirect effects related to the immune response to HCV [30].

The relationship between HCV and these oral manifestations is underpinned by both direct viral effects and the virus's impact on the immune system, leading to inflammatory and autoimmune responses within the oral cavity [31]. The advent of direct-acting antivirals (DAAs) has begun to change the landscape, with emerging evidence suggesting improvements in oral health outcomes among treated individuals [32].

2.1. OLP

OLP is a chronic inflammatory condition of the mucous membranes, often presenting with white, lacy patches, or red, swollen tissues [33]. A significant body of research has explored the association between OLP and HCV infection, with varying prevalence rates reported globally [1]. This association has been a subject of significant research interest, leading to new insights into pathogenesis and management [34]. The global prevalence of HCV in patients with OLP is reported to be variable, with a recent meta-analysis indicating that OLP patients have a four-fold higher frequency of HCV compared to controls. This prevalence exhibits geographical variability. When analyzing the prevalence of OLP in HCV-infected patients across different geographic regions, the African and Southeast Asian regions showed the highest odds ratios of 8.57 and 7.73, respectively. In contrast, studies from the European region did not demonstrate a significant association (OR 2.08 [0.95–4.52]). On a country level, Iraq and Egypt exhibited nearly ten-fold increases in risk, highlighting significant regional variations [35]. This study also suggested that geographical variability could be due to immunogenetic influences, such as different HCV genotypes and human leukocyte antigens (HLA). HCV genotypes 1a and 1b are most common in LP patients with HCV, varying by region. For example, in India, 70% of LP patients had genotype 1b compared to 34.1% in donors [35]. Genotype 3 is predominant in the UK, and genotype 4 is prevalent in Egypt.

Moreover, the association is strong in the Eastern Mediterranean (OR 5.51) but not in Europe (OR 1.47). Some studies detected HCV RNA in skin and oral mucosa, suggesting possible epithelial tropism. The lymphotropic nature of HCV, causing B-lymphocyte expansion and autoimmune responses, might contribute to LP. Increased oxidative stress in HCV patients also plays a role [35].

The pathogenesis of OLP in HCV-infected patients is complex and not fully understood. It is suggested that HCV replicates in the oral mucosa, leading to a localized immune response. The presence of HCV-specific T lymphocytes in the oral mucosa of OLP patients implies the potential involvement of HCV in its pathogenesis. There is also evidence of circulating antibodies to epithelial antigens in some patients with HCV-associated OLP, although their precise role in disease development remains unclear [8]. A recent review suggested that the pathogenesis of OLP involves a complex interplay of immune responses, with dysbiosis in the oral microbial community and altered immune pathways potentially playing a significant role. In particular, pathways involved in defense against bacterial infection and inflammatory responses are activated in OLP-associated microbiomes [36]. Molecular studies have found HCV RNA in oral lichen tissue, indicating sporadic HCV replication in these lesions. However, the exact mechanism by which HCV contributes to OLP remains to be fully elucidated [37]. In fact, the association between HCV and oral lichen planus (OLP) may be due to the virus's ability to replicate in the skin and oral mucosa. While HCV replication is predominantly observed in hepatocytes, some studies have detected viral RNA in the skin and oral mucosa of patients with chronic hepatitis C, regardless of the presence of lichen planus (LP) lesions. However, other studies have failed to find HCV RNA in these tissues, indicating that evidence supporting the epithelial tropism of HCV is currently insufficient [38].

The cytokine profile in HCV-associated OLP suggests an immune response characterized by excessive production of Th1 cytokines following an ineffective antiviral immune response [39].

Various studies have examined the roles of different cytokines in this context:

a. Th1 cytokines and immune response: El-Howati et al. emphasize the role of CD8+ cytotoxic and CD4+ Th1 polarized T-cells in OLP, noting the involvement of other Th subsets such as Th9, Th17, and Tregs in the disease's pathogenesis. They suggest that both direct effects of HCV on the immune system and broader dysregulation contribute to OLP [40]. Studies have consistently shown an increased production of Th1 cytokines, including TNF-alpha, which indicates a strong Th1-mediated immune response [39].
b. Role of CD8+ cytotoxic T-cells: CD8+ T-cells are crucial for targeting HCV-infected cells. However, the high mutation rate of HCV often leads to immune escape, resulting in chronic infection. This mechanism is well-documented and highlights the challenges in clearing the virus [41].
c. Helper T-cells and sustained Th1 response: Helper T-cells assist in maintaining the function of CD8+ T-cells and in cytokine production. In chronic HCV infection, this leads to a sustained Th1 response, which can become dysregulated over time. This prolonged response contributes to the pathology observed in OLP [42].
d. Th9, Th17, and regulatory T-cells (Tregs): Th9 and Th17 cells are associated with inflammation and tissue damage, which are characteristic of chronic infections. Studies have shown that these cells contribute to the immunopathogenesis of OLP [42]. Tregs help maintain immune tolerance and prevent autoimmune responses. Their altered function during HCV infection is a significant factor in the disease progression [42].
e. Salivary cytokine profiles in OLP patients: Research on salivary cytokine profiles in OLP patients has found higher concentrations of IL-2, IL-23, and TGF-β, suggesting these cytokines play a role in OLP pathogenesis [43]. Askoura et al. reported elevated levels of IL-33, IL-17, and IL-25 in HCV patients, indicating their involvement in inflammation and the progression of fibrosis [44].
f. Cytokines and disease prognosis: Zhu et al. highlighted a set of cytokines/chemokines correlated with disease prognosis in chronic liver disease, which is relevant for understanding OLP associated with HCV [45]. Vičić et al. reviewed the immunopathogenesis of lichen planus, emphasizing the complex interplay of immune cells and inflammatory pathways in HCV-associated OLP [46].
g. Impact of HCV eradication on cytokine profiles: Radmanić et al. evaluated the impact of HCV eradication on cytokine and growth factor profiles, providing insights into potential changes in the cytokine environment in OLP following HCV treatment [47].

In summary, as shown in Figure 1, while different studies focus on various cytokines and immune responses, the overarching theme is the multifaceted immune dysregulation driven by both antiviral and inflammatory responses in HCV-associated OLP.

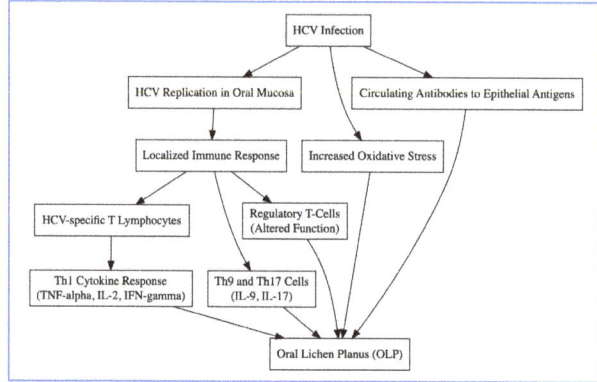

Figure 1. Aetiopathogenic hypotheses of the relationship between HCV infection and OLP.

The variable effect of antiviral therapy, including interferon-alpha (IFN-alpha) with or without ribavirin on OLP has been noted, with some patients experiencing an improvement in OLP lesions following HCV treatment [48]. This suggested a potential direct role of HCV in the pathogenesis of OLP, although this is not a consistent finding across all patients. In fact, some studies reported that OLP occurred, exacerbated, and persisted during IFN treatment for hepatitis C, even when serum HCV RNA became negative. The improvement of the lesions of OLP after the discontinuation of therapy suggests a role of IFN in inducing or worsening these lesions in some patients [45,49]. Moreover, the combination of interferon (IFN) and ribavirin (RBV) achieve sustained virological response (SVR) rates of only 40–50% in patients with genotype 1 and is associated with significant side effects (gastrointestinal, hematological, and psychiatric). The currently developed IFN-free, direct-acting antivirals (DAAs) used to treat HCV infection have low side effect profiles and high efficacy (SVR > 90) [50]. Some recent studies have reinforced the notion that modern DAAs improve OLP clinical outcomes in HCV-infected patients. This evidence supported the hypothesis that successful antiviral therapy against HCV led to improvements in OLP symptoms [4,51]. A study conducted by our research group emphasized that OLP-HCV patients displayed more severe clinical symptoms at baseline and greater erosive areas compared to non-HCV-OLP patients. Post-DAA treatment, the clinical progression in OLP-HCV patients mirrored that of the non-HCV-OLP group, reinforcing the detrimental impact of HCV on OLP. Interestingly, ulcerative lesions increased temporarily after DAA treatment but improved significantly thereafter. Following HCV eradication, some patients achieved complete mucosal healing, underscoring the potential of DAAs to improve both hepatic and extra-hepatic manifestations of HCV. These findings suggest that HCV acts as a pathogenic cofactor in OLP, advocating for routine HCV testing in severe OLP cases, especially in regions with high HCV prevalence like Italy. Further research with larger samples is needed to validate these results and explore the underlying mechanisms [4].

2.2. Xerostomia and Sjögren's Syndrome-like Manifestations

The molecular mechanisms underlying xerostomia associated with HCV infection involve a multifactorial process. Lymphocytic infiltrates in the salivary glands of HCV-infected patients are typically diffuse and predominantly consist of CD8+ T-cells, although some studies have reported a predominance of CD4+ T-cells, but to a lesser extent than in Sjögren's syndrome (SS) [52].

HCV-infected individuals present a higher prevalence of liver involvement and cryoglobulinemia compared to SS patients. Patients with HCV-related salivary gland dysfunction usually lack primary SS antibodies, such as anti-SSA and anti-SSB, showing, on the other side, high levels of other autoantibodies like ANA, ACA, dsDNA, and RF [52]. In a very preliminary study, Aceti et al. have explored the relationship between HCV and Sjögren's syndrome (SS), searching for a potential overlap in clinical features between HCV-related salivary gland dysfunction and SS, concluding that HCV may have no role in the autoimmune organ damage responsible for Sjogren's syndrome [53]. On the other side, another early study by Arrieta et al. reinforced the hypothesis that HCV infects and replicates in the epithelial cells of salivary glands of patients with Sjogren's syndrome or chronic sialadenitis, although the underlying pathogenic mechanisms were not clear [54]. The study conducted by Brito-Zerón et al. investigates how the hepatitis C virus (HCV) influences the immunological profile of Sjögren's syndrome (SS) patients, analyzing 783 cases. The findings reveal that SS patients with HCV exhibit distinct immunological characteristics. In fact, the prevalence of HCV infection in patients with Sjögren's syndrome (SS) varies widely based on classification criteria. HCV-driven autoimmune response in SS is marked by a high prevalence of mixed cryoglobulins, positive rheumatoid factor (RF), monoclonal gammopathy, and low C4 levels. Significant differences in serum monoclonal expression were noted, with SS-HCV patients showing a threefold higher prevalence of circulating monoclonal immunoglobulins (mIgs), predominantly mIgMκ, linked to mixed cryoglobulinemia. SS-HCV patients also exhibited a more restrictive monoclonal expression compared to the diverse profiles in SS patients without HCV, indicating HCV's role in clonal B-cell selection [55].

Several authors have already highlighted the absence of HCV infection in primary SS [56]. For this reason, according to the 2016 American-European Consensus Criteria, evidence of HCV infection is an exclusion criterion for the classification of a patient as having primary SS [57]. A recent study by Maldonado et al. highlighted that HCV-infected patients with xerostomia demonstrated diffuse lymphocytic infiltrates in their salivary glands, predominantly composed of CD8+ T-cells. These infiltrates were associated with significant increases in the number of inflammatory cells, suggesting an ongoing inflammatory response. The study observed chronic sialadenitis and salivary gland (SG) fibrosis in HCV-infected patients, indicative of sustained tissue damage and remodeling in response to chronic inflammation. Analysis of saliva composition revealed significant changes in sodium and mucin 5b levels. Saliva alterations suggest that HCV infection impacts salivary gland function and contributes to the sensation of dry mouth. Submandibular glands in HCV patients showed significant ultrasonographic abnormalities relative to the parotid glands, further supporting the presence of glandular pathology. The research indicated that all HCV patients examined exhibited low saliva flow, pointing to SG hypofunction, which explained the xerostomia symptoms. No significant correlation was found between the degree of lymphocytic infiltrates and the duration of HCV chronic infection. However, there was a positive correlation observed between HCV RNA-positive epithelial cells and the years of HCV infection, highlighting a direct viral contribution to SG pathology. Moreover, patients with HCV showed changes in markers of SG acinar and ductal function, consistent with the observed low saliva flow and xerostomia. The study concluded that HCV infection can cause xerostomia through mechanisms distinct from Sjögren's syndrome. This distinct pathophysiology, reported in Figure 2, has implications for the diagnosis and treatment of xerostomia in HCV-infected individuals. Other viruses, such as hepatitis D virus, HIV-1, human T-cell leukemia virus type 1, and SARS-CoV-2, have also been associated with SG pathology and have provided comparative insights into the viral mechanisms affecting the SGs [52].

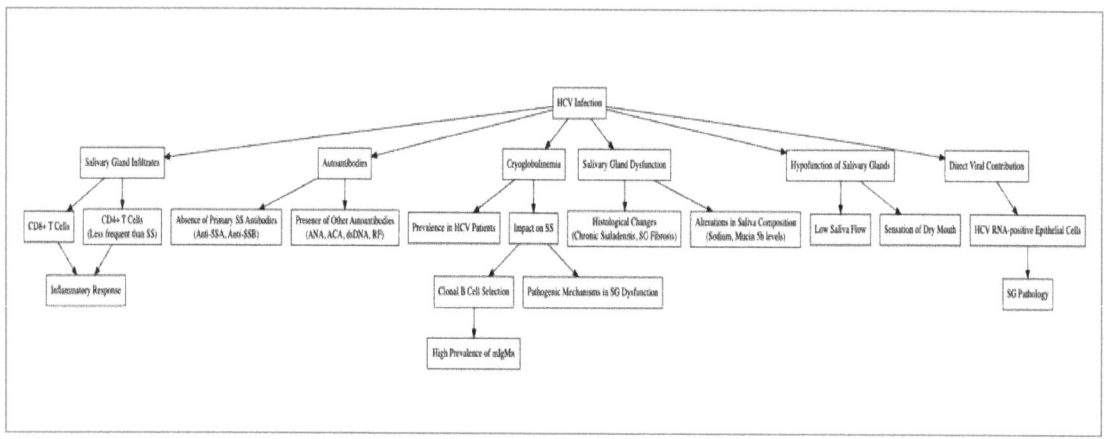

Figure 2. Aetiopathogenic hypotheses of the relationship between HCV infection and Xerostomia and Sjögren's syndrome-like manifestations.

2.3. Periodontal Disease

Some studies have reported that periodontal conditions are exacerbated by HCV infection by an alteration of the immune response, leading to a more severe progression of gum disease [58,59]. The virus exhibits lymphotropism, being traceable in fluids like saliva (though transmission through saliva is debated due to inconsistent detection of viral RNA). The presence of HCV in saliva might be influenced by the periodontal status, with higher

AST levels observed in patients with chronic periodontal disease [60]. Furthermore, HCV antigens and antibodies were studied in gingival crevicular fluid (GCF), with viral RNA and anti-HCV antibodies detected in the GCF of infected patients, suggesting a role as a source of HCV contamination in saliva [61]. Periodontal inflammation increases GCF flow and bleeding, facilitating viral migration from blood to GCF and saliva. Studies have found a high prevalence of HCV RNA in GCF, often higher than in saliva [62]. The presence of HCV in GCF probably involves infected leukocytes, necessitating further research into the molecular and cellular characteristics of GCF in HCV patients [63].

Malone et al. found that periodontal disease increased the risk of developing Alzheimer's disease and related dementias (ADRD) among HCV patients, suggesting a link between oral health and neurodegenerative diseases in the context of HCV infection. The presence of periodontal disease was associated with a higher incidence rate of ADRD and an earlier development of these conditions in HCV patients compared to those without periodontal disease [64]. Nagao and Tsuji investigated the impact of HCV eradication on oral lichen planus (OLP) and the load of periodontal pathogens. Although it can be considered a pilot study, with only four cases presented, they found that the eradication of HCV not only improved OLP lesions but also reduced the number of periodontal pathogens, emphasizing the potential systemic benefits of HCV treatment on oral health [59]. Azatyan et al. explored clinical and morphological lesions of the oral mucosa and periodontium in viral hepatitis C, underlining the significant changes in the dental and periodontal status of patients with HCV. This study directly addresses the oral manifestations in HCV patients, providing clinical insights into the impact of HCV on oral health [65].

Some other studies have expanded our understanding of the etiopathogenetic mechanisms linking periodontal diseases with viral liver diseases, particularly focusing on the role of microbiome and inflammatory processes. Chandran et al. provided a comprehensive review of the role of various viruses in periodontal disease. The review categorizes the impact of viral infections on the etiopathogenesis of periodontal disease, emphasizing the need for a better understanding of viral contributions to disease progression [66]. Gheorghe et al. (2022) discussed the dental and periodontal status of patients with hepatitis B/D. They suggested that maintaining good oral and periodontal health can limit the pathological effects of these liver diseases. They also proposed that a similar interplay could exist in HCV-related liver diseases [67]. All pathogenetic mechanisms are shown in Figure 3.

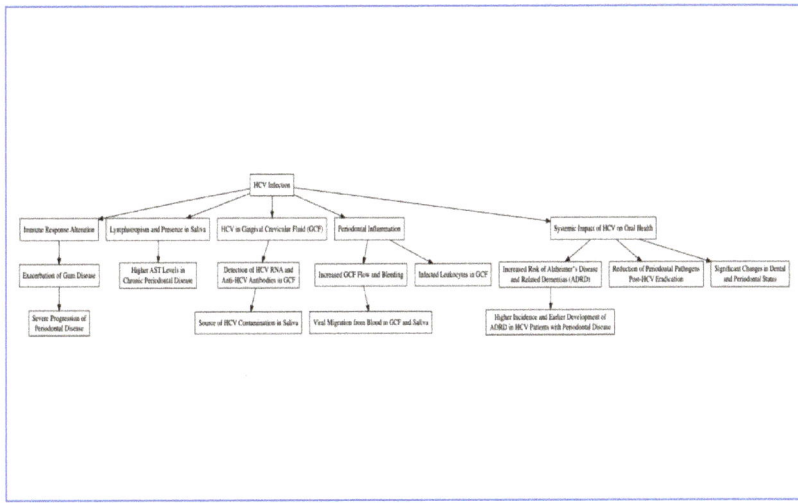

Figure 3. Aetiopathogenic hypotheses of the relationship between HCV infection and periodontitis.

2.4. Head and Neck Squamous Cell Carcinoma

Recent studies have investigated the relationship between OSCC and HCV infection, providing insights into the molecular mechanisms involved and potential impacts on patient survival. Marconi et al. focused on the role of c-Myc in OSCC, indicating its significance in tumor prognosis and stem cell renewal. While it did not directly connect to HCV, the exploration of molecular pathways in OSCC offers insights into potential areas where HCV-related mechanisms might intersect, especially considering the role of c-Myc in various cancers, including those potentially influenced by viral infections [68]. Direct prevalence numbers linking OSCC specifically with HCV infection are less commonly reported and vary significantly based on population studies and the specific criteria used for diagnosing OSCC. However, studies proposed HCV infection as a risk factor for the development of OSCC, potentially due to its role in promoting chronic inflammation and its effects on cellular pathways related to cancer development [69]. In the study of Nagao et al. involving 60 patients, 35% developed multiple primary cancers (MPCs), with a notably higher incidence (62.5%) among those with HCV infection compared to those without (25%). The analysis revealed HCV as a significant risk factor for MPCs alongside primary OSCC, HCC being prevalent among HCV-positive cases. Age over 70, staging IV, and HCV positivity were identified as significant risk factors. The findings underscore the importance of comprehensive medical treatment for HCV-infected OSCC patients in Japan to mitigate the risk of developing HCC and suggest the necessity of monitoring for MPCs beyond the liver, especially given the observed hyperinsulinemia in HCV-positive patients [7]. A study by Fu-Hsiung Su et al. [70] highlighted a significant association between HCV infection and an increased risk of oral cavity cancer. Conducted within a Taiwanese population, this nationwide cohort analysis reveals that individuals with HCV are at a notably higher risk of developing oral cavity cancer compared to those without viral hepatitis. This association is particularly pronounced among adults aged 40–49, underscoring the importance of vigilant oral health monitoring in HCV-infected patients to potentially mitigate cancer risk. The incidence of oral cavity cancers was 2.28-fold higher among patients with HCV alone than non-viral hepatitis group (6.15 versus 2.69 per 10,000 person-years). After adjusting for sociodemographic covariates, HCV alone was significantly associated with an increased risk for oral cancer. However, the study does not specify whether the study population also suffered from liver cirrhosis. This aspect is not negligible when conducting a study of this type and therefore limits the results. In a 2004 study on an Italian cohort of 402 patients with OLP, the relative risk of OSCC for patients with HCV as compared with those without HCV infection was 3.16 (0.8–12.5) [69]. However, although four out of nine patients with OSCC were HCV-infected, the increased risk was not significant, possibly because of low statistical power.

A meta-analysis by Borsetto et al. synthesized evidence on HCV's link to head and neck squamous cell carcinoma (HNSCC), including cancers of the oral cavity, oropharynx, hypopharynx, and larynx. Eight studies were analyzed, showing significant risk associations for oral cavity (RR = 2.13), oropharynx (RR = 1.81), and larynx cancers (RR = 2.57). Hypopharyngeal cancer also showed a trend towards risk elevation (RR = 2.15), though it was not statistically significant. The study underscores the importance of monitoring HCV-infected patients for early HNSCC detection and raises awareness of potential undiagnosed HCV in HNSCC patients [71]. All pathogenetic mechanisms are shown in Figure 4.

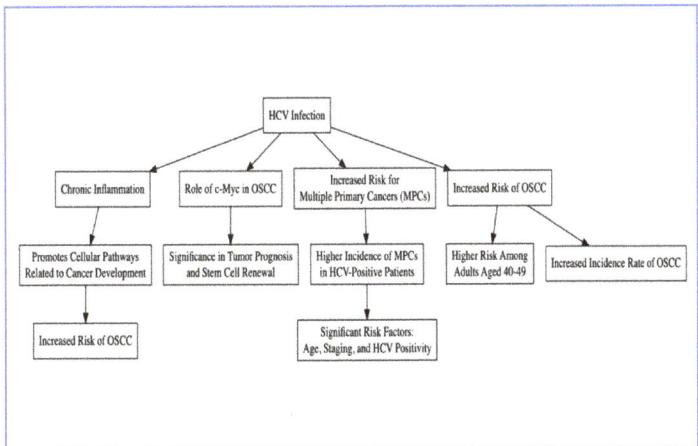

Figure 4. Aetiopathogenic hypotheses of the relationship between HCV infection and HNSCC.

3. Materials and Methods

3.1. Search Strategy

An exploratory literature search was conducted using major scientific databases, including PubMed, Scopus, Web of Science, and Google Scholar, to identify relevant publications on the oral manifestations of HCV infection. The search covered literature published up to April 2023. Search terms used included "hepatitis C virus", "HCV", "oral manifestations", "oral health", "oral lichen planus", "xerostomia", and "periodontal disease", with various combinations of these terms. Boolean operators (AND, OR) were employed to broaden the search.

3.2. Selection Criteria

Given the narrative review's aim to provide a comprehensive overview, studies were selected based on their relevance to the topic of oral manifestations associated with HCV infection. This included original research articles, review papers, case reports, and clinical trials. There were no strict inclusion or exclusion criteria based on study design or language to ensure a broad and inclusive selection of the literature. However, preference was given to studies that significantly contributed to understanding the relationship between HCV infection and oral health outcomes.

3.3. Data Collection

The data collection process involved summarizing key findings from the selected studies, focusing on types of oral manifestations reported, the prevalence among HCV-infected individuals, diagnostic approaches, and treatment outcomes. This process was more qualitative, aiming to capture the breadth of knowledge rather than quantitatively synthesizing data.

3.4. Analysis Method

A narrative synthesis was employed to organize and present the findings. This approach allowed for a flexible interpretation of the diverse body of literature, highlighting themes and patterns regarding oral manifestations of HCV infection, and discussing diagnostic challenges and treatment strategies.

The main results are summarized in diagrams created using RStudio (version 2024.04.2+764).

3.5. Ethical Considerations

As this review is based on the analysis of previously published data, no specific ethical approval was required. Nevertheless, the review was conducted with a commitment

4. Conclusions

The comprehensive review elucidates the potential intricate association between HCV infection and its diverse oral manifestations, notably oral lichen planus, xerostomia, and periodontal disease, underscoring the systemic impact of HCV beyond hepatic involvement. Given the present state of the scientific literature, clinical recommendations of dental practice for HCV patients have to be wide and unspecific, as there is no clear evidence for a specific type of conduct. Such findings encourage the need for heightened vigilance and regular oral health assessments among patients with chronic HCV infections, facilitating early diagnosis and timely intervention. Further studies are yet needed to reach complete scientific evidence. Future research directions should aim at unraveling the underlying pathophysiological mechanisms linking HCV to oral health conditions and refining treatment protocols to encompass comprehensive care strategies that address both hepatic and extrahepatic manifestations of HCV, ultimately enhancing patient outcomes and quality of life.

Funding: This research received no external funding.

Conflicts of Interest: The authors declare no conflict of interest.

References

1. Carrozzo, M.; Scally, K. Oral Manifestations of Hepatitis C Virus Infection. *World J. Gastroenterol.* **2014**, *20*, 7534. [CrossRef]
2. Liu, C.-H.; Kao, J.-H. Acute Hepatitis C Virus Infection: Clinical Update and Remaining Challenges. *Clin. Mol. Hepatol.* **2023**, *29*, 623–642. [CrossRef] [PubMed]
3. Cozzani, E.; Herzum, A.; Burlando, M.; Parodi, A. Cutaneous Manifestations of HAV, HBV, HCV. *Ital. J. Dermatol. Venereol.* **2021**, *156*, 5–12. [CrossRef]
4. Di Stasio, D.; Lucchese, A.; Romano, A.; Adinolfi, L.E.; Serpico, R.; Marrone, A. The Clinical Impact of Direct-Acting Antiviral Treatment on Patients Affected by Hepatitis C Virus-Related Oral Lichen Planus: A Cohort Study. *Clin. Oral Investig.* **2022**, *26*, 5409–5417. [CrossRef] [PubMed]
5. Douam, F.; Lavillette, D.; Cosset, F.-L. The Mechanism of HCV Entry into Host Cells. *Prog. Mol. Biol. Transl. Sci.* **2015**, *129*, 63–107. [CrossRef]
6. Hsu, C.-S.; Chao, Y.-C.; Lin, H.H.; Chen, D.-S.; Kao, J.-H. Systematic Review: Impact of Interferon-Based Therapy on HCV-Related Hepatocellular Carcinoma. *Sci. Rep.* **2015**, *5*, 9954. [CrossRef] [PubMed]
7. Nagao, Y.; Sata, M. High Incidence of Multiple Primary Carcinomas in HCV-Infected Patients with Oral Squamous Cell Carcinoma. *Med. Sci. Monit.* **2009**, *15*, CR453-9.
8. Georgescu, S.; Tampa, M.; Mitran, M.; Mitran, C.; Sarbu, M.; Nicolae, I.; Matei, C.; Caruntu, C.; Neagu, M.; Popa, M. Potential Pathogenic Mechanisms Involved in the Association between Lichen Planus and Hepatitis C Virus Infection (Review). *Exp. Ther. Med.* **2018**, *17*, 1045–1051. [CrossRef]
9. Zeisel, M.B.; Fofana, I.; Fafi-Kremer, S.; Baumert, T.F. Hepatitis C Virus Entry into Hepatocytes: Molecular Mechanisms and Targets for Antiviral Therapies. *J. Hepatol.* **2011**, *54*, 566–576. [CrossRef]
10. Samreen, B.; Khaliq, S.; Ashfaq, U.A.; Khan, M.; Afzal, N.; Shahzad, M.A.; Riaz, S.; Jahan, S. Hepatitis C Virus Entry: Role of Host and Viral Factors. *Infect. Genet. Evol.* **2012**, *12*, 1699–1709. [CrossRef]
11. Nakamuta, M.; Fujino, T.; Yada, R.; Aoyagi, Y.; Yasutake, K.; Kohjima, M.; Fukuizumi, K.; Yoshimoto, T.; Harada, N.; Yada, M.; et al. Expression Profiles of Genes Associated with Viral Entry in HCV-infected Human Liver. *J. Med. Virol.* **2011**, *83*, 921–927. [CrossRef] [PubMed]
12. Bassendine, M.F.; Sheridan, D.A.; Bridge, S.H.; Felmlee, D.J.; Neely, R.D.G. Lipids and HCV. *Semin. Immunopathol.* **2013**, *35*, 87–100. [CrossRef] [PubMed]
13. Song, Y.; Yang, X.; Shen, Y.; Wang, Y.; Xia, X.; Zhang, A. STAT3 Signaling Pathway Plays Importantly Genetic and Functional Roles in HCV Infection. *Mol. Genet. Genom. Med.* **2019**, *7*, e821. [CrossRef] [PubMed]
14. Sansonno, L.; Anna Tucci, F.; Sansonno, S.; Lauletta, G.; Troiani, L.; Sansonno, D. B Cells and HCV: An Infection Model of Autoimmunity. *Autoimmun. Rev.* **2009**, *9*, 93–94. [CrossRef] [PubMed]
15. Ackermann, C.; Smits, M.; Woost, R.; Eberhard, J.M.; Peine, S.; Kummer, S.; Marget, M.; Kuntzen, T.; Kwok, W.W.; Lohse, A.W.; et al. HCV-Specific CD4+ T Cells of Patients with Acute and Chronic HCV Infection Display High Expression of TIGIT and Other Co-Inhibitory Molecules. *Sci. Rep.* **2019**, *9*, 10624. [CrossRef] [PubMed]
16. Roehlen, N.; Crouchet, E.; Baumert, T.F. Liver Fibrosis: Mechanistic Concepts and Therapeutic Perspectives. *Cells* **2020**, *9*, 875. [CrossRef] [PubMed]

17. Park, S.-H.; Rehermann, B. Immune Responses to HCV and Other Hepatitis Viruses. *Immunity* **2014**, *40*, 13–24. [CrossRef]
18. Li, Y.; Liu, S.; Han, M.; Lu, H.; Wang, Q.; Zhang, Y.; Tursun, K.; Li, Z.; Feng, S.; Cheng, J. NS5ATP13 Promotes Liver Fibrogenesis via Activation of Hepatic Stellate Cells. *J. Cell. Biochem.* **2017**, *118*, 2463–2473. [CrossRef] [PubMed]
19. Iwakiri, Y.; Trebicka, J. Portal Hypertension in Cirrhosis: Pathophysiological Mechanisms and Therapy. *JHEP Rep.* **2021**, *3*, 100316. [CrossRef]
20. Latronico, T.; Mascia, C.; Pati, I.; Zuccala, P.; Mengoni, F.; Marocco, R.; Tieghi, T.; Belvisi, V.; Lichtner, M.; Vullo, V.; et al. Liver Fibrosis in HCV Monoinfected and HIV/HCV Coinfected Patients: Dysregulation of Matrix Metalloproteinases (MMPs) and Their Tissue Inhibitors TIMPs and Effect of HCV Protease Inhibitors. *Int. J. Mol. Sci.* **2016**, *17*, 455. [CrossRef]
21. Medvedev, R.; Ploen, D.; Hildt, E. HCV and Oxidative Stress: Implications for HCV Life Cycle and HCV-Associated Pathogenesis. *Oxid. Med. Cell. Longev.* **2016**, *2016*, 9012580. [CrossRef]
22. Premkumar, M.; Anand, A.C. Overview of Complications in Cirrhosis. *J. Clin. Exp. Hepatol.* **2022**, *12*, 1150–1174. [CrossRef] [PubMed]
23. Zanone, M.M.; Marinucci, C.; Ciancio, A.; Cocito, D.; Zardo, F.; Spagone, E.; Ferrero, B.; Cerruti, C.; Charrier, L.; Cavallo, F.; et al. Peripheral Neuropathy after Viral Eradication with Direct-acting Antivirals in Chronic HCV Hepatitis: A Prospective Study. *Liver Int.* **2021**, *41*, 2611–2621. [CrossRef] [PubMed]
24. Kleefeld, F.; Heller, S.; Ingiliz, P.; Jessen, H.; Petersen, A.; Kopp, U.; Kraft, A.; Hahn, K. Interferon-Free Therapy in Hepatitis C Virus (HCV) Monoinfected and HCV/HIV Coinfected Patients: Effect on Cognitive Function, Fatigue, and Mental Health. *J. Neurovirol.* **2018**, *24*, 557–569. [CrossRef] [PubMed]
25. Chemello, L.; Cavalletto, L.; Ferrari, S.; Monaco, S. Impact of Direct Acting Antivirals (DAA) on Neurologic Disorders in Chronic Hepatitis C. *Minerva Gastroenterol.* **2021**, *67*, 234–243. [CrossRef] [PubMed]
26. Cuan-Baltazar, Y.; Soto-Vega, E. Microorganisms Associated to Thyroid Autoimmunity. *Autoimmun. Rev.* **2020**, *19*, 102614. [CrossRef]
27. Retamozo, S.; Quartuccio, L.; Ramos-Casals, M. Crioglobulinemia. *Med. Clin.* **2022**, *158*, 478–487. [CrossRef] [PubMed]
28. Desbois, A.C.; Cacoub, P.; Saadoun, D. Cryoglobulinemia: An Update in 2019. *Jt. Bone Spine* **2019**, *86*, 707–713. [CrossRef]
29. Milovanova, S.Y.; Lysenko (Kozlovskaya), L.V.; Milovanova, L.Y.; Mrykhin, N.N.; Russkih, A.V.; Muchin, N.A. HCV-Associated Mixed Cryoglobulinemia and b-Cell Non-Hodgkin's Lymphoma - Pathogenetically Related Problems. *Ter. Arkh.* **2018**, *90*, 112–120. [CrossRef]
30. Alavian, S.-M.; Mahboobi, N.; Mahboobi, N.; Karayiannis, P. Oral Conditions Associated with Hepatitis C Virus Infection. *Saudi J. Gastroenterol.* **2013**, *19*, 245. [CrossRef]
31. Antonelli, A.; Ferrari, S.M.; Ruffilli, I.; Fallahi, P. Cytokines and HCV-Related Autoimmune Disorders. *Immunol. Res.* **2014**, *60*, 311–319. [CrossRef]
32. Scelza, G. Effect of Hepatitis C Antiviral Therapy on Oral Lichen Planus and Hyposalivation in Inmates. *Ann. Gastroenterol.* **2021**, *35*, 74. [CrossRef]
33. Di Stasio, D.; Guida, A.; Salerno, C.; Contaldo, M.; Esposito, V.; Laino, L.; Serpico, R.; Lucchese, A. Oral Lichen Planus: A Narrative Review. *Front. Biosci.* **2014**, *6*, 370–376. [CrossRef] [PubMed]
34. Mester, A.; Lucaciu, O.; Ciobanu, L.; Apostu, D.; Ilea, A.; Campian, R.S. Clinical Features and Management of Oral Lichen Planus (OLP) with Emphasis on the Management of Hepatitis C Virus (HCV)-Related OLP. *Bosn. J. Basic Med. Sci.* **2018**, *18*, 217–223. [CrossRef]
35. García-Pola, M.; Rodríguez-Fonseca, L.; Suárez-Fernández, C.; Sanjuán-Pardavila, R.; Seoane-Romero, J.; Rodríguez-López, S. Bidirectional Association between Lichen Planus and Hepatitis C—An Update Systematic Review and Meta-Analysis. *J. Clin. Med.* **2023**, *12*, 5777. [CrossRef]
36. Jung, W.; Jang, S. Oral Microbiome Research on Oral Lichen Planus: Current Findings and Perspectives. *Biology* **2022**, *11*, 723. [CrossRef]
37. Nagao, Y.; Sata, M.; Noguchi, S.; Seno'O, T.; Kinoshita, M.; Kameyama, T.; Ueno, T. Detection of Hepatitis C Virus RNA in Oral Lichen Planus and Oral Cancer Tissues. *J. Oral Pathol. Med.* **2000**, *29*, 259–266. [CrossRef] [PubMed]
38. Baek, K.; Choi, Y. The Microbiology of Oral Lichen Planus: Is Microbial Infection the Cause of Oral Lichen Planus? *Mol. Oral Microbiol.* **2018**, *33*, 22–28. [CrossRef] [PubMed]
39. Wang, L.; Wu, W.; Chen, J.; Li, Y.; Xu, M.; Cai, Y. MicroRNA Microarray-Based Identification of Involvement of MiR-155 and MiR-19a in Development of Oral Lichen Planus (OLP) by Modulating Th1/Th2 Balance via Targeting ENOS and Toll-like Receptor 2 (TLR2). *Med. Sci. Monit.* **2018**, *24*, 3591–3603. [CrossRef] [PubMed]
40. El-Howati, A.; Thornhill, M.H.; Colley, H.E.; Murdoch, C. Immune Mechanisms in Oral Lichen Planus. *Oral Dis.* **2023**, *29*, 1400–1415. [CrossRef]
41. Hofmann, M.; Tauber, C.; Hensel, N.; Thimme, R. CD8+ T Cell Responses during HCV Infection and HCC. *J. Clin. Med.* **2021**, *10*, 991. [CrossRef] [PubMed]
42. Kondo, Y.; Ninomiya, M.; Kimura, O.; Machida, K.; Funayama, R.; Nagashima, T.; Kobayashi, K.; Kakazu, E.; Kato, T.; Nakayama, K.; et al. HCV Infection Enhances Th17 Commitment, Which Could Affect the Pathogenesis of Autoimmune Diseases. *PLoS ONE* **2014**, *9*, e98521. [CrossRef] [PubMed]
43. Humberto, J.S.M.; Saia, R.S.; Costa, L.H.A.; Rocha, M.J.A.; Motta, A.C.F. Salivary Cytokine Profile in Patients with Oral Lichen Planus. *Odovtos Int. J. Dent. Sci.* **2023**, 188–200. [CrossRef]

44. Askoura, M.; Abbas, H.A.; Al Sadoun, H.; Abdulaal, W.H.; Abu Lila, A.S.; Almansour, K.; Alshammari, F.; Khafagy, E.-S.; Ibrahim, T.S.; Hegazy, W.A.H. Elevated Levels of IL-33, IL-17 and IL-25 Indicate the Progression from Chronicity to Hepatocellular Carcinoma in Hepatitis C Virus Patients. *Pathogens* **2022**, *11*, 57. [CrossRef]
45. Grossmann, S.d.M.C.; Teixeira, R.; de Aguiar, M.C.F.; do Carmo, M.A.V. Exacerbation of Oral Lichen Planus Lesions during Treatment of Chronic Hepatitis C with Pegylated Interferon and Ribavirin. *Eur. J. Gastroenterol. Hepatol.* **2008**, *20*, 702–706. [CrossRef] [PubMed]
46. Vičić, M.; Hlača, N.; Kaštelan, M.; Brajac, I.; Sotošek, V.; Prpić Massari, L. Comprehensive Insight into Lichen Planus Immunopathogenesis. *Int. J. Mol. Sci.* **2023**, *24*, 3038. [CrossRef] [PubMed]
47. Radmanić, L.; Zidovec-Lepej, S. The Role of Stem Cell Factor, Epidermal Growth Factor and Angiopoietin-2 in HBV, HCV, HCC and NAFLD. *Life* **2022**, *12*, 2072. [CrossRef]
48. Nagao, Y.; Sata, M.; Suzuki, H.; Kameyama, T.; Ueno, T. Histological Improvement of Oral Lichen Planus in Patients with Chronic Hepatitis C Treated with Interferon. *Gastroenterology* **1999**, *117*, 283–284. [CrossRef]
49. Nagao, Y.; Sata, M.; Ide, T.; Suzuki, H.; Tanikawa, K.; Itoh, K.; Kameyama, T. Development and Exacerbation of Oral Lichen Planus during and after Interferon Therapy for Hepatitis C. *Eur. J. Clin. Investig.* **1996**, *26*, 1171–1174. [CrossRef]
50. Cacoub, P.; Desbois, A.C.; Comarmond, C.; Saadoun, D. Impact of Sustained Virological Response on the Extrahepatic Manifestations of Chronic Hepatitis C: A Meta-Analysis. *Gut* **2018**, *67*, 2025–2034. [CrossRef]
51. Carrozzo, M. A Personal Journey through Oral Medicine: The Tale of Hepatitis C Virus and Oral Lichen Planus. *J. Oral Pathol. Med.* **2023**, *52*, 335–338. [CrossRef]
52. Maldonado, J.O.; Beach, M.E.; Wang, Y.; Perez, P.; Yin, H.; Pelayo, E.; Fowler, S.; Alevizos, I.; Grisius, M.; Baer, A.N.; et al. HCV Infection Alters Salivary Gland Histology and Saliva Composition. *J. Dent. Res.* **2022**, *101*, 534–541. [CrossRef]
53. Aceti, A.; Taliani, G.; Sorice, M.; Amendolea, M. HCV and Sjögren's Syndrome. *Lancet* **1992**, *339*, 1425–1426. [CrossRef]
54. Arrieta, J.J.; Rodríguez-Iñigo, E.; Ortiz-Movilla, N.; Bartolomé, J.; Pardo, M.; Manzarbeitia, F.; Oliva, H.; Macías, D.M.; Carreño, V. In Situ Detection of Hepatitis C Virus RNA in Salivary Glands. *Am. J. Pathol.* **2001**, *158*, 259–264. [CrossRef] [PubMed]
55. Brito-Zerón, P.; Gheitasi, H.; Retamozo, S.; Bové, A.; Londoño, M.; Sánchez-Tapias, J.-M.; Caballero, M.; Kostov, B.; Forns, X.; Kaveri, S.V.; et al. How Hepatitis C Virus Modifies the Immunological Profile of Sjögren Syndrome: Analysis of 783 Patients. *Arthritis Res. Ther.* **2015**, *17*, 250. [CrossRef]
56. Marrone, A.; Di Bisceglie, A.M.; Fox, P. Absence of Hepatitis C Viral Infection among Patients with Primary Sjögren's Syndrome. *J. Hepatol.* **1995**, *22*, 599. [CrossRef] [PubMed]
57. Shiboski, C.H.; Shiboski, S.C.; Seror, R.; Criswell, L.A.; Labetoulle, M.; Lietman, T.M.; Rasmussen, A.; Scofield, H.; Vitali, C.; Bowman, S.J.; et al. 2016 American College of Rheumatology/European League Against Rheumatism Classification Criteria for Primary Sjögren's Syndrome: A Consensus and Data-Driven Methodology Involving Three International Patient Cohorts. *Arthritis Rheumatol.* **2017**, *69*, 35–45. [CrossRef]
58. Tang, B.; Yan, C.; Shen, X.; Li, Y. The Bidirectional Biological Interplay between Microbiome and Viruses in Periodontitis and Type-2 Diabetes Mellitus. *Front. Immunol.* **2022**, *13*, 885029. [CrossRef]
59. Nagao, Y.; Tsuji, M. Effects of Hepatitis C Virus Elimination by Direct-Acting Antiviral Agents on the Occurrence of Oral Lichen Planus and Periodontal Pathogen Load: A Preliminary Report. *Int. J. Dent.* **2021**, *2021*, 8925879. [CrossRef] [PubMed]
60. Gheorghe, D.N.; Foia, L.; Toma, V.; Surdu, A.; Herascu, E.; Popescu, D.M.; Surlin, P.; Vere, C.C.; Rogoveanu, I. Hepatitis C Infection and Periodontal Disease: Is There a Common Immunological Link? *J. Immunol. Res.* **2018**, *2018*, 8720101. [CrossRef] [PubMed]
61. Nagao, Y.; Kawahigashi, Y.; Sata, M. Association of Periodontal Diseases and Liver Fibrosis in Patients with HCV and/or HBV Infection. *Hepat. Mon.* **2014**, *14*, e23264. [CrossRef] [PubMed]
62. Albuquerque-Souza, E.; Sahingur, S.E. Periodontitis, Chronic Liver Diseases, and the Emerging Oral-gut-liver Axis. *Periodontol. 2000* **2022**, *89*, 125–141. [CrossRef]
63. Açıkgöz, G.; Cengiz, M.İ.; Keskiner, İ.; Açıkgöz, Ş.; Can, M.; Açıkgöz, A. Correlation of Hepatitis C Antibody Levels in Gingival Crevicular Fluid and Saliva of Hepatitis C Seropositive Hemodialysis Patients. *Int. J. Dent.* **2009**, *2009*, 247121. [CrossRef] [PubMed]
64. Malone, J.; Jung, J.; Tran, L.; Zhao, C. Periodontal Disease and Risk of Dementia in Medicare Patients with Hepatitis C Virus. *J. Alzheimer's Dis.* **2022**, *85*, 1301–1308. [CrossRef] [PubMed]
65. Azatyan, V.; Yessayan, L.; Khachatryan, A.; Perikhanyan, A.; Hovhannisyan, A.; Shmavonyan, M.; Ghazinyan, H.; Gish, R.; Melik-Andreasyan, G.; Porksheyan, K. Assessment of Pathomorphological Characteristics of the Oral Mucosa in Patients with HBV, HCV and HIV. *J. Infect. Dev. Ctries.* **2021**, *15*, 1761–1765. [CrossRef]
66. Chandran, D.W.; Dharmadhikari, D.S.; Shetty, D.D. Viruses in Periodontal Disease: A Literature Review. *Int. J. Appl. Dent. Sci.* **2022**, *8*, 242–245. [CrossRef]
67. Gheorghe, D.N.; Bennardo, F.; Popescu, D.M.; Nicolae, F.M.; Ionele, C.M.; Boldeanu, M.V.; Camen, A.; Rogoveanu, I.; Surlin, P. Oral and Periodontal Implications of Hepatitis Type B and D. Current State of Knowledge and Future Perspectives. *J. Pers. Med.* **2022**, *12*, 1580. [CrossRef]
68. Marconi, G.D.; Della Rocca, Y.; Fonticoli, L.; Melfi, F.; Rajan, T.S.; Carradori, S.; Pizzicannella, J.; Trubiani, O.; Diomede, F. C-Myc Expression in Oral Squamous Cell Carcinoma: Molecular Mechanisms in Cell Survival and Cancer Progression. *Pharmaceuticals* **2022**, *15*, 890. [CrossRef]

69. Gandolfo, S.; Richiardi, L.; Carrozzo, M.; Broccoletti, R.; Carbone, M.; Pagano, M.; Vestita, C.; Rosso, S.; Merletti, F. Risk of Oral Squamous Cell Carcinoma in 402 Patients with Oral Lichen Planus: A Follow-up Study in an Italian Population. *Oral Oncol.* **2004**, *40*, 77–83. [CrossRef]
70. Su, F.-H.; Chang, S.-N.; Chen, P.-C.; Sung, F.-C.; Huang, S.-F.; Chiou, H.-Y.; Su, C.-T.; Lin, C.-C.; Yeh, C.-C. Positive Association Between Hepatitis C Infection and Oral Cavity Cancer: A Nationwide Population-Based Cohort Study in Taiwan. *PLoS ONE* **2012**, *7*, e48109. [CrossRef]
71. Borsetto, D.; Fussey, J.; Fabris, L.; Bandolin, L.; Gaudioso, P.; Phillips, V.; Polesel, J.; Boscolo-Rizzo, P. HCV Infection and the Risk of Head and Neck Cancer: A Meta-Analysis. *Oral Oncol.* **2020**, *109*, 104869. [CrossRef] [PubMed]

Disclaimer/Publisher's Note: The statements, opinions and data contained in all publications are solely those of the individual author(s) and contributor(s) and not of MDPI and/or the editor(s). MDPI and/or the editor(s) disclaim responsibility for any injury to people or property resulting from any ideas, methods, instructions or products referred to in the content.

MDPI AG
Grosspeteranlage 5
4052 Basel
Switzerland
Tel.: +41 61 683 77 34

Journal of Clinical Medicine Editorial Office
E-mail: jcm@mdpi.com
www.mdpi.com/journal/jcm

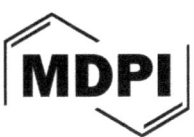

Disclaimer/Publisher's Note: The statements, opinions and data contained in all publications are solely those of the individual author(s) and contributor(s) and not of MDPI and/or the editor(s). MDPI and/or the editor(s) disclaim responsibility for any injury to people or property resulting from any ideas, methods, instructions or products referred to in the content.

www.ingramcontent.com/pod-product-compliance
Lightning Source LLC
LaVergne TN
LVHW070046120526
838202LV00101B/817